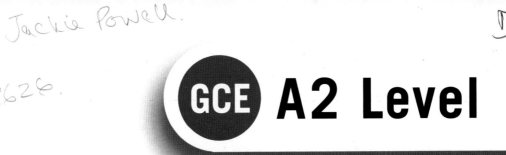

GCE A2 Level

D0543130

A2 Level for **AQA**

Health &
Social Care

Series editor: Neil Moonie

www.heinemann.co.uk

✓ Free online support
✓ Useful weblinks
✓ 24 hour online ordering

01865 888058

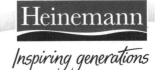

Inspiring generations

Heinemann Educational Publishers
Halley Court, Jordan Hill, Oxford OX2 8EJ
Part of Harcourt Education

Heinemann is the registered trademark of Harcourt Education Limited

First published 2006
10 09 08 07 06
10 9 8 7 6 5 4 3 2 1

British Library Cataloguing in Publication Data is available
from the British Library on request.

10-digit ISBN: 0 435 35292 X
13-digit ISBN: 978 0 435352 92 9

Edited by Diane Chandler

Typeset by Macmillan, India

Original illustrations © Harcourt Education Limited, 2006

Illustrated by Tek-Art, Croydon

Cover design by Peter Stratton

Printed in the UK by Bath Press

Cover photo: © OSF

Websites
Please note that the examples of websites suggested in this book were up to date at the
time of writing. It is essential for tutors to preview each site before using it to ensure that
the URL is still accurate and the content is appropriate. We suggest that tutors bookmark
useful sites and consider enabling students to access them through the school or college
intranet.

Crown copyright material reproduced with permission of the Controller of Her Majesty's
Stationery Office and the Queen's Printer for Scotland.

Tel: 01865 888058   www.heinemann.co.uk

Contents

Introduction   vi

Unit 11 — Working in Health and Social Care   01

11.1   Employment sectors   03
11.2   Roles and conditions   17
11.3   Meeting individual needs   23
11.4   Legislation   30
11.5   Quality assurance   32
11.6   Interview techniques   37
11.7   Ethical issues   42

Unit 12 — Human Development: Factors and Theories   49

12.1   Factors affecting development   51
12.2   Theories of cognitive development   59
12.3   Theories of personality development   76

Unit 13 — The Role of Exercise in Maintaining Health and Well-being   91

13.1   Exercise-related fitness   93
13.2   Physical, social and psychological benefits of regular exercise   101
13.3   Standard monitoring methods and tables   106
13.4   Safety in physical activity   113
13.5   Barriers to participation in regular exercise   118
13.6   Exercise and disease prevention   121
13.7   Exercise programmes for different clients   125

Unit 15 — Service Users with Disabilities   137

15.1   What is disability?   139
15.2   Causes of impairments   141
15.3   Disability conditions   144

15.4 Practitioners and provision   163
15.5 Barriers   174
15.6 Aids and adaptations   180
15.7 Legislation   182

Unit 16 Early Years Education   191

16.1 The roles of learning, child-rearing, genetics and maturation   193
16.2 How early years learning takes place   197
16.3 Techniques for enabling learning   199
16.4 Theories of development, learning and education   205
16.5 Assessment in early years education   218
16.6 Issues in early years learning and education   223

Unit 19 Physiological Aspects of Health   231

19.1 Physiological measurements of service users   233
19.2 Control mechanisms   245
19.3 Structure and functions   253

Unit 21 Research Methods and Perspectives   273

21.1 Methods of research   275
21.2 Sampling   292
21.3 Ethical issues   295
21.4 Data processing and presentation   298

Answers to Assessment Questions   309
Glossary   317
Index   327

Acknowledgements

The authors and publisher would like to thank the following individuals and organisations for permission to reproduce photographs:

Alamy/Frances M.Roberts pp**234**; Alamy/Mediacolor's pp**27**; Alamy/Photofusion Picture Library pp**179, 285**; Alamy/SHOUT pp**204**; Alamy/Steve Skjold pp**137**; Comstock Images pp**109**; Corbis pp**195, 231**; Education Photos/John Walmsley pp**224**; Eyewire pp**91**; Getty Images/PhotoDisc pp**1, 95, 151, 158, 219** left, **219** right, **273**; Harcourt Ltd/Devon Obugenga Shaw pp**284**; Harcourt Ltd/Gareth Boden pp**220**; Harcourt Ltd/ Martin Sookias/Mencap pp**26**; Harcourt Ltd/Peter Evans pp**196**; Harcourt Ltd/Jules Selmes pp**49, 148, 191, 194, 197, 203, 206, 207, 212, 221**; Harcourt Ltd/Tudor Photography pp**144**; Richard Smith pp**15, 167**; Science Photo Library/Adam Gault pp**33**; Science Photo Library/Antonia Reeve pp**112**; Science Photo Library/Lauren Shear pp**153**; Science Photo Library/De Repentigny, Publiphoto Diffusion Science Library pp**182**; Visuals Unlimited/ Corbis UK Ltd pp**261**

The following organisations and individuals contributed towards Unit 11:

The London Borough of Sutton
Sutton and Merton Primary Care Trust
Epsom and St Helier University Hospital Trust
Age Concern
The Stroke Association

Every effort has been made to contact copyright holders of material reproduced in this book. Any omissions will be rectified in subsequent printings if notice is given to the publishers.

Introduction

This book has been written to support students who are studying for the GCE A2 AQA award. The book includes the following A2 Units of the award:

Unit 11	Working in Health and Social Care
Unit 12	Human Development: Factors and Theories
Unit 13	The Role of Exercise in Maintaining Health and Well-being
Unit 15	Service Users with Disabilities
Unit 16	Early Years Education
Unit 19	Physiological Aspects of Health
Unit 21	Research Methods and Perspectives

This book has been organised to cover each of these units in detail. Headings are designed to make it easy to follow the content of each unit and to find the information needed to support achievement. As well as providing information each unit is designed to stimulate the development of the thinking skills needed to achieve an advanced award.

Assessment

Each unit will be assessed by coursework or by an external test set and marked by AQA. Detailed guidance for coursework assessment and external test requirements can be found in the unit specifications and at AQAs web site (www.aqa.org.uk). This book has been designed to support students to achieve high grades as set out in AQAs guidance available during 2005.

Special features of this book

Throughout the text there are a number of features that are designed to encourage reflection and to help students make links between theory and practice. In particular, this book has been designed to encourage a depth of learning and understanding and to encourage students to go beyond a surface level of understanding, characterised by a reliance on memorising and describing issues.

The special features of this book include:

What if?

Thought provoking questions or dilemmas are presented in order to encourage reflective thinking. Sometimes these questions might provide a basis for reflection involving discussion with others.

Did you know?

Interesting facts or snippets of information are included to encourage reflective thinking.

Try it out

Practical activities or tasks that might be undertaken by individuals or groups are suggested. These activities may encourage a deeper level of exploration and understanding.

Scenario

We have used this term in place of the more traditional term 'case study' because the idea of people being perceived as 'cases' does not fit easily with the notion of empowerment – a key value highlighted by government policy and AQA standards. Scenarios are presented throughout the units to help explain the significance of theoretical ideas to health, social care and early years settings.

Consider this

Each author has designed a 'consider this' feature at the end of each section of each unit. Each 'consider this' involves a brief scenario followed by a series of questions. The first easy questions ask students to simply identify issues. The next questions ask students to go into greater depth and analyse issues using theory. Finally, there are questions that ask for an in-depth understanding of issues. At this level the questions require students to access a wide range of learning in order to make an appropriate judgement or evaluation about an issue. This 'thinking skill' will contribute towards the achievement of high grades at Advanced (A2) level.

Key concept

Because the authors believe that the development of analytic and evaluative skills requires the ability to use concepts, they have identified key concepts and offered a brief explanation of how these terms might be used.

Section summary

Schematic diagrams, tables or other systems for providing an overview of theoretical content are used at the end of sections in order to help clarify the theory in each section.

Assessment guidance

At the end of each unit there is a 'how you will be assessed' section that provides either sample test material for externally assessed units or outline guidance and ideas designed to help students achieve the highest grades when preparing internally assessed coursework.

Unit test

Internally assessed units also feature questions that can be used as a learning check for the content of that unit.

Glossary

This book contains a useful glossary to provide fast reference for key terms and concepts used within the units.

References

There is a full list of references used within each unit together with useful websites at the end of each unit.

Author details

Beryl Stretch, former Head of Health and Social Care in a large College of Further Education. Currently part of the senior examining board for Edexcel, GCE and GCSE Health and Social Care. Former external and internal verifier for VCE, GNVQ, NVQ programmes and Examiner for GCSE human biology. Contributor to several best-selling textbooks on health and social care at all levels.

Dee Spencer-Perkins, began her social services career in research, moving on to become a trainer and then a training manager. She is a Chartered Member of the Chartered Institute of Personnel and Development, and now works as an independent trainer, consultant and writer specialising in language and communication. Dee also has a keen interest in disability issues.

Karen Hucker, has worked in post-16 education for 17 years and is now currently a College Principal. During her career, she has been Head of Health and Social Care and has considerable experience in the delivery of vocational education as well as academic studies. She has been an examiner and external verifier for a range of courses in the health and social care field. She is also a part time inspector for OfSTED. Karen has been an author for several years and has contributed to texts as well as writing several books independently.

Louise Sutton, fitness specialist and dietitian, is a principal lecturer in the Carnegie Faculty of Sport and Education at Leeds Metropolitan University. She has contributed to several best-selling textbooks on sport, health and fitness.

Neil Moonie, former Deputy Director of the Department of Social Services, Health and Education in a College of Further and Higher Education. Chartered Psychologist, part-time lecturer and contributor to a wide range of textbooks and learning resources in the field of health and social care. Editor of Heinemann's GNVQ Intermediate and Advanced textbooks on health and social care since 1993 and editor of the 2000 Standards AVCE textbook.

Sylvia Aslangul has been involved with health and social care all her working life. She has a nursing background and she then moved into teaching vocational and degree courses in Further and Higher Education. She is an Associate Lecturer in Health with the Open University. She was an External Verifier for Health and Social Care courses for Edexcel for 15 years. She has been editor and contributor to a range of textbooks on health and social care. Sylvia represents the voluntary sector on health and care committees that organise and develop services in her local area.

Working in health and social care

Unit

11

This unit covers the following sections:

11.1 Employment sectors

11.2 Roles and conditions

11.3 Meeting individual needs

11.4 Legislation

11.5 Quality assurance

11.6 Interview techniques

11.7 Ethical issues

Introduction

This unit aims to increase your understanding of the world of work in health and social care. It also helps you reflect on your own suitability for different job roles.

This unit requires you to use knowledge of service provision, life quality factors and caring skills described in the AS level Unit 1 Effective Caring.

This unit provides knowledge on which the following AS units are built. Unit 1 Effective Caring, Unit 2 Effective Communication, Unit 7 Needs and Provision for Elderly Clients, Unit 8 Needs and Provision for Early Years' Clients, Unit 9 Complementary Therapies, Unit 10, Psychological Perspectives, Unit 21 Research Methods and Perspectives.

Unit assessment

You need to produce a report describing and evaluating two contrasting job roles in health and social care. The report should also include an evaluation of your own suitability for these roles. A more detailed guide to the assessment is given at the end of the unit. You will also need to refer to the guidance given on the AQA website (www.aqa.org.uk).

11.1 Employment sectors

Working in health and social care

There are many jobs in health and social care; some of these require specialist skills and training. However in many jobs there are common skills required. The list below shows the qualities and skills that a group of health and care workers identified as being essential for many roles. In the list personality traits as well as skills are identified. However suitable your skills are for any job, they need to be underpinned by knowledge. Health and social care workers need to know the reasons why they do certain tasks. Also, in health and social care work, technology is continually changing. Technology isn't simply about clinical procedures and drugs, but it also includes the use of information technology. For example, one initiative that is currently being developed is the use of electronic patient records for all patients. These records will be accessible to all health and social care workers supporting a patient or service user.

As we go through this section, you need to think about the skills you would need for the jobs we discuss and perhaps check your skills against this list. Some skills develop as we gain more experience in work and through training, but some people may feel they could never do a particular job as they feel unsuited to it because of their personality. For example, during nurse training, students gain experience in a variety of placements. When they have finished their foundation year, they will enter the specialism they have chosen. However, some nurses find they could not work with certain groups, such as people with mental health problems. Some people are better suited to certain jobs because of aspects of their personality or experience.

Think it over

Look at the following list of skills that were drawn up by workers in health and social care. These are core skills that would be needed by almost anyone working in health and social care.

* good communication skills: verbal, written, non-verbal

* good telephone manner

* clear handwriting

* able to write reports

* computer skills

* can work as part of a team

* can work independently

* can make decisions

* able to drive

* observation skills

* assessment skills

* numeracy skills

* aware of health and safety

* good record keeping

* listening skills

* can supervise others.

Even if you had all these skills, there are certain personal qualities that could be very important in any job. What personal qualities would you list as being important? Do you think these qualities are innate (that is you are born with them) or do you think you can develop them?

Look at the list of personal qualities below and decide whether these qualities are innate or could be learned.

Are there any others you could add to the list? What personal qualities do you think you have that you could bring to a job in health or social care?

* sense of humour

* patience

* tact

* sympathy

* respect for others

* politeness

* ability to maintain confidentiality

* ability to work under pressure

* confidence

* friendliness.

Can you think of any more? Sometimes having a sense of humour can be useful to the team when working under pressure, but we need to know when a joking approach is inappropriate – for example, when you are discussing serious matters with relatives.

What are the qualities you could bring to a job in health or social care? What situations do you feel you might not cope with? Sometimes it is important to be aware of our weaknesses as well as our strengths. For example, if you prefer to work in a team, you might not be happy working on your own. In job interviews you may be asked about your strengths and weaknesses, so it is useful to make sure you know how to answer this question.

The employment sectors in health and social care

This section covers the main employment sectors in health and social care. Health and social services have been traditionally provided by three sectors shown in Figure 11.1.

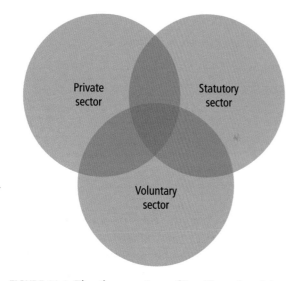

FIGURE 11.1 *The three sectors of health and social care*

The public or statutory sector

The statutory sector includes the NHS (National Health Service) and local authorities who have a legal **duty** to provide health and social care services.

The NHS

The NHS provides services in hospitals and in the community. There are many different areas of work within the NHS. Some jobs involve close contact with patients. Some jobs are to do with the organisation and management of the service, and others are back up services. Over one million staff work for the NHS in the UK at the present time. NHS trusts spend 60–70 per cent of their budget on staff costs.

Staffing of the NHS was a key issue in *The NHS Plan* (2000). There was a commitment to recruiting more staff and to retaining staff that were already working for the NHS. The NHS aimed to recruit:

* 7,500 more consultants

* 2,000 more GPs

* 20,000 more nursing staff

* over 6,500 more allied health professionals.

Allied Health Professionals: this group was called PAMS (Professions Allied to Medicine). They are a group of staff who support clinical services. They include dieticians, physiotherapists, orthoptists, occupational therapists, and speech and language therapists.

More details of this group are available on the Internet (www.nhscareers.nhs.uk).

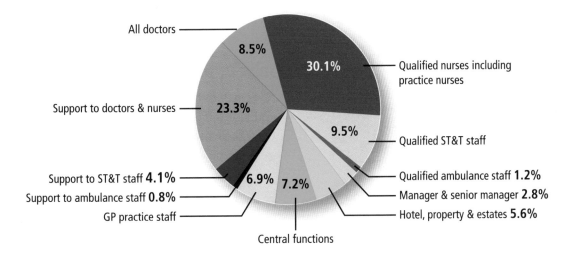

All doctors — 8.5%

30.1% Qualified nurses including practice nurses

Support to doctors & nurses — 23.3%

9.5% — Qualified ST&T staff

Support to ST&T staff **4.1%**

Support to ambulance staff **0.8%**

GP practice staff

6.9% 7.2%

Qualified ambulance staff **1.2%**

Manager & senior manager **2.8%**

Hotel, property & estates **5.6%**

Central functions

ST&T: Scientific, therapeutic and technical
Source: Wellards **NHS** Handbook *(2004)*

FIGURE 11.2 *Staff numbers working in the NHS in 2003*

Think it over

Look at the website and identify the range of Allied Health Professionals that contribute to patient and client care.

When we think of who works for the NHS we tend to think about doctors and nurses who may work in hospitals or in the community. However there are many other workers who contribute their skills to the running of the NHS. Table 11.1 shows

INDIRECT CARE	DIRECT CARE	GENERAL SUPPORT
Practice Manager	GPs	Caretaker
Receptionists	Practice Nurses	Security Staff
Secretary	Health Visitors	Cleaners
Booking Clerk (Clinics)	District Nurses	Maintenance Staff
Clerical Staff	Podiatrist	
	Asthma Nurse	
	Counsellor	
	Community Midwives	

TABLE 11.1 *The staff at a GP's surgery*

an organisation chart for a GP's surgery. Everyone at the practice contributes towards caring for the patient either directly or indirectly.

'Improving Working Lives' (IWL) was an important aspect of the NHS Plan to do with offering better working conditions for all staff. The following areas are being developed by all Primary Care Trusts (PCTs) and Hospital Trusts:

* job security
* working conditions
* model employment practice
* the work/life balance (the ability to balance life in and outside work)
* lifelong learning through continuous updating of skills and training
* fair pay
* staff involvement
* good communication skills.

Many NHS staff have caring responsibilities, either for children or other family members. It is important that there should be a flexible approach to work, including job sharing opportunities and flexible hours.

Apart from midwifery, there is a national shortage of trained nurses, so many trusts try to encourage skilled nurses back to work. These nurses may include people who have stopped work to have a family who now want to come back to nursing. Many hospital trusts run 'Back to Nursing' courses which have been very successful. If we cannot find enough nurses in the UK, nurses may be recruited from overseas.

We can see from this example that cultural differences may cause problems if the NHS recruits staff from other countries. In this trust there is an on-going training programme that includes cultural differences and expectations.

Jobs in the NHS

NHS staff work in the community (primary care) and also in hospitals (secondary care). In England in 2003–04 there were:

* 325 million consultations with GPs or nurses in primary care

* 13.3 million outpatient consultations

* over 5.4 million people admitted to hospital for planned treatment

* 13.9 million people who attended Accident and Emergency (A&E)

* 4.2 million emergency admissions.

(*Source: www.nhscareers.nhs.uk*)

These figures show that many staff are needed to support the NHS.

Nursing and midwifery

Nursing is organised into four branches. When nurses enter training for the Registered Nurse (RN) qualification, there is a Common Foundation programme in the first year of training which gives a general introduction to all four branches. In the second and third year of training, nurses focus on the branch they want to specialise in. The four branches are:

* adult nursing

* children's nursing

* mental health nursing

* learning disability nursing.

Midwifery and health visiting are seen as separate professions, although they are still within the nursing category. There are a variety of routes into midwifery. In health visiting registered nurses complete additional training.

Health care assistants

Health care assistants (HCAs) work with nurses and other professionals, helping with treatment and patients' comfort and well-being. They can work in the hospital or community setting. In the hospital they might make beds and assist patients with washing, feeding and toileting. Therapy assistants could be attached to various therapy workers, such as occupational therapists or physiotherapists. They help patients with mobility aids or exercises. In podiatry, they may help patients by cutting toe-nails and changing dressings.

SCENARIO
Rosemary

Rosemary is a health care assistant attached to a GP practice in South London. She runs a clinic where she checks patients who are on medication for high blood pressure. At each session she takes patients' blood pressure, weighs them and offers advice. She has had specialist training to do this. If she is concerned about a patient she will ask the practice nurse or doctor to see them. She works under the supervision of the practice nurse. She enjoys the job as she gets to know the patients who are regular visitors.

Social services

Local authorities provide a wide range of services related to health and social care. Larger councils are responsible for organising social services. Parish councils have limited responsibilities and social services in their area would be operated by larger district councils. Local authorities employ workers in social services and education, and this includes early years services and special education. Local authority social service staff are employed by the council.

Social workers

This term describes staff who work with families and individuals who need assistance with practical, personal and emotional problems. Some social workers are generic workers, and work with a range of service user groups. Others are 'specialist social workers' who work with a specific service user group, such as children, or people with learning disabilities. With current policy changes, most local authorities have a separate children and families department.

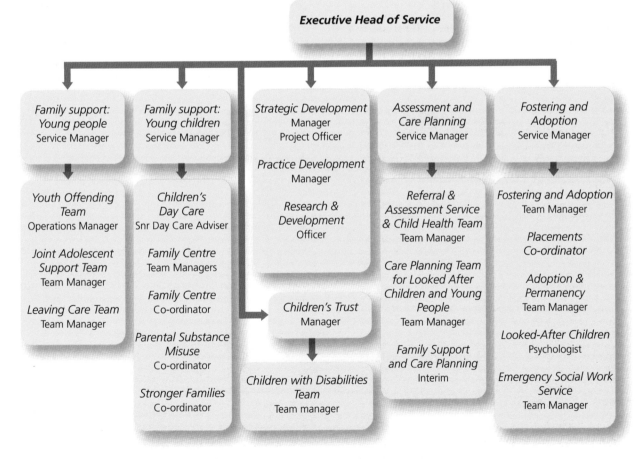

FIGURE 11.3 *A children and families department*

Training of social workers

Since 2003, the three-year degree in social work has replaced the two-year diploma in England. The DipSW is being phased out, but people with this qualification will still be recognised social workers.

Social care workers

Social care workers do not need qualifications or training to start a job in social care, however they will be given initial training. This training is called an 'induction' and will cover health and safety, manual handling (safe lifting practice) and anything else that the employer thinks is necessary to do the job. Most councils offer staff the chance to study for an NVQ at Levels 1 to 4, although in practice, staff start at Level 2. Managers would be expected to work towards Level 4 and also an additional management qualification. Table 11.2 shows the range of jobs in social care providing services for certain service user groups.

Education – early years and special needs

Much of the budget spent by local councils goes on social services and education.

As a result of legislation and policy, social services are working more closely with NHS organisations and with the voluntary sector. **Sure Start** is an example of this way of working in the context of early years provision.

Sure Start

This is a government initiative to support families, carers, parents-to-be and children under five who are living in poverty. The support to families is provided by health and social care professionals as well as voluntary organisations. As part of the Sure Start programme (2002), extended schools (which provide care and education to children of pre-school age, as well as pre- and post-school

OLDER PEOPLE	PEOPLE WITH DISABILITIES	BABIES AND YOUNG CHILDREN
Social worker for older people	Benefits officer – direct payments and other benefits	Family support worker
Social worker for older people with special needs	Home adaptation officer	Nursery nurse
Domiciliary care worker	Domiciliary care worker	'Portage' service officer
Day centre care worker	Equipment officer – occupational therapist	Fostering and adoption social worker
Incontinence support worker	Transport officer – drivers	Child protection officer
Finance officer	Respite care worker	Social worker * emergency * family support * special needs
Equipment manager – occupational therapist	Social worker/specialist	
Sheltered housing warden		
Housing officer		

TABLE 11.2 *The range of jobs in social care*

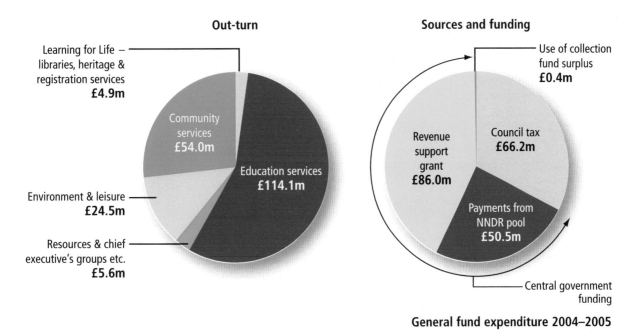

Out-turn

Learning for Life –
libraries, heritage &
registration services
£4.9m

Community
services
£54.0m

Education services
£114.1m

Environment & leisure
£24.5m

Resources & chief
executive's groups etc.
£5.6m

Sources and funding

Use of collection
fund surplus
£0.4m

Revenue
support
grant
£86.0m

Council tax
£66.2m

Payments from
NNDR pool
£50.5m

Central government
funding

General fund expenditure 2004–2005

NNDR: National non-domestic rates (central government funding)
Source: London Borough of Sutton finance department

FIGURE 11.4 *Income and expenditure of a local authority*

resources for school age children). **Sure Start Centres** are developing multi-disciplinary teams to work in these centres. Figure 11.5 shows that workers at these centres come from both statutory and voluntary sectors of health and social care.

The independent sector

The independent sector is divided into the private sector and the voluntary sector.

The private sector in health and social care

Private health and social care services cover a wide range. They include private hospitals and clinics which provide secondary care and specialist services; individual practitioners such as chiropractors and osteopaths who offer alternative therapies, as well as state registered therapists such as physiotherapists. Many dentists are now private practitioners. There are private nursing

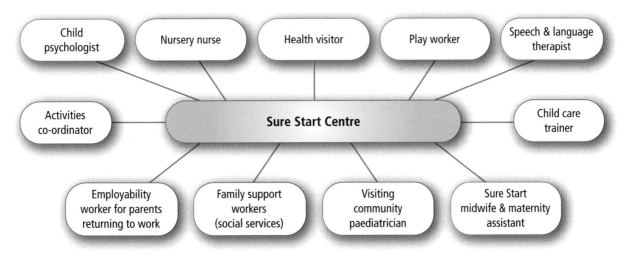

Child
psychologist

Nursery nurse

Health visitor

Play worker

Speech & language
therapist

Activities
co-ordinator

Sure Start Centre

Child care
trainer

Employability
worker for parents
returning to work

Family support
workers
(social services)

Visiting
community
paediatrician

Sure Start
midwife & maternity
assistant

FIGURE 11.5 *A multi-disciplinary team at a Sure Start Centre*

NHS SERVICES	SOCIAL SERVICES	COMMUNITY	EDUCATION SYSTEMS
Speech and language therapist	Family and children social worker	Nanny	Early years teacher
Health visitors	Residential care worker	Childminder	Teaching assistant
Children's nurse	Family support worker	Playgroup worker	Special needs teacher
Nursery nurse	Portage worker		Educational psychologist
Hospital play specialist	Adoption officer		Nursery nurse
Care assistant	Fostering officer		
Behavioural psychologist			

TABLE 11.3 *The range of jobs in early years' and special needs services*

agencies that provide nurses for hospitals, nursing homes and individuals. In social care there are private residential homes and agencies employing social care workers. Adoption and fostering agencies are commissioned by social services to provide services. Social services also buy in care workers from agencies to look after people in their own homes. Since the NHS and Community Care Act (1990) there has been an increase in the mixed economy of care, where more and more services are provided by the independent sector rather than by the statutory sector. Private providers of services are mostly profit-making bodies.

Private not-for-profit providers

Not-for-profit organisations are set up as charitable trusts, where any surplus income is fed back into the organisation. Examples of these can be residential homes, sheltered housing and other housing associations. Many not-for-profit providers have developed into large voluntary organisations, dependent for much of their income on contracts with the statutory sector. Jobs in the private sector are similar to those in the statutory sector of health and social care.

The voluntary sector

The voluntary sector is becoming increasingly important as a provider of services in health and social care since the 1990 NHS and Community Care Act. Voluntary organisations were often set up

to look after the interests of a particular service user group, for example older people (Age Concern), children (National Children's Home), people with learning disabilities (Mencap). They acted as pressure groups and tried to influence government policy. Now many of these organisations depend on the money earned from the services they provide for social services, PCTs and hospital trusts. Many of the larger organisations operate at a national level where they represent their particular service user group and provide information through leaflets, websites and brochures.

Local branches of voluntary organisations, such as Age Concern, provide a range of services and are also represented on local committees in health and social care. As the role of the voluntary sector has increased, the numbers of staff they employ has also risen. In 2004 it was estimated that the voluntary sector employed 500,000 people. Compared with the statutory sector, the voluntary sector employs more women than men; more ethnic minorities, and more part-time workers (quote from Stuart Etherington, Chief Executive of the National Council for Voluntary Organisations 2005). Voluntary organisations are seen to provide services in the community for hard to reach groups. In one area, the local voluntary organisations have provided services for refugees, for teenagers at risk of offending, for families which include children who are at risk of abuse, and for older isolated people. Voluntary organisations are seen as being more flexible than statutory services and disadvantaged people feel less threatened by them.

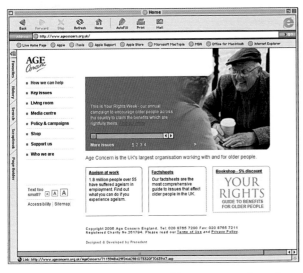

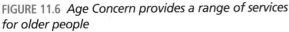

FIGURE 11.6 *Age Concern provides a range of services for older people*

All voluntary organisations depend on volunteers who give their time freely, but they also employ professionals who raise funding, negotiate contracts with health and social care services, and co-ordinate services. One of the most successful schemes developed by a branch of Age Concern is the hospital discharge scheme which is organised by a trained member of staff. The scheme uses volunteers to help with shopping and encourage older people to regain their independence when they return home from hospital. The need for this service became apparent when many older people found that they did not qualify for social services care, but were nervous about coping after returning home. Many older people live alone and have little contact with family or neighbours.

Think it over

Look at the extract from the person specification for the post of Hospital Discharge Co-ordinator (on page 12).

What qualifications and skills are needed for the post?

Are there any other qualities and experience that you think you would need for the job?

Funding of health and social care

Funding of the NHS

The NHS budget in England and Wales is planned to reach £105.6 billion by 2007–8. Central taxation and National Insurance Contributions provide 95 per cent of the funding. Patient charges account for 2 per cent of the overall funding. The majority of the NHS budget is spent on:

* staffing costs
* IT systems
* care, upkeep and replacement of existing buildings
* equipment
* policy changes (for example, the decision to invest in a big new IT system, can have a major effect on how the budget is spent).

SCENARIO

Age Concern

Age Concern acts as a lobbyist for older people but also provides a range of services commissioned and paid for by social services or by the NHS. In the annual report of a local Age Concern you will find a list of the services they offer and also the sources of funding. In one London borough, Age Concern offers services including the following:

* Information and advice on benefits, housing and other issues
* Ageing well project: assists people to prevent accidents in the home and to promote healthy living and exercise
* Healthy living project: offers healthy meals in a café, exercise classes and advice on health
* Home security service: provides smoke alarms and security locks and chains as well as testing electric blankets
* Hospital discharge scheme: supports people who have left hospital and need help with shopping and confidence building
* Advocacy scheme: supports older people.

Hospital Discharge Co-ordinator

Purpose of the post

To be responsible for, and deliver, the day-to-day management of the hospital discharge support scheme. The scheme provides a supportive service to people aged 65+ who are not eligible for social services care packages. Users of the service will be referred via A&E, the wards, or immediately before discharge. The aim of the post is to befriend, enable and promote independence following an illness or injury for a limited time. The post holder will assess the needs of the older person and arrange for support from either volunteers, or other appropriate agencies.

Personal specification

1. At least two years experience in the health, social service, or voluntary sector.

2. Experience of client assessment.

3. Experience of working on your own without direct supervision.

4. Awareness of the issues facing older people and a commitment and determination to see that people have access to services they need.

5. The ability to challenge inappropriate discharge.

6. A friendly and open personality with the ability to communicate with older people.

7. Experience of recruiting and supporting volunteers.

8. Ability to manage your own work load and meet deadlines.

9. Car owner/driver essential

10. IT skills including Microsoft Word and Excel.

Mixed economy of care

This term refers to the provision of care from a range of service providers. The Conservative government of the 1980s felt that by introducing competition between service providers, the services provided would be cost effective and of high quality. Instead of most services being provided by the local social services, the majority of services would be commissioned from the private or voluntary sector but social services

would continue to provide services to service users who had complex needs. Since the 1980s this trend has continued.

Key concepts

Providers of services: could be NHS trust hospitals, private agencies or the voluntary sector.

Commissioners of services: could be Primary Care Trusts (PCTs), all other NHS trusts (such as hospital trusts) and social services departments.

As a result of the NHS and Community Care Act (1990), hospitals were able to arrange contracts with private agencies, particularly for catering and cleaning, instead of employing people directly to do this work.

What if?

If you were going to buy a new mobile phone, would cost be the main factor or are there other factors that you would consider to be important?

Is buying the cheapest always a good idea?

Can you think of any problems that might be introduced by developing the idea of a market in care?

Funding local authority social services

Central government funds local councils through the Standard Spending Assessment (SSA) formula. The amount of money given to local councils is based on the population profile of the area, and includes factors such as the number of older people and single parents, types of housing, ethnic groupings and population density. Apart from the SSA, local councils raise funds from the local council tax and from fees and charges for their services. The local council provides social care services to those who are assessed as being in need. However, many services provided by the council are means

PEOPLE IN HOSPITAL	OLDER PEOPLE IN THE COMMUNITY	BABIES/CHILDREN IN THE COMMUNITY	PEOPLE WITH LEARNING DISABILITIES AND THEIR CARERS
Discharge support worker	Lunchclub organiser	Nursery nurse	Family support worker
Counsellor	Podiatrist	'Homestart' organiser	Respite care worker
Advocate	Occupational therapist	Health visitor	Leisure club manager
Organiser of car service	Recreation assistant	Family support officer	Day care manager
Bereavement support worker	Project worker for: ✳ advocacy ✳ befriending ✳ home support ✳ equipment store ✳ healthy living centre	Playgroup leader	Care worker
	Domiciliary care	Toddlers clubs and after school support worker	Social worker
	Transport officer	Benefits worker	Special needs assistant
	'Safe Home' organiser	Social worker	
	Residential care worker	Adoption officer	
	Day centre manager	Teaching assistant	
	Benefits officer		
	Sensory impairment officer (RNIB, RNID)		

TABLE 11.4 *The range of jobs in the voluntary sector for different client groups*

tested – that is, people who apply for social services have their needs assessed, but they also have their income assessed. After income assessment, which would include benefit payments such as the Disability Living Allowance, social services will decide the amount they should pay for services.

Social services provide a range of services to many client groups, but changes in policy have led to social services becoming purchasers of services rather than direct providers (see Mixed economy of care, page 12). Voluntary organisations and private agencies provide services such as personal care, adoption and fostering services, but the local

authority retains responsibility for ensuring that the services are of a high quality. Social services provide care 24 hours a day, seven days a week and there is a duty social worker on call for emergencies at all times.

Funding the voluntary sector

Funding of the voluntary sector comes from a range of sources. Most income is derived from contracts with statutory providers who pay for services supplied by the organisation, as described above. Lottery funding may be applied for but there are strict requirements – usually the project would need to address a particular disadvantaged group, such as refugees. Grants can be obtained from charitable trusts, but these are usually one-off payments. Voluntary organisations are finding that charitable donations have reduced in recent years, so they are competing with private organisations in offering services to the statutory sector and to individuals who can pay for the service

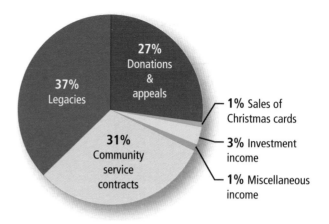

Source: The Stroke Association Annual Review 2005

FIGURE 11.7 *Funding of the Stroke Association of England and Wales*

paying for services; by payments received from the statutory sector and by health insurance companies if individuals belong to an insurance scheme.

Factors affecting the availability of jobs

There are many factors affecting the availability of jobs, including national and local factors.

> ### SCENARIO
> ### Cleaning service
> Many older people or people who have disabilities find cleaning their homes a problem. One voluntary organisation has set up a service to provide cleaning. The organisation advertised for self-employed cleaners. These were interviewed and passed through the CRB (criminal records bureau) police check. They were introduced to possible clients. The contract for cleaning is between the client and the cleaner. The organisation is paid a weekly agency fee by the cleaner. The service has proved very popular. Clients feel they have the support of the organisation and feel confident about the person they are letting into their home. The organisation is receiving an income for the service.

As funding patterns and legislation continue to change, voluntary organisations will need to adapt to new methods of obtaining funds in the future. All voluntary organisations produce an annual report in which they show how the organisation is funded for the year. Most funding is through income paid by the statutory sector for services provided.

> **Think it over**
>
> Look at Figure 11.7 and describe the pattern you see.
>
> Where does the funding come from?

Funding the private sector

The private sector of health and social care services is funded directly by patients or service users

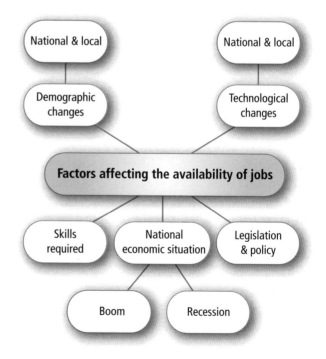

FIGURE 11.8 *Factors affecting the availability of jobs in health and social care*

UK economic situation

If the country is in an economic recession, unemployment levels will rise and job vacancies will decrease. If the country has a growing economy, unemployment will be limited and there will be an increase in job vacancies as services expand, especially in the private sector. Government spending on the statutory sector will increase and this will mean expansion in this sector as well.

Local economic factors

Between 2003 and 2004, house prices rose very fast in many areas of the UK. This meant that some essential workers in health and social care could not afford to buy homes in areas where they wished to work. Many hospitals and social service departments in south east England have difficulty filling posts because of the cost of accommodation. Workers in health and social care have lower levels of pay compared with the business sector.

Development of new technology

Continued changes in technology in health and social care will impact on jobs in the sector. More people with IT skills will be employed to develop the way in which records are kept. For example, the electronic patient record will mean that each patient will have a lifelong record accessible by staff in health and social care services in hospitals and in the community. Technology has also changed operating procedures and this has affected the average length of stay in hospital. Many patients have day surgery and then go home. New technology also includes changes in drug therapy that can mean patients with mental health problems can be looked after in the community instead of in hospital. These examples show that technology can affect the number, type and the location of staff required.

Skills

Skills are closely related to technological changes. With the NHS *Agenda for Change*

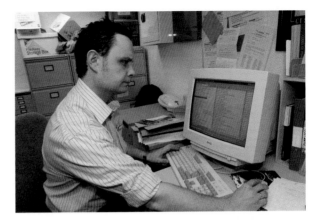

FIGURE 11.9 *Technology has changed record keeping*

proposals (published in 2004) the skills used by NHS staff in their jobs will be evaluated and payment may change as a result. Skills that were important in the past – such as the importance of taking patients' histories and diagnosing medical conditions on the basis of a detailed physical examination – are still important, but with the use of more sophisticated scans and blood tests, it is easier and quicker to make diagnoses of most conditions. However, skills are still needed to interpret the results of scans and other tests. Certain new skills have developed as the result of these technological changes, but some jobs have been deskilled so tasks previously undertaken by trained nurses are now done by health care assistants. These changes affect the nature of jobs in health and social care.

Demographic changes

The population profile affects the availability of jobs in health and social care. Many doctors and nurses in the NHS are aged over 55 and there are concerns about a shortage of trained staff after they retire. The population in the UK is ageing, there are many jobs caring for older people, but there are staff shortages in this area. The declining birth rate in recent years means the number of younger people entering health and social care in the future will also decline.

Political factors

The 2005 European Directive means that NHS staff can work for up to 48 hours a week. This has had an impact on jobs in the NHS and affects staff in areas such as A&E, where cover is required 24 hours a day. It has also affected out-of-hours cover in the community now that GPs are not required to provide 24-hour-a-day care for their patients. Out-of-hours care is provided by doctors' co-operatives who work as agencies. To cover staff shortages in the community, some PCTs have recruited doctors from Europe as EU nationals can now work in the UK. There is a shortage of NHS dentists in 2005 and dentists have been recruited from Poland to help fill the gaps.

National policies

Since 1997, national policies such as the NHS Plan have set targets for the number of staff required to deliver care. National Service Frameworks (NSFs) covering the care of older people, coronary heart disease and diabetes have impacted on the staffing levels needed and the skills required from staff.

> ### SCENARIO
> ### Stroke units
> In the NSF for Older People, one of the targets is to set up a specialist stroke unit in every acute hospital (one containing an AXE department and specialist services). This unit would need a specialist stroke consultant and stroke nurses to staff the unit. There is a shortage of these skills, and training staff to take on these posts takes time. One acute hospital trust has set up a stroke unit and this has improved the treatment of stroke patients dramatically, but staffing the unit is still a problem.

Summary

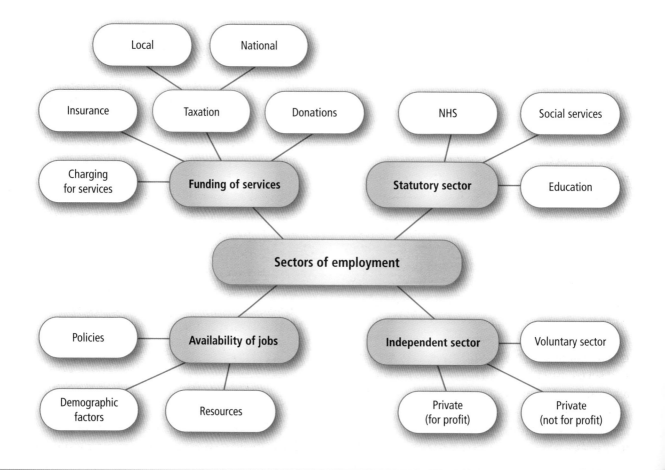

1. Define the term 'mixed economy of care'.

2. If you have a range of service providers in health and social care and early years services, what could be the benefits:

* for service users?

* for purchasers of services?

Can you think of any problems?

3. Many local councils have sold their residential homes to private companies. Can you think of advantages and disadvantages of this practice:

* for staff working in the service?

* for service users receiving the service?

* for commissioners of the service?

11.2 Roles and conditions

In this section you will learn about employment in health and social care and the qualifications needed for different jobs. Jobs in health and social care vary both in status and in the nature of the work being done.

Roles in health and social care

If you look at an organisation chart, like the one for a social services children's department in Table 11.1, you will see that the chart shows the roles within the organisation rather than the names of individual people. If a person leaves, their role will usually remain the same, but someone else will carry it out. It is very important that people are clear about their role – in other words, they must know what is expected from them in their work. This is why a detailed summary of a person's role is usually included within their job description.

Some organisations have a very clear management structure, with directors at the top and social care teams at the bottom. This is called a hierarchical bureaucratic structure. In a smaller organisation, such as a care home, the team is likely to be much smaller. In smaller teams, roles may not be so clearly defined because with staff

sickness or shortage, workers may be required to perform a wider variety of tasks.

Key concepts

Roles: the expected pattern of behaviour associated with a particular position in society. In health and social care the roles of doctors, nurses and other workers are clearly defined and upheld by codes of conduct.

Responsibilities: the term 'responsibilities' relates to the duties, accountability and authority attached to a particular job role. In any job description you will find that the responsibilities of the job are clearly identified.

Conditions of employment

Many employers recognise that staff are their greatest asset. When you are appointed to a post you will receive a summary of the conditions of employment of the post. Conditions of employment will include the following:

* *details of your salary:* this will include the employer's package of pay and employment benefits which includes contractual sickness and maternity leave, allowances and special leave. Under recent legislation, paternity leave would also be included.

* *travel arrangements:* some employers in health and social care are encouraging staff to use transport effectively. Depending on your job you may be offered various schemes such as bicycle loan, car-hire scheme, motor vehicle loan, or travel expenses

* *annual leave:* will be stated in your contract. This depends on the job you have and the hours you work. Annual leave tends to increase once you have been with the employer for five years continuous service

* *pension benefits:* in statutory health and social care services you will be able to join the pension scheme. Private and voluntary organisations may also have their own pension scheme

* *flexible working:* in some jobs it is possible to have flexible working hours, including special

If you look at the following job description you will see that the role of the social care worker has certain responsibilities.

Job description

Care Manager (hospital service)
Report to: Senior Care Manager

Main purpose of the job

1. To assess the needs of individuals and their carers

2. Together with the service users and carers, to devise and implement care plans according to their needs

3. To provide counselling and continuing support to users and carers when appropriate

4. To monitor, review and evaluate services in order to ensure that they are provided effectively and in accordance with need

Responsibilities and duties

1. Provide an assessment service to individuals, their carers and other agencies

2. Initiate and co-ordinate care plans for and with individual service users and their carers, liaising with professional colleagues and representatives of voluntary and private agencies

3. Supervise and support staff as agreed with the Care Manager

4. Offer support, counselling and advice as required to service users and their carers

5. Through the assessment and prioritisation of need, purchase appropriate services within the budget constraints

6. Monitor the efficiency and effectiveness of care plans

7. Review the needs of individual service users and their carers

8. Identify and report unmet need and service shortfalls in the construction of care plans

9. Maintain client records in accordance with council policy

10. Respond to and, where possible, resolve complaints using the councils complaints policy

11. Advise the manager on the quality and value for money of purchased services

12. Participate in multi-disciplinary and inter-agency meetings and working groups and represent the department as required

Look carefully at the job description and draw up a list of the skills required in this post

What knowledge do you think this person would need to do this job?

What previous experience would be helpful in this job?

arrangements such as job sharing, home working, term time only jobs, flexible locations and shift patterns, and overtime arrangements

* *training and staff development:* most statutory services in health and social care offer an annual training programme so that staff can develop skills relevant to the job.

Conditions of service include the period of notice that has to be given by either staff or employer and also will include probationary periods and disciplinary procedures. Conditions of service are important for both employers and staff as they can increase job satisfaction among staff and reduce staff turnover. It is expensive for employers to advertise, recruit and appoint staff, so a stable happy workforce benefits everyone – including patients and clients.

Qualifications and employment

Training in health and social care has become an important issue and is upheld by government policy. Since December 2005 there has been a requirement for all care workers to be qualified to at least NVQ Level 2. In practice this may be difficult to achieve, but staff should be working towards the qualification, and training is one aspect that would be checked by inspectors.

Training and personal development plans are in place for all doctors, nurses and other staff working in the NHS. The higher qualifications you have, the greater opportunity you have for career progression and promotion.

JOB TITLE	QUALIFICATIONS REQUIRED	SERVICE USER GROUP	JOB ROLE
Health care assistant (HCA)	No national minimum requirements Good general education and/or experience NVQs available	Service users in hospital and community of all ages	Personal care Supporting patients Supporting qualified nurses and therapists
Social care worker	No national minimum requirements Initial training given NVQs available	Service users in community of all ages and disabilities	Supporting users in their home and in the community Domiciliary care Residential care
Registered nurse (RN) * children * adult nursing * mental health * learning disabilities	Different qualifications Degree or diploma entry requirements set by each higher education institution	Specialist groups depending on training All ages and disabilities in hospital and community	Depends on nature of post Could be specialist in stroke care, theatre work or district nursing
Health visitor	Registered nursing qualification and health visitor training	Children aged 0–8 Extended to include all age groups	Support children and families in the community
Teaching assistant * early years	No national minimum standards Experience and ability to get on with children NVQs available	Children aged 3–7	Support individual children with special needs Support the whole class or class groups with numeracy, literacy and IT
Nursery nurse	Certificate in childcare and education (CACHE) Diploma in childcare and education	Children aged 0–5	Support individual children and groups in schools, family centres, nurseries, private families
Paramedic	Some GCSEs or A levels, or NVQ Level 3	Users who need emergency services	Support patients to provide medication and other interventions when required
Physiotherapist	Degree in a relevant subject	Users in hospital and community of all ages and disabilities	Provide rehabilitation to post-operative patients to prevent loss of independence by encouraging exercise to restore body function

continued on next page

TABLE 11.5 *Jobs in health and social care*

JOB TITLE	QUALIFICATIONS REQUIRED	SERVICE USER GROUP	JOB ROLE
Occupational therapist	Degree in a relevant subject	All ages working in community and hospital People with disabilities, mobility and sensory problems	Recommend and supply equipment and aids to support patients' lifestyles Promote independent living
Management positions in health and social care	Range of qualifications including graduate entry, NVQs at level 4 and other professional qualifications	Indirect contact with service users, in most cases service users of all ages in community and hospital	Supervise staff to ensure local and national targets are met Plan delivery of services
Practice manager in GP practice	Diploma in primary care management NVQ level 3 or A levels	Indirectly responsible for patients within the practice	Organise delivery of services Train new members of staff (receptionists) Manage finances in the practice
Practice nurse	Registered nurse and additional training	Patients registered with the practice	Support GPs in practice Deliver specialist clinics: diabetes, asthma, hypertension (high blood pressure) Administer immunisations Provide routine services: ear syringing, changing dressings, etc.
Speech and language therapist	Degree	Service users of all ages who have difficulty with communication and/or swallowing problems	Support carers and other workers Help people with problems using exercises and techniques to improve speech and swallowing

TABLE 11.5 *Jobs in health and social care*

Job satisfaction

In many health and care organisations staff have opportunities to express their views about the job they are doing. Job satisfaction can be measured in various ways. In one hospital trust there is an annual review of staff attitudes to gauge job satisfaction. In most jobs there is an annual appraisal system when the worker meets with their line manager to discuss how they feel about their job, what they have achieved in the past year and the training they would like to do in the following year.

Sickness levels and staff turnover can also be seen as indicators of job satisfaction. The Healthcare Commission carries out an annual survey of NHS staff which includes questions covering job satisfaction. The 2004 survey showed that NHS staff are generally fairly satisfied. (You can find the results of the survey on www.healthcarecommission.org.uk).

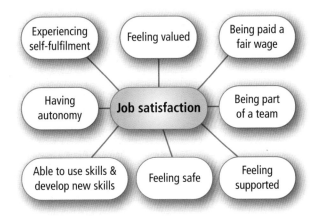

FIGURE 11.10 *The factors that may contribute to job satisfaction*

> **Think it over**
>
> Think about a job you have done – it could be part-time or it could be voluntary work or babysitting. What makes the job worth while? Is it just the money you receive?

Research studies have shown that some people who do repetitive jobs have limited job satisfaction. At the same time, it also depends on the worker's expectations of the job. Some women want limited responsibility in what could be seen as boring work, because much of their satisfaction comes from outside work in their family life. Other part-time workers in care enjoy the work they do because they feel they are using skills they have, although the work is low paid and low status. Job satisfaction is individual to each person.

Different jobs in health and social care have different outcomes. In some, there may be limited contact with patients, for example, working in a records department or an operating theatre. In others, the contact with service users and their families is ongoing.

> **SCENARIO**
>
> **Denise**
>
> Denise is a health visitor. She is attached to a GP practice. She enjoys her job because she has contact with the same families over a long period. She will support the family from when the midwife hands over responsibility to her, to when the child starts school. Much of the satisfaction she gets from her job is from seeing the babies growing into children and being able to support them

How might Denise feel about her job if she was part of a Sure Start team on a run-down estate and saw many families stuck in a spiral of poverty and social exclusion in spite of the best efforts of the team?

> **SCENARIO**
>
> **Audrey**
>
> Audrey works as a phlebotomist (taking blood) in a cancer hospital. She goes round the wards and also sees patients when they attend clinics. She enjoys her job as she sees some patients on a regular basis when they come for check ups. However, she finds it stressful when some patients do not recover and she sees them becoming weaker.

If you are thinking about applying for a job in health and social care you need to consider how you would feel about working with people who may not recover.

What do you think could be the pros and cons of working in the following areas of health and social care:

* working in a residential home for the elderly and mentally confused

* working in a nursery attached to a hospital

* working in a hospice

* working in a GP's surgery as a receptionist

* working in a hospital as a porter on shift work

All these jobs provide an important service but you may feel that some would be more suitable for your personality and abilities.

Job status

Some jobs in health and social care have higher status than others. People are more impressed if you tell them you are a brain surgeon and less impressed if you tell them you are a health care assistant. Status is linked to the prestige given by society to groups or individuals. Some people are concerned to have a job that gives them high status. Many high status positions are linked to

professions such as medicine, but the status given to different roles can be a reflection of the values of society.

Currently in the UK, footballers and celebrities are given high status.

Why do you think this is?

What do they represent that gives them high status?

Summary

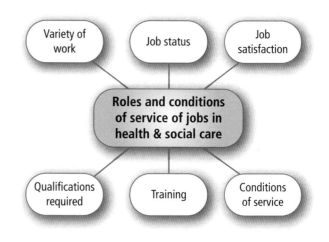

1. In this section we have looked at the skills required in certain jobs. Look again at the list of skills and personal qualities (pages 3 and 4) and decide which of these are relevant for the following jobs:

* a person working as an escort in a bus taking children with learning disabilities to their special school

* a midwife

* a care assistant working in an old people's residential home.

2. If you were thinking of working part time in your local care home at the weekends, what factors about the job and conditions of service would be important to you?

3. Different jobs have different social status. High status jobs in health and social care attract high salaries but they also tend to be filled by white males, whereas low status jobs such as care assistants tend to be filled by women and ethnic minorities. Can you think why this is the case?

11.3 Meeting individual needs

In this section you need to refer to the quality of life factors and caring skills and techniques listed in the AS Unit 1 Effective Caring, so that you can learn how practitioners in health and social care apply these to meet the needs of service users. This section also covers how different practitioner roles and conditions of service lead to the fulfilment of practitioner's needs. The factors shown in Figure 11.11 underpin the planning of care for service users and patients in social care.

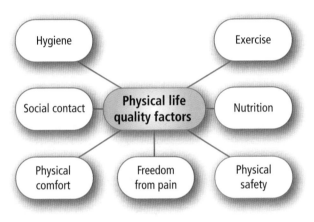

FIGURE 11.11 *The physical quality of life factors*

Meeting the needs of service users

There are three important aspects that are covered in this section:

* the process of care planning and its components
* the care planning cycle
* assessment of service provision; identifying needs, monitoring and reviewing of care plans and the importance of involving service users and carers in the process.

The process of care planning and its components

Care planning should be needs led and should benefit the service user's health and well-being. If there is a carer, their needs should also be included in the care planning.

The process of care planning in the community

With the development of closer working between health and social care services in the community, care planning has become more streamlined. In the past, service users often had to deal quite separately with different health and social care services in order to have their needs met. This meant a lot of duplication of effort and waste of time, as service users often had to give the same information to each service separately. The different services often failed to communicate effectively with each other, which resulted in less efficient care for the service user. However, with the development of IT systems, many care assessments are sent by email to different practitioners involved in the person's care. It is hoped that with the development of multi-disciplinary working, the service user will not have to continually respond to the same questions from different health and social care services.

Care planning based on the needs of the individual was seen as a cornerstone of the NHS and Community Care Act (1990). However with increasing demands on the service (partly caused by the increasing numbers of older people in the population) social services have had to develop criteria which determine who will receive care services and how these will be delivered.

In 2003, the Department of Health produced a document called *Fair Access to Care Services: Guidance on Eligibility Criteria for Adult Social Care*. According to the Fair Access to Care Services (FACS) initiative, councils should assess an individual's presenting needs and decide which are most important. An assessment would be made of the risks that may occur for the person if care is not provided. Councils should focus on those in greatest immediate or longer term need. The idea behind the guidance is that there should be a more consistent approach to needs assessment in all parts of England and Wales, as up until these new proposals, different councils operated different systems when assessing need. For example, if you had two relatives living in different parts of the country with the same levels of disability, you could find they were offered

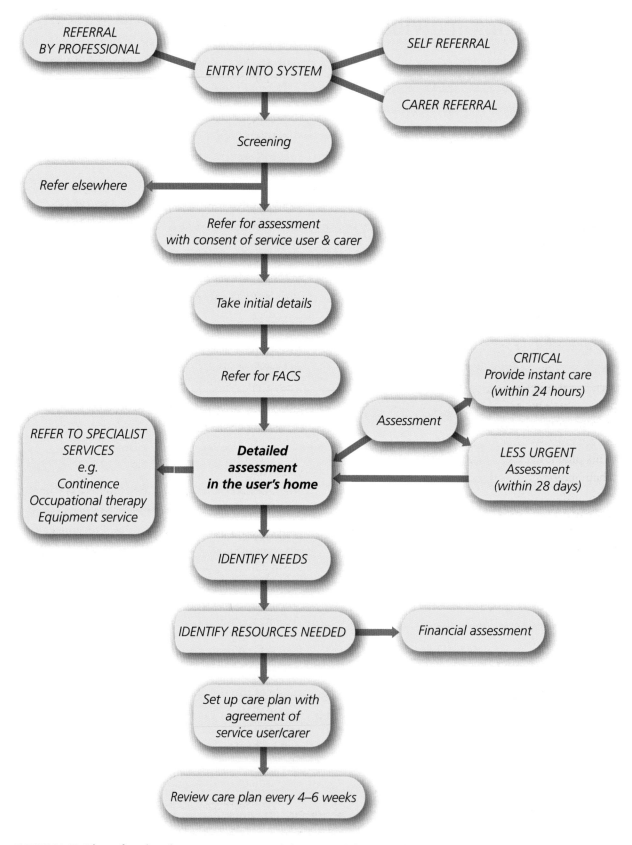

FIGURE 11.12 *The referral and assessment approach in one social service department*

different levels of services, and one might pay nothing for a service while the other would be means tested.

The care plan cycle in social care

Referral for assessment of need

In social services there has been an increase in joint working with the local PCT so that a person coming to social services for assessment may be referred for health services to the PCT. In some areas there is a single phone number to call for referral for all types of assessment, and the referral may be done by a health or social care professional or by the user or carer.

Assessment of need

With more joined-up working between health and social care, a key worker (sometimes called the lead professional) who could either be a health worker or from social services, would assess the needs of the person, usually visiting them at their home, or in hospital if they are about to be discharged or in a rehabilitation unit. Although the guidance focuses on the user, carers should also be involved in the assessment process. The FACS eligibility criteria for service are graded into four bands, which describe the seriousness of the risk to independence or other effects if needs are not addressed. The bands are:

* *critical:* this band includes cases where life is, or will be, threatened, or serious abuse or neglect has occurred or may occur, or serious health problems have developed

* *substantial:* this band covers less critical factors but there is still a substantial risk to the person if care is not delivered

* *moderate and low:* these bands have a lower level of risk.

The full details of FACS are available (www.doh.gov.uk/seg/facs). The FACs assessment is based on the physical life quality factors but psychological factors are also important. For example, giving a service user choice and treating them with respect is also significant.

Care planning – after assessment of need

Once the assessment of need has been carried out, the process continues.

Deciding eligibility for service
Does the person fit the criteria used by the social services?

Drawing up a care plan
This identifies who will do what and when, and may include targets where appropriate.

Identifying services that will be provided
The person and/or their carer should have contact details of everyone involved in their care.

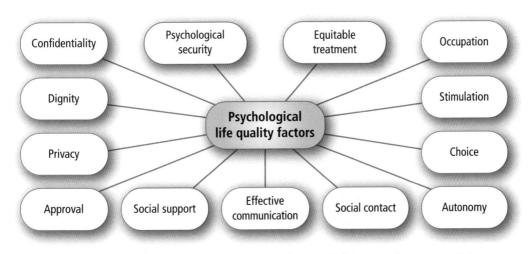

FIGURE 11.13 *The factors that affect the quality of life for both users and providers in health and social care*

Review of the care plan and service provision

This may take place 4–6 weeks after the start of the care plan, or it may be less frequent depending on the situation. If there is a sudden change in the health or mobility of the person, reviews may be more frequent.

In all stages of the process of care planning service users and carers should participate. The patient or service user is seen as central to the care planning process; however, in some cases the service user may be unable to understand the process and they may need to help of an **advocate.**

> ### Key concept
>
> *Advocacy:* when someone speaks on behalf of someone else who is unable to voice their views because of learning difficulties, mental health problems or other reasons. The advocate can be a professional, a volunteer or a relative.

Care planning has to take account of the diversity of the individual related to culture, language, intellectual ability, and mobility. Councils should be aware of the rights of service users and have regard for the Sex Discrimination Act (1975), the Disability Discrimination Act (1995), the Human Rights Act (1998) and the Race Relations (Amendment) Act (2000).

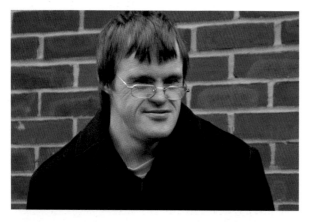

FIGURE 11.14 *A disabled person may need an advocate to help present their views*

SCENARIO
Mrs Brown

Mrs Brown is 80 years old. She is being discharged from hospital following a fall in which she fractured her hip. She lives on her own and is concerned about how she will manage at home. A social worker visits her in hospital and discusses the support she will need when she gets home. An occupational therapist goes home with Mrs Brown before her discharge and identifies the adaptations she will need if she is to be able to cope independently when she comes home. Mrs Brown is very worried and 'takes it out' on all the workers she meets. She is terrified 'they' will put her in a home without her consent. The care plan has been drawn up and involves the practice nurse visiting to monitor Mrs Brown's diabetes; a care worker will come each day to help Mrs Brown with her personal care; a volunteer from Age Concern will do her shopping and social services have arranged for a cleaner to come in twice a week. Two days after her return from hospital the practice nurse comes to check on Mrs Brown. Mrs Brown says she doesn't want anyone in the house; she can manage; she becomes very abusive.

Try it out

Care plans are only one part of the process of caring for people. The caring skills and techniques used by workers can help to ensure that the service user is kept safe and that the care plans are put into practice.

Look at the quality of life factors that could affect Mrs Brown's recovery. What physical life factors could be at risk if Mrs Brown refuses to let people help her? What skills and techniques could care workers use to overcome these problems? Figure 11.15 shows the caring skills and techniques used.

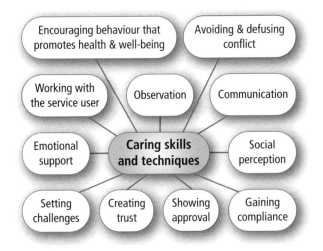

FIGURE 11.15 *Caring skills and techniques*

1. Recognition of a problem
2. Initial assessment and investigation
3. Assessment and planning
4. Implementation and review
5. Rehabilitation.

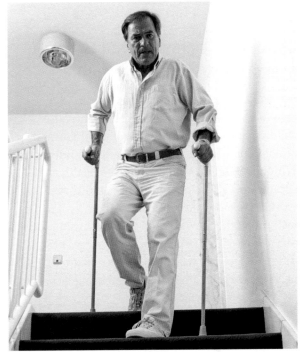

FIGURE 11.16 *Tony on his crutches*

Care planning in health care

Care planning in social care is often about supporting service users whose needs are long term. As time goes by, the care plan will be reviewed on a regular basis and additional needs may develop due to increasing age, disability or lack of mobility. However in care planning in the acute setting of a hospital, the care plan may go through several stages:

SCENARIO

Tony

Tony is 50. He has suffered from severe osteo-arthritis after a sports injury to his knee when playing football. He is finding it difficult to walk far, to manage stairs and he has had to change to an automatic car as he cannot manage using the clutch pedal. He is in a great deal of pain. He goes to see his GP who looks at his knee and sends him for an X-ray. The X-ray confirms that Tony has severe arthritis in his knee joint and the doctor also notices that he has muscle wastage in his thigh muscle. He refers Tony to the consultant orthopaedic surgeon who examines Tony and decides he needs a total knee replacement. He is put on the waiting list and meanwhile he attends Physiotherapy for exercises to improve his muscles. After six months, Tony enters hospital and has his operation. 24 hours after the op,

Tony is walking with a zimmer frame and starting physiotherapy. He has painkillers for the pain and other drugs to reduce the danger of deep vein thrombosis. After six days Tony is discharged from hospital to his home. The OT has advised him to use a helping hand to pick things up from the floor and use a high bar stool in the kitchen. For three weeks he manages on crutches and then he is able to walk with a stick. He continues to do his exercises to strengthen his leg. After six weeks he sees the consultant again. He starts driving again and goes back to work eight weeks after the surgery. The pain is getting better and he can do more and more each week. He sees the consultant six months after the operation and is discharged from hospital. He is now able to lead a normal life and do most of the activities he has always enjoyed in the past.

> **Try it out**
>
> Look at the scenario and identify the stages in Tony's care cycle
>
> Look again at Tony's story and identify which caring skills and techniques health workers would use to support him in his treatment and recovery.

Children's issues related to assessment in the community

Services for children in health and social care are often managed differently. This is because children are seen as particularly vulnerable and also because their needs may change rapidly. With increased integration between health and social care services and education, multi-agency working is more likely. A child will be assigned a lead professional who could be from health, social services or education. Figure 11.17 shows how different agencies work together to ensure that the needs of children are met through using a common assessment approach. Specialist assessments may also be used in more complicated cases.

The Common Assessment Process (CAP) for children

This common assessment is a standardised approach to assessing the needs of children and young people. It was developed in 2005 and came out of the Green Paper *Every Child Matters*. The framework can be viewed online (www.everychildmatters.gov.uk/key-documents). The common assessment approach is used for babies, children or young people. There is a checklist the professional will use to decide whether a common assessment is needed. The parents are involved throughout the process.

Stages of CAP for children and young people from the perspective of the lead professional

Stage 1 Preparation

Talk to child/young person and their parent. A pre-assessment checklist may be used. You may

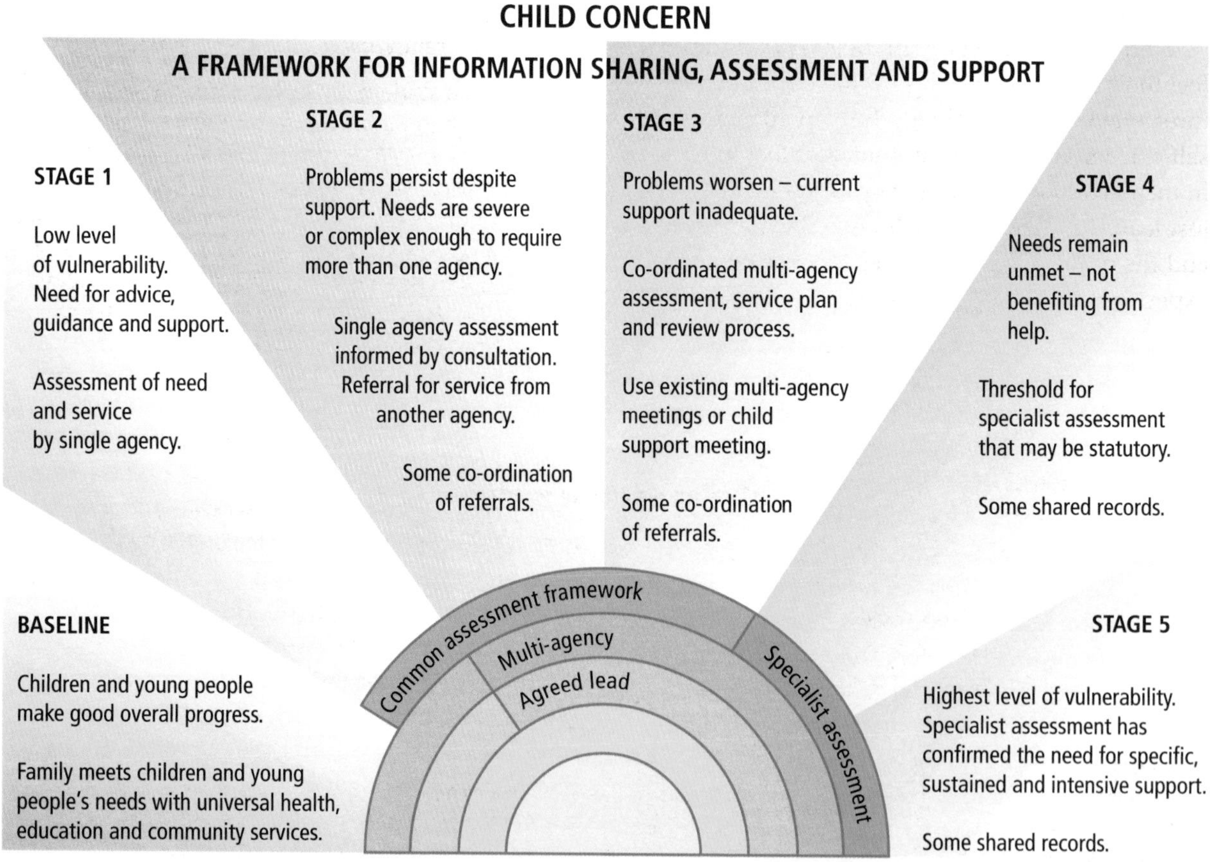

CHILD CONCERN
A FRAMEWORK FOR INFORMATION SHARING, ASSESSMENT AND SUPPORT
STAGE 1
Low level of vulnerability. Need for advice, guidance and support.
Assessment of need and service by single agency.
STAGE 2
Problems persist despite support. Needs are severe or complex enough to require more than one agency.
Single agency assessment informed by consultation. Referral for service from another agency.
Some co-ordination of referrals.
STAGE 3
Problems worsen – current support inadequate.
Co-ordinated multi-agency assessment, service plan and review process.
Use existing multi-agency meetings or child support meeting.
Some co-ordination of referrals.
STAGE 4
Needs remain unmet – not benefiting from help.
Threshold for specialist assessment that may be statutory.
Some shared records.
BASELINE
Children and young people make good overall progress.
Family meets children and young people's needs with universal health, education and community services.
STAGE 5
Highest level of vulnerability. Specialist assessment has confirmed the need for specific, sustained and intensive support.
Some shared records.
Common assessment framework
Multi-agency
Agreed lead
Specialist assessment

FIGURE 11.17 *Assessment and review of children*

decide a fuller assessment is not needed at this point but if you decide it is appropriate, you need to seek the agreement of the child/young person so that you may talk to colleagues about them.

Stage 2 Discussion

You complete the assessment with the child/parent or family. You use the information from all sources (school, GP, etc.). You agree the actions that the service and the family will deliver and record this.

Stage 3 Service delivery

You deliver on your actions. You refer to other services depending on the needs of the child. You monitor progress. If a range of agencies are used, identify a lead professional who is the contact at all times.

Meeting the needs of workers in health and social care

Just as service users have needs that should be met through the provision of services, workers in health and social care also have needs. Quality of life factors are just as important to workers.

Staff can feel unhappy in their work if they feel their efforts are not appreciated. If they feel threatened or undervalued, this can affect their self-esteem. It is important that staff feel fulfilled in their work. If they don't say anything but just leave, the problems will never be addressed and the next person who takes their place may experience the same difficulties.

Summary

Try it out

Look again at Figures 11.11 and 11.13. The way we experience our lives is affected by both emotional and physical factors. The following scenarios show workers experiencing problems because of various factors in their work. In your groups discuss how the problem could be put right.

1. Sedina works at night in A&E. The department is often short staffed. On Fridays there are often groups of drunken youths who frighten Sedina.

2. Louise works in a care home. She feels the manager doesn't like her. She has asked her if she can study for her NVQ Level 2. Other staff who have only just joined the care home have started on their NVQs already.

3. Ann works as a receptionist in the X-ray department. She has to do a lot of work on the computer. Ann has been having trouble with her eyes and her back as the chair she uses is very old.

4. Mark works as a porter in a local hospital. He enjoys the work and likes to keep busy. He is supposed to have a one-hour lunch break, but his manager says they are short staffed. Mark grabs a sandwich from the snack bar.

5. Sam is a student nurse. His current placement is in a drop-in day centre for mental health patients who have severe mental illness. He has been allocated a mentor, Phil, but Sam never sees him. He feels very isolated. Last week he set up a game of football with some of the service users. Phil arrived at the end of the session and said he shouldn't have organised the activity without clearing it with him first.

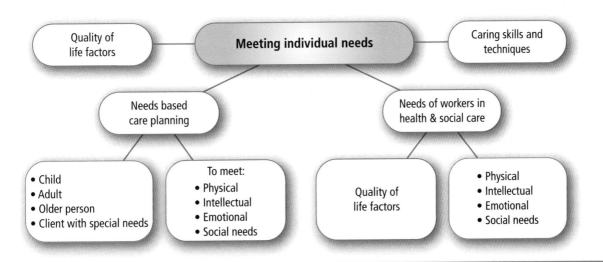

1. Mary is 50. She has been blind since birth. She lives on her own in a flat. You are Mary's lead professional and you are assessing her needs. Identify the four main categories of need that Mary has and describe how you could meet these needs.

2. Mark (25) has recently started his new job working as a night nurse in A&E. What are Mark's needs and how could these be met in the work situation? Safety aspects are a key consideration. What could his line manager do to ensure his safety needs are met?

3. Quality of life factors affect the level of satisfaction in every job. Look at Ann's story. How could her experience at work be improved?

   Ann (44) works in a busy operating theatre in a general hospital. She works shifts. The manager draws up the shift timetable each month in advance. Staff who have young children are given shift patterns that fit in with the school day and school holidays. Ann is single but lives with her elderly father. She is his main carer. Ann finds she is often working weekends and late evening shifts. Ann finds it difficult to arrange any social life for herself and to take her father to appointments. She finds her life is becoming exhausting and she is worried she will make mistakes at work. Her manager is very difficult to talk to when Ann tries to discuss her hours.

11.4 Legislation

Legislation changes affecting provision of health and social care can arise for a variety of reasons. The main factors are:

* *economic:* the need to reduce government spending

* *political:* views about the role of the state and how far it should support families and individuals in society

* *technological:* changes in the organisation of services and of society

* *demographic changes:* e.g. an ageing population

* *the influence of the European Courts:* e.g. the European working time directive limits the hours that may be worked by all health and social care staff.

There have been many changes in legislation in the last 20 years that have effected changes in the provision of health and social care.

The NHS and Community Care Act (1990)

This important act changed the way services are provided. The key aspects of the act include:

1. The focus on a needs-based approach: this meant that the fundamental priority was meeting the needs of service users.

2. The mixed economy of care: services were to be provided by a range of agencies. The role of the statutory sector in providing services would be reduced and the role of the independent sector, including both private agencies and voluntary organisations, would increase.

3. People would be encouraged to remain in their own homes, supported by community services, rather than be cared for in residential homes.

4. Social services became purchasers of care (or commissioners) rather than providers. As we have already seen, the voluntary sector and other agencies already provide a range of services that have been paid for by the council.

Further developments in policy that affect the provision of health and social care services

1. Social services and health care organisations have limited budgets. These budgets are controlled by central government. PCTs buy in services from acute hospitals and other providers with funding directly from the Department of Health.

2. Current government policy encourages a close partnership between health and social care agencies. This partnership includes joint funding of services by health and social services – such as intermediate care services and children's services; and joint funding of posts in local areas – for example, a strategic director who plans integrated services.

3. Limited funding of the statutory sector has encouraged the development of the role of the

voluntary sector in providing cost effective services.

4. Joint care planning to meet the needs of individual members in the community is another effect of closer working between health and social services. We have already seen an example of this in the care planning cycle outlined on page 25.

The 1998 White Paper *Modernising Social Services*

This White Paper set out the programme for change for social services. Staff were to be trained and standards of care would be improved. A national register of care staff would be set up. Protection of vulnerable client groups, such as older people, people with learning disabilities, people with mental health problems and children was seen as a key issue and all staff had to receive training on Protection issues related to abuse. This was in response to news stories of abuse taking place in social care.

The Children Act (2004)

This legislation placed a duty on people working with children and young people to have systems in place that would protect children from abuse and other problems. Each local authority had to appoint a Director of Children's Services who would work in partnership with education and health services. Multi-disciplinary teams have been set up to work with children.

Legislation has encouraged closer partnerships between health, social services and early years services. In the past, health and social care workers worked in isolation from each other and there seemed to be a clash of cultures between health and social care. Health professionals

Key concept

Multi-disciplinary team (MD teams): workers from different specialist professions who work together to provide care for patients or clients. Multi-disciplinary teams work in the community or in the hospital. They can work with a particular client group, such as children, or people with mental health problems.

SCENARIO
Multi-disciplinary working

In a Sure Start Circle there is a central office where all the team work together to support children and families in the area (see Figure 11.17). Referrals to the team may come from school nurses, voluntary groups, GPs or families can self-refer. Sara, the team leader, is a social worker and the nominated child protection officer for the centre. She organises team meetings to discuss particular concerns. Members of the team have regular training as child protection issues are constantly developing. The midwife on the team advises pregnant women and encourages them to give up smoking. The health visitor visits families and keeps records on any issues of concern. The family support worker visits families in their homes and offers advice. She also runs parenting groups, and gives advice on benefits. There are several Tamil families on the estate so the team runs a drop-in coffee morning to advise families on health and other issues, and an interpreter attends these sessions. Sara feels that Sure Start multi-disciplinary teams are making a great difference to the lives of families and children in deprived areas. Working in a team has benefits for the staff as well as they can discuss problems with colleagues and refer clients quickly so that they can receive the support they need.

addressed clinical needs and social care workers tended to look at social needs, including offering advice on managing incomes and applying for benefits. With the single assessment process developed through the National Service Framework (NSF) for Older People, health and social care workers assess clinical and social needs, although there is often a separate financial assessment. Single assessments are being developed for other groups, including children through CAP (see page 28). This is a further example of how legislation has changed practice.

In this section we have seen that legislation has effected many changes in the ways health and social care services are organised and delivered.

Summary

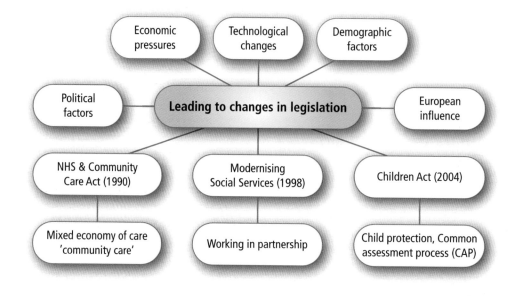

- Economic pressures
- Technological changes
- Demographic factors
- Political factors
- **Leading to changes in legislation**
- European influence
- NHS & Community Care Act (1990)
- Modernising Social Services (1998)
- Children Act (2004)
- Mixed economy of care 'community care'
- Working in partnership
- Child protection, Common assessment process (CAP)

11.5 Quality assurance

In this section you will learn about ways in which the service user's experience of treatment provided by practitioners can be assessed. These include the measurement of service delivery against performance indicators such as waiting times and clinical outcomes, as well as the use of service user satisfaction questionnaires and interviews.

Standards

Standards can be set nationally; such as the National Service Frameworks (NSFs) or they can be set locally by health and social care organisations. Very often, standards are also part of the code of conduct that workers in particular organisations should follow when delivering a service.

Key concepts

Standards: can be defined as the level and quality of service or performance that conforms to a recognised model.

Governance: is the organisation and delivery of services so that they meet the standards required by the inspection bodies and by the Board or governing body of an organisation.

In NHS Trusts there is a clinical governance committee that audits performance in the Trust. A similar process is carried out in all health and social care organisations. Governance can also be seen to be part of the function of scrutiny committees in local councils and of trustee boards in the voluntary sector.

Quality control: systems that are put in place by health and social care organisations to ensure that services are of a high quality.

Monitoring service delivery is part of quality control. For example, waiting times and cleanliness are monitored in NHS trusts. Care provision in social care may be monitored using feedback from service users. League tables are seen as one aspect of quality control in early years education. Media reports and complaints and comments received from patients and service users can also have an effect on how the services are organised.

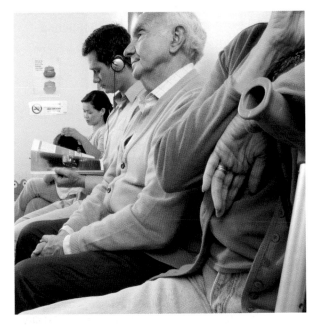

FIGURE 11.18 *Waiting times in hospitals are now monitored*

Quality in the NHS

One of the key aims of the NHS Plan is to improve quality services and to reduce errors. The model for delivering quality services is set out in the 1998 Department of Health Paper *A First Class Service: Quality in the new NHS.* The model includes clear standards of service, patient and public involvement, and ways of monitoring services.

The Healthcare Commission

This body was set up under the Health and Social Care (Community Health and Standards)

Many complaints were received by a local PCT about access to chiropody services. There was a shortage of chiropodists or podiatrists, and this meant long waiting lists. In an area with a high proportion of older people with foot problems there was no toenail cutting service. The problem was highlighted by a letter to the local paper. As a result the local Age Concern provided a toenail cutting service and health care assistants are being trained to cut nails. Podiatry assistants are also being trained to do more skilled work so that fully trained podiatrists can concentrate on the more advanced techniques.

Act (2003) and came into being on 1 April 2004. The role of the **Healthcare Commission** is to encourage improvement in the provision of health care by and for NHS organisations in England and Wales. It also deals with complaints from patients. The Commission has the power to inspect all premises used to provide NHS health care and it can also interview any person working for the NHS or any patient receiving health care. Patients' views are seen as an important aspect in monitoring the quality of services.

Commission for Patient and Public Involvement in Health (CPPIH)

This was set up to work at national, regional and local levels in England to monitor the NHS and to involve the public in decision making about the provision of health services. This was done through setting up **Patient and Public Involvement Forums** (PPIFs) in 2003. Every NHS trust in England has a PPIF and its members are often ex-patients of the trust who can contribute their experience.

Patient and Public Involvement Forums (PPIFs)

These are independent organisations and they have the powers to inspect all premises used by NHS patients, including the private sector, and they consider the quality of the services from the patient's viewpoint. If there is a planned change to service, the PPIF will be involved in the consultation process. PPIFs hold several meetings a year in public and these should be advertised in the local newspapers.

Think it over

The NHS and the services it provides are varied and complex. It is led by highly trained professionals. Can you think of any problems that could arise for patients and other lay members on the patients' Forum who do not have extensive medical knowledge?

Independent Complaints Advocacy Services (ICAS)

These were also established after the Health and Social Care Act (HSCA, 2001). They are independent bodies which help patients pursue a complaint about a particular NHS service. They also offer information and advice and will act as advocate for the patient (i.e. they may write letters, attend meetings and speak on the patient's behalf). They also advise patients of the options open to them if they wish to complain. Citizens Advice Bureaux can tell people the location of their local ICAS.

PALS (Patients Advice and Liaison Services)

All trusts have to have a PALS service. As is suggested by the title, PALS offers advice to patients. In a hospital you will usually find the PALS office near the main reception and all patients using the Trust should be advised of their existence. PALS try to resolve problems on the spot – this could be dealing with a complaint about cleaning on a ward or the quality of the food. PALS give information to patients, their carers and their families about local health services, and put people in touch with local support groups. They direct people to ICAS or to the trust's own complaints service and they may refer issues of concern to the hospital management and to the PPIF. PALS produce a leaflet telling people about their service and these are usually easily available in the Trust.

Monitoring service delivery using patients views

All NHS Trusts have to have a complaints system set up to record, monitor and review complaints. A manager at senior level is appointed to lead on the process. Complaints are reported to the trust board four times a year and any significant patterns are monitored. As well as complaints monitoring, hospital trusts administer the 'UK In-patient Survey' to everyone who has been an inpatient for at least one night. The survey is part of the monitoring process and is required by the Healthcare Commission. It consists of 68 questions and covers seven key areas:

* emergency and planned admissions
* the environment and facilities
* care and treatment, especially pain relief
* doctors and nurses
* adequacy of patient information
* discharge
* overall impression.

Here are some of the questions patients are asked:

1. After arriving at hospital, how long did you wait for admission to a room or a ward?

2. During your stay in hospital, did you ever share a room or bay with a member of the opposite sex?

3. How clean was the hospital room or ward that you were in?

4. How clean were the toilets and bathrooms that you used?

5. How would you rate the courtesy of the doctors?

In one trust the scores were good for emergency care, number of nurses on duty and explanation of test results. However the trust scored badly on information and communication, food, and the use of mixed sex wards. As a result of this survey the trust has drawn up a plan to improve these areas. Surveys like this are a useful tool to identify areas of poor quality, but as we have seen with all research tools, you have to be aware of the sample size and the scoring system. In this postal survey 481 patients took part, with a 61.6 per cent response rate from the sample. Patients' responses can be affected by a range of factors – as you know yourself. For example, different people have different ideas about what is a 'good meal'.

National Patients' Surveys take place every year. In 2004, the following National Patients' Surveys took place:

✳ children and young people survey

✳ ambulance trusts survey

✳ service users in mental health trusts.

The surveys are collated by the NHS survey advice centre and are used as part of the mechanism for the performance ratings of trusts.

Involving service users in the NHS

Section 11 of the Health and Social Care Act (2001) places a duty on NHS trusts to make arrangements to involve and consult patients and the public in service planning and operation, and in proposals for change. This is a new duty for trusts, as before they involved the public only when there was a planned change to service provision.

Patient prospectuses

All PCTs have to produce a patient prospectus entitled *Your guide to local health services*. These guides are available at GPs' surgeries, and in some areas they have been delivered to people's homes.

Think it over

Obtain a copy of the guide produced by your local PCT and make a list of all the services provided. How do you think the quality of these services could be monitored?

Quality assurance in social care

Regulation and inspection in social services has also been developed. The **Commission for Social Care Inspection** (CSCI) was set up in April 2004. It is responsible for:

✳ carrying out inspections of all social care organisations – statutory, private and voluntary – against national standards, and publishing reports

✳ registering services that meet national minimum standards

✳ carrying out inspections of local social service authorities

✳ publishing an annual report to Parliament on progress in social care and an analysis of where money has been spent

✳ publishing star ratings for local authorities.

The CSCI sets out regulations and information about specific social care standards (see www.csci.org.uk).

Quality in Early Years' Services: OFSTED

OFSTED (the Office for Standards in Education) was set up in 1993 and was responsible for the quality of education in all maintained schools and nursery schools. It has developed its inspection role to cover childminding and out of school care for children up to the age of eight. It carries out four main functions in order to ensure that day care providers and childminders meet the national standards.

Registration

Childminders and day care providers have to be registered by OFSTED. Premises are also checked.

Inspection

OFSTED inspects childcare providers every three years to judge the quality and standards of the childcare provided.

Investigation

OFSTED investigates any complaints or concerns voiced by parents or members of the public, and issues raised in inspection reports.

Enforcement

OFSTED can take action if there is a risk to children in the service provided. This may lead to the cancellation of the registration of the childminder or care provider. For more details on OFSTED look at the website (www.ofsted.gov.uk).

Factors affecting access to services

There are many factors affecting access to health and social care services (see Figure 11.19).

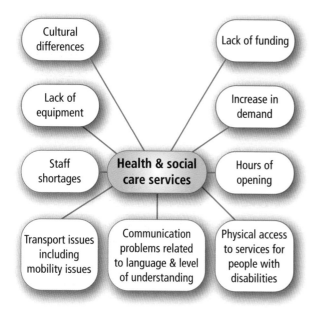

FIGURE 11.19 *Factors which affect access to health and social care services*

The government is aware that many patients and relatives do not want to travel long distances to hospital. By 2008 it is proposing that there should be more local care centres that can treat people nearer their homes. There will be fewer acute hospitals dealing with emergencies and complicated surgery, and more local centres looking after people who do not have complex

needs. People who have most difficulty accessing health and social care services are:

* older people
* mothers with young children
* ethnic minorities – especially those who do not have good spoken English
* disabled people – including those with learning disabilities.

SCENARIO
Retinal screening

In one PCT a retinal screening clinic was set up for diabetic patients so that the condition of their eyes could be monitored. These patients tend to be older people. In the first few months of the service it was found that the 'did not attend' rate was very high. When patients were asked why they did not attend they said that transport was a problem as the centre was not served by a bus.

As a result of this, the voluntary sector organised volunteer drivers and the PCT began discussions with the local bus company to see if they could provide a route nearer the clinic.

SCENARIO
Antenatal clinic

It was noted that the infant mortality rate among Bangladeshi and Pakistani families was higher than the average. When the community midwife investigated this, she found that women from these groups did not feel comfortable coming to the antenatal clinic. They had problems communicating with health staff and they did not wish to be examined by male staff.

As a result, an interpreter met the women and came with them to the clinic. Female staff examined them and problems were identified at an early stage.

Sometimes insufficient provision leads to difficulties with access (as we have already seen with the complaints about chiropody services, page 33). A sudden increase in demand can also affect access.

SCENARIO
Drop-in clinics
Many local sexual health clinics have been unable to meet the demand for their services. Changes in sexual lifestyles among young people have led to an increase in sexually transmitted diseases (STDs). Sometimes people have to wait six weeks for an appointment and the drop-in clinics have to turn people away. In order to meet the demand, increased funding and additional resources – both staff, laboratory services and equipment – will have to increase, and this change will take time to come about.

Apart from these examples, many factors affect access to services. Shortage of specialist staff is a key issue, and very often a form of rationing takes place. There has been an increase in mental health problems among children, but no increase in specialist staff. In one PCT, children will only be referred to the mental health team if they are suicidal.

Access to social care services

Many centres and nurseries offering day care are difficult to access. This can be a particular problem in rural areas. Transport is often a key issue in accessing services. Resources, staff and equipment are also a key concern for all aspects of social care. If the demand for a particular service increases, additional staff will be needed. For example, PCTs and local councils are working together to provide equipment in the community through the ICES (Integrated Community Equipment Service). Equipment for children with special needs (such as a wheelchair or car seat) can be expensive and as the child grows the equipment needs to be replaced. Specialist beds and other equipment for people with sensory problems are also provided through ICES.

Budgets for equipment are very tightly controlled in social care, and this can affect provision. For example, the continence service in one area only allows a certain number of pads for each client in order to keep within the budget.

Summary

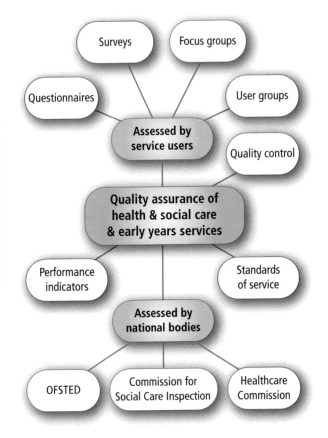

Consider this

1. Quality of services can be assessed by external inspection and by the views of users of the service. Discuss the advantages and disadvantages of each approach.

2. Service users' questionnaires are seen as a useful tool for assessing quality. What are the problems of using questionnaires in this way?

3. Access to services can affect the experience of users. Discuss the problems that may occur:

✳ in urban areas

✳ in rural areas.

11.6 Interview techniques

In this section you will learn how to design an interview schedule to measure satisfaction. This section prepares you for the report you will write for your assessment for this unit. Because the subject of this unit is working in health and social care, we focus mainly on devising an interview schedule to find out how satisfied someone is in their job. If you refer to Unit 21 you will find detailed guidance on research which will help you with this unit, particularly if you decide to interview service users about their experience.

Measuring job satisfaction

Staff attitudes are known to affect patient care, both directly and indirectly. For example, staff with a positive attitude are more likely to work effectively and efficiently. Staff who feel overworked are more likely to suffer from stress and be away from work as a result, increasing the workload of others. One healthcare organisation that measures job satisfaction is the Healthcare Commission who have been conducting annual national NHS staff surveys since 2003.

More details about the national NHS staff survey can be found on the Healthcare Commission website, and there is also a summary of the key findings of the 2004 survey. This is useful for you to look at, as it shows you how the survey was done and the type of questions that were asked.

Measuring satisfaction with a service received

Questionnaires can be a useful tool to provide information about satisfaction with a service in health and social care. Figure 11.20 shows an example of a questionnaire used in GPs' surgeries. Look at it carefully. Can you think of the advantages and disadvantages of using a questionnaire like this?

Structured interviews with service users, as part of your work for this unit, would need to be arranged with care. You would need to make it clear to the respondent that you are finding out about their experience but you would not be able to act as an advocate for them or to intervene in their care.

Structured interviews

Interviews involve the researcher meeting with individual subjects and collecting data directly from them. Interviews can be formally structured, following a schedule which has been drawn up

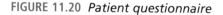

FIGURE 11.20 *Patient questionnaire*

in advance, and this would be an appropriate approach to use in your study.

Structured interviews are well defined and clearly structured. Interviewers follow an interview schedule, which contains a list of questions similar to a questionnaire, but unlike a questionnaire, it is the interviewer who asks the questions and records the subject's answers. They enable the interviewer to stay in control of the conversation and find out answers to specific questions, while at the same time offering opportunities for the interviewee to have his or her say.

Key concept

Interview schedule: the order and content of the questions you will ask in your interview.

Closed and open questions

In both questionnaires and interviews, questions can be either closed or open. Closed questions usually have a limited response and can cover basic data about the person, such as age, marital status, number of children, type of work done, etc.

Examples of closed questions would be:

* what is your name?

* how old are you?

* do you have any children?

This type of information is easily analysed and presented. However, many questionnaires and structured interviews also make use of open questions. Examples of these would be:

* how do you feel about coming to this hospital/clinic?

* can you tell me about the care you received while you were in hospital?

* could the service be improved in any way?

* why did you choose to apply for this job?

How and *what* are useful words to use in order to gain a full response from your interviewee. Very often the interviewer may prompt the subject for further information such as:

* why do you say that?

* is there anything else?

* can you tell me more about that?

Open questions require skill on the part of the interviewer, especially if personal and sensitive issues are being covered. They give a great deal of useful information, but both open and closed questions must be relevant to the purpose of the study rather than an excuse for the interviewer to be intrusive and nosy.

Rating scales

Rating scales are used a great deal in questionnaires and interview schedules. Sometimes the interviewer will give the respondent a card which has the range of responses written on it. Sometimes the interviewer will sit next to the respondent and work through the questions with them.

Here are some sample questions showing how job satisfaction could be measured.

Example 1 Balance between work and personal life

For each statement below, indicate whether you agree or disagree with the statement made. Use a scale where 1 is 'strongly agree' and 10 is 'strongly disagree'.

I am able to work flexibly when I have existing personal commitments. ☐

My manager is very approachable and I am able to talk to her/him about my workload. ☐

Ratings like this can be useful, but they give limited information when used on their own. You can immediately see from these examples that these questions may need clarification from the interviewer – do interviewer and interviewee both understand the terms used in the question in the same way? You would probably want to ask another question such as 'why do you say that?' in order to gain more information.

Example 2 Opportunity for flexible working

Does your company offer any of the following options? Please tick those that apply.

* flexitime ☐

* part-time hours or a reduced working day ☐

* working from home. ☐

Think it over

What are the problems here? Although the employer may offer these options, we don't know whether the respondent uses these or finds them helpful.

Look at the following example, to do with staff satisfaction.

Example 3 Satisfaction at work

Please indicate whether you agree or disagree with the statements below relating to your level of satisfaction at work. Use a scale where 1 is 'strongly agree' and 10 is 'strongly disagree'.

I get praise from my manager when I perform well at work. ☐

My manager is good at supporting me during busy or stressful times. ☐

I know that my work is appreciated and that I play an important role within my company. ☐

Can you think of any problems with these ratings? Will these responses give you sufficient information? Would you need additional questions? Ratings on their own give limited information and may not reflect the true experience of the respondent. In addition, concern about who may see the replies may make respondents unwilling to give a true response. That is why it is useful to use additional evidence as well. Ratings are useful, however, in that they are easy to analyse and to identify particular patterns of response.

Life quality factors include physical safety issues. Many workers in health and social care services may work with aggressive or difficult people, and the way this is dealt with by the organisation is an important aspect of job satisfaction.

Example 4 Awareness of action taken to deal with violence or harassment in the workplace

Please indicate whether you feel that your employer would take effective action to protect you from the following scenarios by marking either yes, no or don't know against each one.

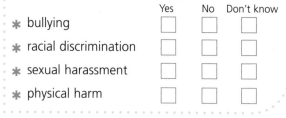

	Yes	No	Don't know
✳ bullying	☐	☐	☐
✳ racial discrimination	☐	☐	☐
✳ sexual harassment	☐	☐	☐
✳ physical harm	☐	☐	☐

Again, you may want to know more details. Scoring the responses could be difficult if there are a lot of 'don't knows'. Therefore it would make sense to have additional questions that would give more details. We can see from these examples that ratings can be useful in some circumstances but if you are trying to understand someone's experience of work they have limited validity.

Some pitfalls to avoid in interview questions

Avoiding bias

Bias can affect the interview if you allow your own feelings to affect the type of questions asked and the way you ask the questions. You need to concentrate on the purpose of the interview and make sure all the questions relate directly to that. You also need to avoid asking leading questions such as:

✳ 'the meals are awful, aren't they?'

✳ 'they never see you on time, do they?'

Try it out

Think how you could rephrase the leading questions above using an open ended approach.

It is very important that you avoid bias in your assessment. When you interview someone, don't make assumptions about their job or the service they have received, and don't reveal your own feelings. For example, if you interview someone who works in a hospice, don't say, 'it must be awful working with dying people.' Many hospices offer respite care, and not all patients die in hospices.

Multiple questions

Multiple questions involve asking more than one question at the same time, and can be confusing. For example:

✳ 'how often have you been coming here and do you always see the same doctor?'

✳ 'how long have you had home care and what do the carers do?'

✳ 'are you in charge of this clinic and who do you work with?'

It is always better to reword questions like this so that you are only asking one question at a time.

Setting up your structured interview

Preparing the interview questions

Before you begin preparing the questions to go in your interview schedule, you need to think carefully about the purpose of the interview. Whether you interview a job-holder or a service user, the main purpose of your interview is to find out how their needs are being met – in the case of a job-holder, you need to find out how the job meets their needs, and in the case of a service user, you need to find out how well their personal needs were met in the service they experienced. A good way to start is to look at the life quality factors outlined in Figures 11.11 and 11.13, and use these as a starting point for your questions.

Planning the questions

Think of a range of questions you could ask that are relevant to finding out the level of satisfaction. Look at the list and make sure there are no repetitions or questions that go off the point. Consider whether you could use a rating scale or pre-coded number values in some of your closed questions. You might choose one of the formats below:

> Examples
> How would you rate aspect X of the service you received?
> poor   adequate   good   excellent
>
> Rate aspect Y of the service you received, where 1 is poor and 5 is excellent:
> 1   2   3   4   5

When you have done this, put the questions in order. Begin with an introduction stating the purpose of the research and then go onto easy, general questions. The respondents need to be set at ease before you move onto more specific questions.

Checking the questions

When you have completed the interview schedule, check the questions again.

* Are there too many questions, which might put the respondents off, or too few?
* Will your respondents know the answers?
* Could the questions upset or embarrass the respondent?
* Are any questions too long and confusing?
* Are the questions clear?
* Have you used words that the respondents will understand?
* Are there any leading questions?
* If you give a range of options, do they cover all possible answers?

Testing the questions

It may be a good idea to test your questions on a fellow student to see if they find any of the questions difficult to understand or repetitive, or if they have any other problems.

Setting up the interview

You need to decide when and where the interview will take place. At this stage it is also useful to think about the information you will give to the subject, e.g. the reason for the interview, how long it will take, etc. In some cases it may be useful to give the subject an information sheet about the research and at the same time give them a consent form to sign (see Figure 11.21). See also Unit 21, page 295, for general guidance on setting up interviews and getting informed consent.

Recording an interviewee's responses

In most structured interviews the responses will be written down on the interview sheet. If the interview is very long and complex and you are asking a lot of supplementary questions, you may think about using a tape recorder. If you tape record the interview, you need to include consent for this and you should also explain to the interviewee that the tape will be destroyed after your study is complete.

Summary

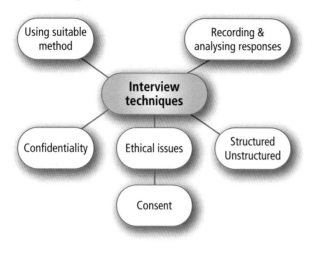

11.7 Ethical issues

There are important ethical considerations that you need to be aware of when interviewing respondents.

Avoiding embarrassment and distress in the interview

It is important that anyone you interview is not caused any distress or embarrassment. For example, if you interview someone about their job, they may find it difficult to tell you what salary scale they are on. One way of getting round this is to have a list of bands of salary and they can tell you which band they come into. Examples of how this is done can be found in the annual report of an NHS trust when the salaries of senior directors are itemised using bands, so you do not know the exact sum. This is one way of avoiding embarrassment.

When you are preparing the interview schedule, you need to look at the questions and areas you have decided to cover. If you are interviewing a service user about their satisfaction with services, you need to be careful not to go into too much detail if they are becoming distressed because they had a bad experience. One way services can be improved is by finding out how services users and carers feel about their experience, but this has to be done sensitively. Practise your interview on someone first and ask them if they find any of the questions offensive, too personal or difficult to understand. You should make clear to the person

you are interviewing that they do not have to answer all the questions (see Figure 11.21).

Maintaining confidentiality

In research interviews it is important to be aware of confidentiality. Information about the interviewee, and any information you gain from them, is confidential. This needs to be explained before the interview takes place and when you gain the interviewee's consent. You must not give any information in the research report that could identify the person. This can be difficult if the patient you interview had a particular operation, or the staff member you interviewed has a particular role that could be identified – for example, the nursing director of a hospital in your area. You would need to give the person and also the hospital a different name so they could not be identified.

It is important to think about where and when you will conduct the interview. You need some privacy where you will not be interrupted and where people cannot overhear you. If you tape record the interview you need to tell the subject what you will do with the tapes afterwards.

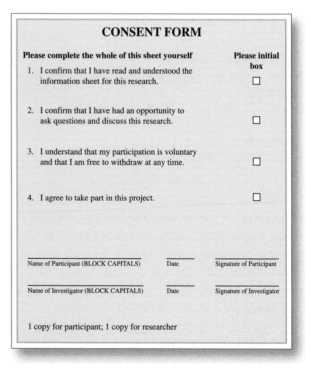

FIGURE 11.21 *Consent form*

Seeking informed consent

You need to make sure that the person you interview gives his or her consent to the research. There are several standard forms you can use to do this (see Figure 11.21).

Informed consent means that the interviewee is fully aware of what you are going to do; what you will do with the information obtained; and how long you will keep the data.

Some people are unable to give informed consent because they lack the mental capacity to understand what you propose to do; either because of illness, such as Alzheimer's disease (see page 145), or because of lack of intellectual maturity. This would include children and people who have learning disabilities. Some researchers would also exclude people who do not speak English fluently as they may not fully understand what you are asking them to do.

Informed consent can be a difficult ethical issue. If you were a district nurse and you wanted to interview your patients about their satisfaction with their care, they may find it difficult to refuse you as they may worry that refusal could affect their care. In consent forms there is usually a section that states that refusal to participate will not affect their care in any way. Consent has to be freely given with no coercion.

Right to withdraw

In the preparation for the interview, you should always state that the person has the right to withdraw at any time. A patient may initially consent and then change their mind. In the example of the district nurse quoted above, patients might feel if they withdrew from a study they would get poor treatment from the district nurse. It must be explained that withdrawal from a study will not affect the care given to them. As long as you follow these ethical guidelines and explain the research fully, giving the person plenty of time to think about what you are asking them to do and answering any questions they may have, you hope that interviewees will not withdraw. It is your responsibility to make sure you have fully explained the interview process. Sometimes it is useful to give the person a copy of the questions you are going to ask in advance so that nothing comes as a great surprise.

Summary

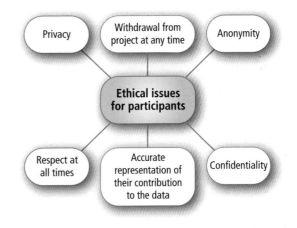

Consider this

1. You decide you are going to interview some parents about their experience of a local nursery school. Think about the following issues and decide how you would address them:

   * permission for the study

   * confidentiality

   * type of interview you would use and when and where you would conduct the interview.

2. What are the advantages and disadvantages of the following?

   * closed questions

   * open questions

   * tape-recorded interviews

   * writing down the responses given.

3. Informed consent is an important issue in research. How would you gain informed consent with the following subjects?

   * a person whose first language is not English?

   * an older man who has the early stages of Alzheimer's disease?

   * a child of eight?

UNIT 11 ASSESSMENT

How you will be assessed

For this unit you must produce a report describing and evaluating two job roles in health and social care. The report should also include an evaluation of your own suitability for these roles. Your report should be wholly your own work and not based on a shared exercise. The report may contribute to your key skills communication evidence. When writing your report you should include sections under each of the following headings:

* A Introduction

* B Evidence

* C Evaluation

* D Appendix.

Assessment preparation

A Introduction
Your introduction should describe each job role you have chosen and include the following four aspects for each role:

* sector (statutory, voluntary or private)

* role of the job (the main duties of the job)

* status of the job

* conditions of work.

You need to decide which job roles you are going to evaluate. Your decision could be based on the access you have to information and to health and social care practitioners. The following list of people and information may give you some ideas on how you can access information on jobs:

* the practice manager of your local GP surgery

* the Patient and Public Involvement manager of your local hospital of PCT

* the Internet

* jobs advertised in the local or national press
  (e.g. *Community Care Magazine*).

You could write to these people for the job descriptions of positions advertised:

* the manager of a residential care home

* the manager of the local social services department or the human resources department of the council

* a 'Sure Start' manager

* the manager of a nursery

* the head teacher of an infant school

* people you know personally

* the college careers adviser

* the school 'Connexions' adviser.

The choice of the jobs you select is very important as you may need to interview someone in one of these posts for Section B of the assessment.

B Evidence

This section should include the interview you carried out with one person who is either someone who works in health and social care in one of the jobs you have described, or else with a service user who has received health or social care from one of the practitioners whose job you have described. For both types of interview you need to ensure that the materials you have designed reflect the requirement of the assessment. Look carefully at the guidance given in the unit specification. Once you have decided who you are going to interview you need to decide how you will approach them so that they understand what you are proposing to do. You may decide to write an introductory letter explaining the purpose of the research. Once you have gained their consent you may decide to give them a list of the areas you are going to cover in the interview so that they are not surprised in any way. Use the following checklist to remind yourself of what you need to decide:

* type of method used – are you just going to have a list of topic areas you will cover or will you prepare a set of questions?

* how will you record their responses – will you use a tape recorder or will you write their responses down?

* if you use a tape recorder, how will you make sure your interviewee is comfortable with this?

* how will you gain consent and record that consent was given?

* what confidentiality issues may arise and how will you deal with these?

* how much time will you need to:
    * prepare the interview
    * carry out the interview
    * write up the interview?

Time factors are a crucial aspect of the research process. It may be helpful to devise an action plan with set dates for completing each section of the assessment process.

C Evaluation

This section should include an evaluation of the two job roles you have described and an evaluation of your own suitability for these job roles. It may be helpful to draw up lists of the key points so that you can compare and contrast the two roles. You may find there are more similarities than differences. You need to refer to the sections in this unit that refer to the roles and conditions of employment – including such factors as conditions of service, team working and opportunities for training. Depending on the job roles you have chosen, certain aspects may be very important. When you evaluate your own suitability for the two job roles you have compared, you need to decide what skills you have. Look back at the lists of skills and qualities on pages 3 and 4. These may remind you of what are seen as important skills and qualities in health and social care. You also need to identify your own physical, intellectual, emotional and social needs and whether these could be met in the roles you evaluate.

D Appendix

This should include references to sources you have used in developing your report. It could also include letters written to managers and others when you were setting up the interview. It may be an idea to keep a file of materials you have used. This file could include:

* copies of the job descriptions/roles you have chosen

* the interview schedule used

* the consent form

* written transcripts of the responses given at the interview

* a list of skills appropriate for health and social care workers.

It could also include your work plan for the assessment showing how you have planned the assessment and the time taken on producing the work.

Grading of the assessment

AO1 Knowledge and skills
In order to achieve a high grade you need to give a detailed description of two job roles and show understanding of the sector of employment, the role of the job, the status of the job and the conditions of service attached to the job. This section must be well written using vocabulary relevant to the sector.

AO2 Application
In order to achieve a high grade you must show you have the ability to apply the knowledge you have gained from studying the unit and researching job roles to discuss and analyse the two job roles you have chosen, using a comprehensive and well-structured approach.

AO3 Research and analysis
In order to achieve a high grade the report needs to be fully documented and detailed. When you discuss your own aptitudes for particular job roles you need to show insight using a systematic approach. The work should be written in a fluent style using appropriate specialist language showing well-developed analytical skills.

AO4 Evaluation
In order to achieve a high grade the evaluations of the two job roles need to be complete and comprehensive and reflect the level of presentation in the rest of the report. Evaluation should include a well-developed analytical approach, showing lack of bias.

References and further reading

Guide to the Social Services in 2004/05 (2000)
London: Waterlow Publishing

Health Care Commission (2005) *NHS Staff Survey 2004 Summary of Key Findings*

HM Government (1997) *The New NHS Modern Dependable* London: HMSO

HM Government (1998) *Modernising Social Services* London: HMSO

HM Government (1998) *A First Class Service* London: HMSO

HM Government (2000) *The NHS Plan* London: HMSO

HM Government (2003) Green Paper *Every Child Matters* London: HMSO

HM Government (2003) *Fair Access to Care Services* London: HMSO

HM Government (2004) White Paper *Every Child Matters: Next Steps* London: HMSO

HM Government (2005) Green Paper *Independence, Well-being and Choice* London: HMSO

Moonie, N. (2000) *Advanced Health and Social Care* Oxford: Heinemann

Moonie, N. (2004) *GCE AS Level AQA in Health and Social Care* Oxford: Heinemann

Wellards NHS Handbook 2004–2005 (2004)
Wadhurst East, Sussex: JMH Publishing Ltd.

Useful websites

www.communitycare.co.uk

www.csci.org.uk
Commission for Social Care Inspection

www.dh.gov.uk
Department of Health

www.gsci.org.uk

www.healthcarecommission.org.uk
Health Care Commission

www.nhscareers.nhs.uk
Careers in the National Health Service

www.nhs.uk
National Health Service

www.ofsted.gov.uk
Office for Standards in Education

www.show.scot.uk

www.surestart.gov.uk
Outlines the first Sure Start programme introduced in 2002

www.wales.gov.uk.

Human development: factors and theories

This unit covers the following sections:

12.1 Factors affecting development

12.2 Theories of cognitive development

12.3 Theories of personality development

Introduction

Each human being is unique. There is no one in the past, alive now, or in the future who will have exactly the same biology, life experience, or thoughts that you have. But what are the factors that result in the unique nature of each person? This unit explores some of the influences that may impact on human development. The second section of this unit looks at some theories of cognitive development and learning theory, including the work of Piaget, Skinner's learning theory and Bandura's social learning theory. The third section explores some famous psychological theories relevant to personality development, including the work of Freud, Bowlby and Maslow.

Unit assessment

This unit will be assessed by a two-hour external test. A more detailed guide to the assessment is given at the end of the unit.

12.1 Factors affecting development

Genetic factors

Each living cell in the human body has a nucleus with 23 pairs of chromosomes inside it. In each pair of chromosomes one chromosome comes from the father and one from the mother. Each chromosome carries units of inheritance known as genes and the genes on each chromosome interact to create a new set of 'instructions' to make a new human being. Genes are made of a substance called deoxyribonucleic acid or 'DNA' for short. It is this DNA that actually contains instructions for producing proteins that regulate physiological processes.

> **Think it over**
>
> Reece is 44 years old and seriously overweight. He is well informed about the health risks associated with his weight but he says that he can't do anything about it because his problem is caused by genetics. Reece explains: 'You see, I know people who are as thin as a rake and they don't eat any less than I do – I am meant to be this way, it runs in the family, I have tried but I just can't loose weight.'Is Reece right – do inherited influences make us what we are?

Although half of your chromosomes come from your mother and half from your father, your genetic pattern can differ from that of your mother or father. When a sperm fertilises an egg to create a baby, new combinations of genes occur. The pattern of genetic instructions that results from the interaction of your mother's and father's genes is called your genotype.

An individual person results from the interaction of their genetic pattern and their environment. It has become fashionable for journalists to talk about 'genes for' criminal behaviour, or intelligence, or certain illnesses. But it is extremely unlikely that complex social behaviours can be explained purely in terms of the biochemical instructions in your DNA for building cell structures.

> **Key concepts**
>
> *Genes:* units that contain the information and instructions that control the development of living organisms. Genes influence individual differences such as our gender, hair and eye colour, height and skin colour.
>
> *Genotype:* the type of genetic pattern that an individual inherits. Your genotype will influence issues such as your height, hair, eye colour and so on.

As we learn more about the emerging science of genetics it is widely accepted that genetic influences interact and are interlinked with environmental influences. So genetics may influence how we put on weight – but it is unlikely that genetics will be the only reason why a person becomes overweight. It might be impossible to be overweight if there was little food available. Genetics may influence the development of our physiology and this may in turn influence behaviour; however, our genetics do not control or cause our actions directly.

> **Key concept**
>
> *Phenotype:* the outcome of the interaction of a person's genotype with the environment that they experience. For example, although genes may influence height and body shape, your height and body shape will also be influenced by diet and lifestyle. What you end up looking like will result from the interaction of genetics and environment.

It is important to recognise that in Reece's story at the beginning of this section, Reece may be right – his physiology may be different from many other people's, and he may indeed find it harder to maintain a healthy body weight than some other people do. Even so, Reece's genetics do not directly create excessive body weight. If Reece had experienced different environmental and socio-economic influences – if he had developed a different self concept – he might have found a way of managing his physiology and weight.

Socio-economic factors

Genetic and socio-economic issues interact in the two scenarios below; can you see how different socio-economic circumstances can alter the outcomes of a person's genetic inheritance?

Income

The economic resources that an individual or family has can make a major difference to the quality of life a person leads. A person's weekly income enables him or her to pay for a house or flat, and to buy food and clothes. Income mainly comes from:

* wages from employment
* profits from business if you are self-employed
* benefits paid by the government
* money from invested wealth, such as interest on bank accounts or bonds
* money raised through the sale of property you own.

Income is not distributed equally in the UK. The top 20 per cent of households get around 15 times more money each year than the poorest 20 per cent of households. Income is subject to taxation and other forms of redistribution. This means that the highest paid have to pay tax on their income, whilst many poorer households receive benefits that increase income. After tax and benefits have been paid out, the richest 20 per cent are only four times better off than the poorest 20 per cent of households (*Social Trends* 2004).

Did you know?

Approximately 10 per cent of the UK population have no savings or investments at all. Among the 20 to 34 age group, 20 per cent of people have no savings or investments and among young people aged 16 to 24, 56 per cent of people have no savings (Paxton and Dixon 2004).

SCENARIO

Jack and Maxwell

Jack and Maxwell are brothers and both share a genetic tendency to become dependent on alcohol. They are born to parents who rent accommodation in a deprived housing estate. Jack and Maxwell's parents split up and Jack goes to live with his grandmother.

Maxwell's story

Maxwell remains at home and his father re-marries. Maxwell does not get on with his stepmother and spends a lot of time playing with the children on the estate where he lives. Maxwell's friends hate school and are impressed by the status and wealth of the drug dealers who supply people in the neighbourhood. By the age of 11 Maxwell has tried a range of drugs including alcohol. His concentration at school is impaired through lack of motivation and the effects of substances he has tried. As Maxwell grows older he frequently drinks alcohol and finds that he 'needs to drink'. By 17 he spends many evenings drinking and cannot manage to cope either with education or with the idea of getting a job. By early adulthood Maxwell is unemployed, has few friends, no qualifications and serious health problems.

Jack's story

Jack grows up with his grandmother who takes a close interest in his development. At school Jack mixes with friends who are interested in computers. Jack does not play out on the street but often goes to a friend of the family in the evening where he can play on the computer. Jack is able to join in on a weekend project at school to develop IT skills. Jack imagines a future where he can make a career out of information technology. He does not mix with people who drink alcohol or take drugs. At 16 years of age Jack believes that drinking is unhealthy and decides to avoid alcohol because he adopts the religious views of his grandparents. By early adulthood Jack has good educational qualifications and decides to study for a degree. He is in good health and has a range of supportive friends and relatives and believes he has few problems in life.

Nowadays households with an income that is less than 60 per cent of 'median' income in the UK are considered to be living in poverty. A median is the middle value in a range of numbers so 'low income' means that you have an income that is only worth 60 per cent of the middle income level. This measure is used by the government's Social Exclusion Unit and also by the European Union for making comparisons between member countries. People with a very low level of income are poor relative to the expectations of most people.

Just over a sixth of Britain's population (17 per cent) were estimated, by the Institute for Fiscal Studies, to be living on a low income in the period 2001–2002 (*Social Trends 2004*). If a measure of income after housing costs is used then 22 per cent of households live in income poverty (Paxton and Dixon 2004).

Key groups of people who have to live on very little money include:

* one-parent families
* people who are unemployed
* elderly people
* people who are sick or disabled
* unskilled couples (where only one person works in an unskilled job).

Social Trends (2004) estimates that around 30 per cent of children (3.8 million children) live in low-income households (after housing costs). It states that 'children living in workless families or households have a much higher risk of low income than those in families with one or more adults in full-time work'. Around three-quarters of children living in 'workless' or lone-parent families live in low-income households (*Social Trends* 2004).

The impact of low income

Paxton and Dixon (2004) quote research conclusions which show that: 'Children who grew up in poverty during the 1970s did worse at school, were six times less likely to enter higher education, and one-and-a-half times more likely to be unemployed – and earned 10 per cent less during their lifetimes than those who did not experience poverty as children.' They cite the following disadvantages of poverty:

* *Poverty is associated with being a victim of crime.* '4.8 per cent of people who earned under £5,000 a year were burgled in 2003–4 compared to only 2.7 per cent of people who earned over £30,000.'

* *Poorer communities are more likely to live in polluted areas.* 'In 2003 there were five times as many industrial sites in the wards containing the most deprived 10 per cent of the population and seven times as many emission sources as in wards with the least deprived 10 per cent.'

* *Low social class is associated with an increased risk of dying young.* 'In 2003 children of fathers in the lower social class were twice as likely to die within one year of birth, five times more likely to die in a traffic accident and 15 times more likely to die in a house fire than those in the highest social class.'

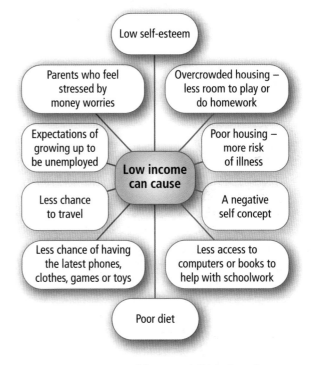

FIGURE 12.1 *Some problems a child belonging to a low-income family may face*

Housing

People with high incomes often feel confident about their future and their ability to take out a mortgage to buy their own home. These people can also choose where and how they would like to live.

People on low incomes tend to have less choice. People on low incomes may often rent property in more densely populated housing areas. Wealthier people will often live in more spacious and less stressful conditions than low income families.

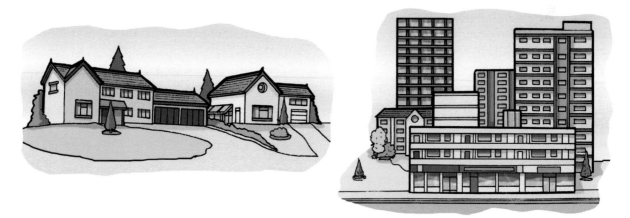

FIGURE 12.2 *Your home can have a great effect on your health and well-being*

According to the Acheson report (1998), 'Poor quality housing is associated with poor health.

What if?

Look the hazards listed in Figure 12.3. How do you think living in poor housing might influence a person's self-esteem?

Dampness is associated with increased prevalence of allergic and inflammatory lung diseases, such as asthma.' The report also noted, '40 per cent of all fatal accidents happen in the home. Almost half of all accidents to children are associated with architectural features in and around the home. Households in disadvantaged circumstances are likely to be the worst affected by such accidents.'

Older properties are often less well insulated than modern properties. Many older people on low incomes worry about the cost of heating in their homes. Older, poorly-maintained homes are likely to cost more to heat than recently built properties. For some people who live on a low income in high-density housing the problems shown in Figure 12.4 may create stress.

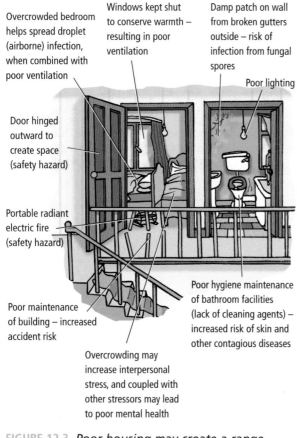

Overcrowded bedroom helps spread droplet (airborne) infection, when combined with poor ventilation

Windows kept shut to conserve warmth – resulting in poor ventilation

Damp patch on wall from broken gutters outside – risk of infection from fungal spores

Poor lighting

Door hinged outward to create space (safety hazard)

Portable radiant electric fire (safety hazard)

Poor maintenance of building – increased accident risk

Overcrowding may increase interpersonal stress, and coupled with other stressors may lead to poor mental health

Poor hygiene maintenance of bathroom facilities (lack of cleaning agents) – increased risk of skin and other contagious diseases

FIGURE 12.3 *Poor housing may create a range of risks*

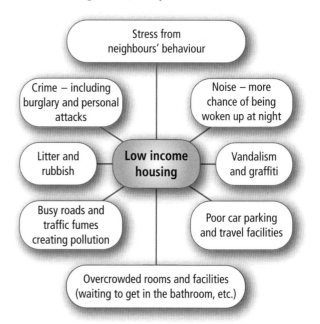

Stress from neighbours' behaviour

Crime – including burglary and personal attacks

Noise – more chance of being woken up at night

Litter and rubbish

Low income housing

Vandalism and graffiti

Busy roads and traffic fumes creating pollution

Poor car parking and travel facilities

Overcrowded rooms and facilities (waiting to get in the bathroom, etc.)

FIGURE 12.4 *High-density housing may create stress*

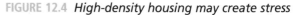

Growing up and living in the most deprived neighbourhoods may greatly restrict an individual's chance of developing their full intellectual, social or emotional potential. The problems of poor facilities and crime may stop employers from starting businesses. Poor facilities and crime may help to cause unemployment. Unemployment may contribute to poor facilities because people have little money to spend. Growing up in a neighbourhood with widespread unemployment, crime and poor facilities may do little to motivate children to achieve a good education. If people do not achieve a good standard of education they may find it harder to get jobs. The problems 'feed off' each other, creating housing estates and areas which are stressful to live in. Neighbourhoods may have a major impact on a person's life chances of growing up to lead a fulfilled life.

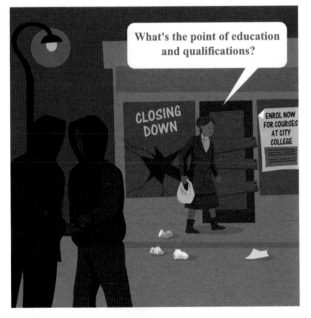

FIGURE 12.5 *The neighbourhood you live in can affect your life chances*

Nutrition

The Acheson report (1998) noted that people in low socio-economic groups 'spend more on foods richer in energy and high in fat and sugar, which are cheaper per unit of energy than foods rich in protective nutrients, such as fruit and vegetables'. 'People on low incomes eat less healthily partly because of cost, rather than lack of concern or information. Therefore increased availability of affordable 'healthy' food should lead to improved nutrition in the least well off.' The report notes evidence that:

* people in low socio-economic groups eat more processed foods containing high levels of salt, thus increasing the risk of cardiovascular disease

* obesity is more prevalent in low socio-economic groups than in higher groups – increasing the risk of ill-health for people in low socio-economic groups

* babies born to mothers in low socio-economic groups are more likely to have reduced birth weights than those in higher groups. Low birth weight is linked with the risk of cardiovascular disease in later life

* women in lower socio-economic groups are less likely to breast feed their babies. Breast feeding helps to protect infants from infection.

People with a low income will find it harder to travel to supermarkets and stock up on cheaper food. Healthy food may cost more than processed food which contains higher amounts of sugar and salt. A low income may push people to choose an unhealthy diet, because it can be harder and more expensive to choose a healthy one.

Many people do not follow government advice on diet. Government guidelines recommend that a healthy diet should include at least five portions of fruit and vegetables a day. A national diet and nutrition survey carried out between 2000 and 2001 found that only 13 per cent of men and 15 per cent of women follow this advice. No young men between 19 and 24 were following this advice. Some people may have been socialised into dietary and health habits that cause them to ignore government advice. People with a low income may have less of a choice when it comes to avoiding processed food.

Education

Although everyone in the UK has the right to education, educational opportunities may not be exactly the same for everyone. In 1998 the Acheson report noted that schools in deprived neighbourhoods were likely to suffer more problems

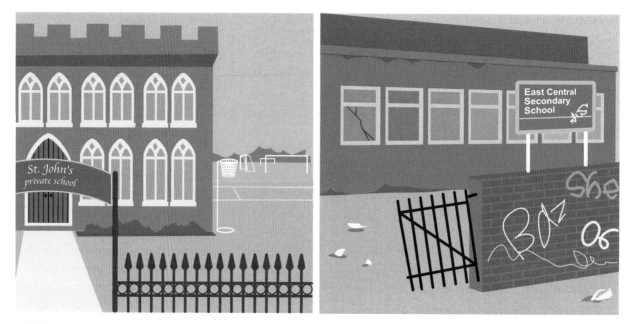

FIGURE 12.6 *Educational opportunities are not the same for all*

than schools in the more affluent areas. 'Schools in disadvantaged areas are likely to be restricted in space and have the environment degraded by litter, graffiti, and acts of vandalism. This contributes to more stressful working conditions for staff and pupils. Children coming to school hungry or stressed as a result of their social and economic environment will be unable to take full advantage of learning opportunities. Stress, depression and social exclusion may reduce parents' capacity to participate in their children's education.'

Education has a link with health in that low levels of educational achievement are associated with poor health in adult life (Acheson 1998). Paxton and Dixon (2004) discuss the links between low income and educational achievement. At primary school level they note 'between 1999 and 2002, pupils in schools where a lower proportion of the intake is eligible for free school meals made more progress at both Key Stage 2 (age 7 to 11) and Key Stage 3 (age 11 to 14) than those in schools where more were eligible for free school meals'. At secondary education level Paxton and Dixon (2004) reported that children from the higher social classes achieved more high-grade GCSEs than children from the lower social classes and lower income families.

It is likely that the combined effects of poor resources, low expectations and the need to earn money often influence young people from low income families to give education a low priority.

Access to health services

Areas with many low-income households may have poorer facilities than more wealthy areas. Several studies have shown that life expectancy is shorter in deprived areas as compared with more affluent areas of housing.

Although the National Health Service (NHS) provides free health care for everyone there are concerns that some groups of people may not receive the same quality of access to GP services and to preventative health as others. Deprived areas may have greater difficulty in recruiting GPs and nurses. The Acheson report documented that some health care premises in poorer areas were of lower quality than in more wealthy areas. This report also identified an 'inverse law' that meant that communities with the greatest need received the lowest level of service and resources, whilst those with the lowest need receive the highest level. The report stated: 'Communities most at risk of ill health tend to experience the least satisfactory access to the full range of preventive services, the so called "inverse prevention law". Prevention services include cancer screening programmes, health promotion and immunisation. While differences are most noticeable amongst socio-economic groups it is likely that, for example amongst Bangladeshi women, additional inequalities in access are experienced. Lack of access to women practitioners can be a deterrent to Asian women taking up an invitation for cervical cancer screening. Local studies have shown that access to female practitioners is poorest in areas with high concentrations of Asian residents and that practices with a female doctor or nurse are more likely to reach the cervical cytology targets set out in the GP contract.'

The report also found that services for people with heart disease were poorer for Asian people, despite higher mortality rates for people in this community.

The quality of health care services and active health promotion may be influenced by the socio-economic characteristics of a neighbourhood. The government now has targets to reduce the gap in life expectancy between health authority areas. There is an *NHS Plan* (2000) that is regularly updated in order to improve the quality of health services. Improved services for heart disease and cancer are a current priority.

The interaction of factors

Just because a person is born with a genetic pattern that might contribute to becoming overweight, it does not mean that that person will become overweight. Just because a person is born into a low income environment does not mean that that person must grow up to be poor and disadvantaged. What happens to people is immensely complicated. Genetic factors interact with socio-economic factors. An individual's understanding of him or herself will also influence the effect that socio-economic factors or genetics may have. One way of understanding these interactions is described in Figure 12.7.

Some theories have assumed that people are passive objects that are fixed and determined by genetic and socio-economic influences. But other approaches stress that even a young infant can influence his or her carers. Once a person develops a sense of self then that person will start to make choices and attempt to influence and control the environment that they find

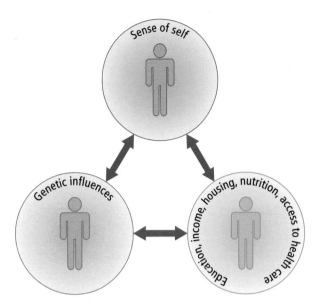

FIGURE 12.7 *Many factors influence an individual's sense of self*

themselves in. A person's understanding of their situation represents a third area of influence on behaviour. People are capable of choices that can affect how socio-economic influences work; for example people have some choice over their diet and over the way they react to education. It may even become possible to avoid the consequences of our genetic structure by accessing modern scientific and medical treatments.

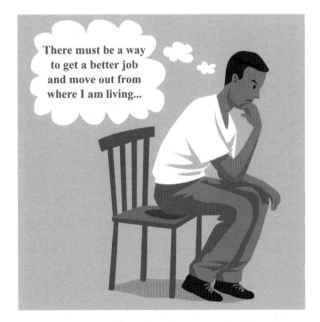

FIGURE 12.8 *The use of imagination may be the first step to breaking away from the consequences of inherited, environmental and socio-economic influences*

Interaction with other people

A sense of self and the ability to make choices develops from a person's interactions with others. Some key influences during childhood and adolescence are set out in Table 12.1.

KEY INFLUENCES	DESCRIPTION
Infancy – attachment	If a child experiences a secure loving relationship with his or her carers, this attachment may be remembered and may influence the person's ability to make loving attachments later in life, (see section on John Bowlby, page 81).
Childhood – play	Play activities may help to develop practical skills such as coordinating muscles and actions. Play may also help an individual to develop social skills and relationships, for example by acting out social roles such as the role of a teacher. Play activity can help a child to find out how something works or what happens if you touch or drop an object. Play activity – often with other children – provides an important learning experience that may influence the person's development.
Adolescence – friendship groups	During adolescence friendship groups can have a major influence on social behaviour and the beliefs and attitudes of an individual. Belonging to a group of friends may be an important part of a person's self concept and social development.

TABLE 12.1 *Influences on childhood and adolescence*

Family experiences of attachment, play and later social experiences with friendship groups may provide a basis for adult self-confidence.

Summary

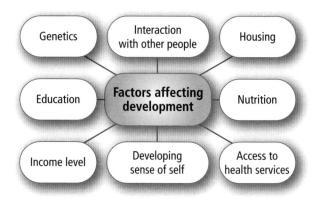

Consider this

Maisie is an 86-year-old member of a reminiscence group at a day centre. Maisie is a happy person who feels in control of her life. During discussion Maisie talks about her life, explaining: 'Life was hard in them days, but everyone looked after everyone else; my family would go without things just so I could grow up fit and healthy. No one could want a better family, and all my life I've been lucky. I've never been rich but I always had enough to get by. Life is what you make it – I enjoy my life. I've got no time for people who moan and grumble. If something's not right in your life then do something about it – that's what I say.'

Maisie appears to have had positive family experiences, but she grew up in a low-income family.

Can you identify some of the disadvantages that growing up on a low income may involve?

Can you identify some other disadvantages that Maisie may have experienced in her development?

Can you identify some positive influences that may have contributed to Maisie's happy and successful life?

Can you explain how different types of influence can interact so that no one influence necessarily determines the quality of life that a person experiences?

12.2 Theories of cognitive development

Piaget's theory of learning

Cognition involves the mental processes involved in thinking about and understanding our experience. Infants and children do not think in exactly the same way as adults.

Jean Piaget (1894–1980) was one of the first people to study the development of human thought and reasoning. He believed that:

* infants, children and adults actively seek to understand the world that they live in. People build mental representations or theories of the world in their minds because it is human nature to do so

* children learn through experience. Teachers can only help with or facilitate learning by helping to create useful experiences

* as children grow older they develop increasingly complex ways of interpreting the world

* developing theories about the world involves processes called **accommodation** (fitting new information into existing **schemas**); **assimilation** (changing schemas, ideas and theories when new information is discovered); and **equilibration** (creating a balance between theory and experience in order to make sense of the world).

Schema theory

A **schema** is a mental organisation of thought patterns. If you were told a story about going shopping, you would already have a lot of knowledge about the way shops are organised; how goods are paid for; conversations with shop assistants and so on. It appears that when we hear complex information we store the information associated with schemas that already exist in our thinking. When we come to recall information, we partly recall what we were told and partly recall the associations that were made with our pre-existing knowledge. We can take in a great deal of new information linked to pre-existing schemas but our memories can become distorted in the process.

When we experience other people's behaviour we will create an internal memory or internal representation of what we experienced. We are likely to bias our memories to fit with our normal way of thinking. Or in more technical language, we reconstruct what we think we saw and heard in terms of our pre-existing schemata ('schemata' is the plural of 'schema').

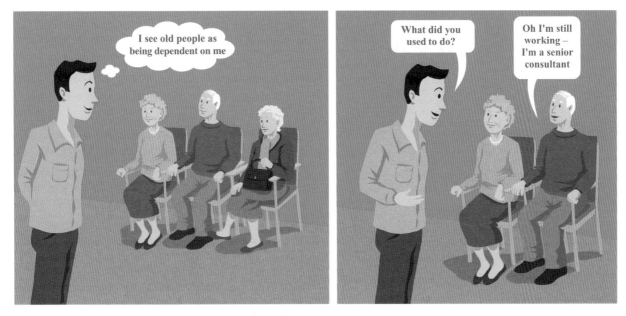

FIGURE 12.9 *We build a set of assumptions based on our experience but the way we think may not always be right*

A simple explanation of Piaget's theory of learning might be based on a young child's experience of animals. Perhaps a child goes to a park and sees ducks for the first time. The child has already seen pictures of animals in books and has seen other animals in real life. The child will 'take in' or assimilate the idea of 'ducks' as a new category of animal. As the child experiences more examples of ducks, the child will need to adapt their idea of what ducks can look like – this is called 'accommodation'. The child will now have a balanced theory of what ducks are, and will be able to identify them effectively.

As the child grows older they will lose their 'equilibration' on this idea when they have to make sense of the idea that ducks are birds and not animals. Life involves constant development and changing of ideas.

In Piaget's theory, learning is a process which is constantly working to enable people to cope with or 'adapt to' their environment. Teachers should never try 'to put ideas into children'. Teachers are most successful when they create useful experiences which stimulate children to make sense, or make new sense, of their experience. Learning is about the changing of mental schemas – only the learner can change the way they think.

Children cannot learn skills before they are maturationally ready. Trying to teach abstract theories (such as psychodynamic theory) to five-year-olds would never work – no matter what teaching skills a person had.

Piaget is also famous for his theory that there are stages of cognitive development. Piaget developed his theory by observing and questioning young children. He believed that children progress through four stages of intellectual development, shown in Table 12.2.

Piaget believed that the four stages were caused by an inbuilt inherited pattern of development. Nowadays research suggests that infants are more able to understand their world than Piaget thought. It also appears that most people take a lot longer than 11 years to become skilled at abstract logical thinking. The development of formal logical thought my also be very dependent on the quality of education that a person receives.

The sensorimotor stage

Babies are born with the ability to see, hear and touch objects – they can sense objects.

Babies are also born with a range of reflexes such as the sucking reflex to enable them to feed.

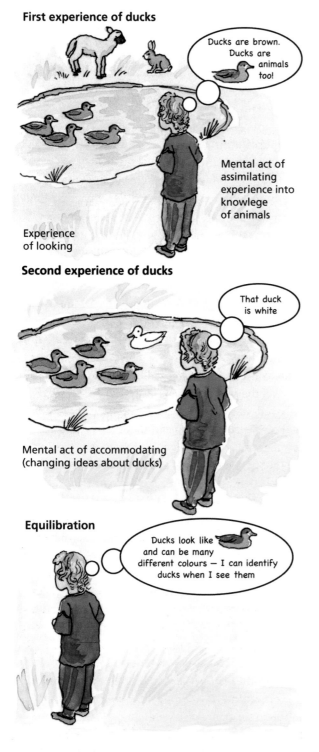

First experience of ducks

Ducks are brown. Ducks are animals too!

Mental act of assimilating experience into knowlege of animals

Experience of looking

Second experience of ducks

That duck is white

Mental act of accommodating (changing ideas about ducks)

Equilibration

Ducks look like and can be many different colours – I can identify ducks when I see them

FIGURE 12.10 *Piaget's theory of building knowledge through assimilation, accommodation and equilibration*

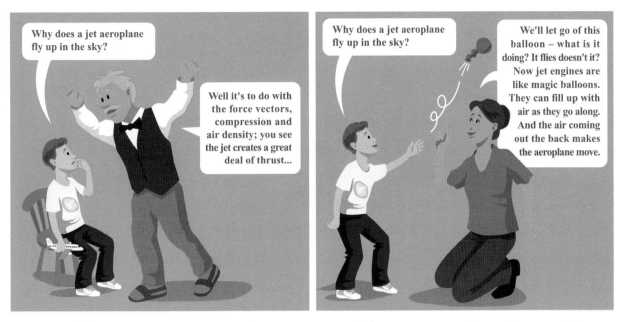

FIGURE 12.11 *A five-year-old child is not ready to understand abstract concepts; but a five-year-old may be able to understand the concrete (practical) experience of letting go of a balloon*

STAGE	DEVELOPMENT
Sensorimotor stage: birth to 1.5 or 2 years	Learning to use senses and muscles – thinking without language
Pre-operational stage: 2 to 7 years	Pre-logical thinking – thinking in language but without understanding logic
Concrete operational stage: 7 to 11 years	Logical thinking is limited to practical situations
Formal operational stage: from 11 years	Thinking using logic and abstract thought processes – adult thinking

TABLE 12.2 *Piaget's stages of cognitive development*

These reflexes lead to 'motor actions' controlling body muscles. The **sensorimotor** stage is a stage when thinking is limited to sensing objects and performing motor actions. Piaget believed that a baby would not have a working system for remembering and thinking about the world until he or she was about 18 months old. So during the sensorimotor stage thought processes are limited to sensing and responding to the world.

Object permanence

Piaget believed that infants would not be able to make sense of the things that they experienced. If a six-month-old child was reaching for a rattle and the rattle was covered with a cloth then the child would act as if the rattle had now ceased to exist. Piaget believed that young infants had great difficulty in making sense of objects and that they were unable to use their imagination in order to remember objects. Towards the end of the sensorimotor period children would begin to internalise picture memories in their minds. Piaget noticed this in his daughter, Jacqueline, at 14 months of age. Jacqueline had seen an 18-month-old child stamping his feet and having a temper tantrum. The next day Jacqueline imitated this behaviour. She must have been able to picture the behaviour in her mind in order to copy it later.

The sensorimotor period ends when a child can understand that objects have a permanent existence (this is called object permanence). The child knows that objects still exist even if he or she is not looking at them. At the end of the sensorimotor period, children will know that their father and mother still exist even if they are not seen. When an infant develops a system of thinking that enables them to imagine events or objects that they cannot see – then they can understand that objects continue to exist even when they cannot be seen.

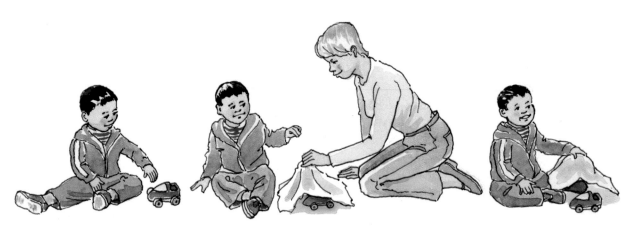

FIGURE 12.12 *Understanding the concept of object permanence (around 18 months)*

As the child loses a toy he or she will start to search for it, because it can be pictured and because the child has learned how objects work. If an object can't be seen, it will have gone somewhere – it will not have just 'gone'. Understanding the permanence of objects was also called 'conserving' objects. The child could keep, or conserve, a memory of the object. The end of the sensorimotor period is also a time when children are beginning to use one- and two-word utterances to recognise and describe things. Piaget believed that language was a powerful tool that we use to organise and construct our understanding of the world.

The pre-operational stage

Pre-operational means pre-logical; during this stage Piaget believed that children could not think in a logical way. Children can use words to communicate but they do not understand the logical implications involved in language. Piaget explained that pre-operational children cannot conserve number, mass and volume. For example, conservation of number involves understanding that ten buttons stretched out in a line involves the same number of buttons as ten buttons in a pile. A young child might agree that there were ten buttons in the line and in the pile, but then the child might say that there are more buttons in the line because it is longer. A child may be able to count to ten but may not understand what the number ten really means. You could test the way a child is thinking (a test of cognitive functioning) by

working with a child and performing a test using counters as described above.

Conservation

Pre-logical children do not understand the logic involved in concepts such as the number ten. Another way of saying this is that they cannot 'conserve' or keep the meaning of the word like ten. They can agree that there are ten sweets in a pile and also in a line but then say that there are more sweets in the line. This means that they cannot 'conserve number' – they don't understand what numbers really mean.

Decentring

Piaget believed that pre-operational children were unable to imagine other people's viewpoints. Piaget believed that children were centred on their own thoughts, that they were, in other words, egocentric.

A test of cognitive functioning — conservation of volume

Work with a child who is under seven years of age and ask the child to fill two identical glasses to the same level with water. Then take one glass and pour the water from it into a different-shaped glass – ideally a wider glass so that the water level will be different. Now ask the child if there is the same amount of water in the first glass as in the wider glass. You may find that the child says that there is more water in the taller glass. Equally possible the child may say that the second glass is fatter so there is more water in that glass. Either way the child will be failing to conserve volume – if it is the same water then there must be the same amount no matter how it looks.

In a famous experiment Piaget showed four- to six-year-old children a model of three mountains. Piaget moved a little doll around the model and asked the children to guess what the little doll might be able to see. Piaget gave the children photographs which showed the different views of the mountains. The children were asked to pick out a photograph that would show what the doll could see. Children were also invited to try using boxes to show the outline of the mountains that the doll could see.

Egocentricity: believing that everyone will see or feel the same things that you do.

Young children couldn't cope with this problem and tended to choose pictures which showed what *they* could see of the model mountains. Piaget believed that the children were centred on their own way of seeing things.

To understand that other people can see things from a different view, a child would need to decentre his or her thoughts. Piaget believed that pre-operational children could not think flexibly enough to imagine the experiences of other people. He believed that young children lived in their own world of limited imagination. Social and emotional maturity comes about because of the development of thought processes that enable a child to decentre. Decentring involves the ability to use language and concepts in order to

Decentring: the ability to imagine the thoughts and feelings of other people when they differ from the thoughts and feelings that you are currently experiencing.

understand that other people's experiences may be different from your own.

The concrete operational stage

Children in the **concrete operational** stage can think logically provided the issues are 'down to earth' or concrete. In this stage children may be able to understand simple logical puzzles. For example, pre-operational children may have difficulty with a verbal puzzles such as, 'if Kelly is Mark's sister, who is Kelly's brother?' But by the concrete operational stage children can work out that Mark must be Kelly's brother if she is his sister. During the concrete operational stage children can work out some logical issues in their minds. Children can think logically provided they can see examples of the problem they are working with.

For example, suppose you ask a question like, 'Samira is taller than Corrine, but Samira is smaller than Leslie, so who is the tallest? You may find that the seven- or eight-year-old has difficulty mentally

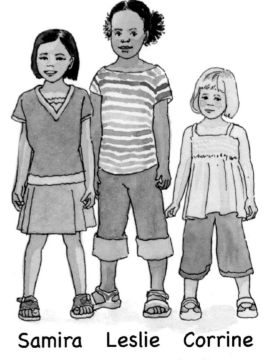

Samira   Leslie   Corrine

FIGURE 12.13 *Samira, Corrine and Leslie*

imaging the information in a way that will enable him or her to answer the question. But if the child can see a picture of Samira, Corrine and Leslie they might quickly point out who is the tallest.

The formal operational stage

With formal logical reasoning an adult can solve complex problems in his or her head. Formal logical operations enable adolescents and adults to use abstract concepts and theories in order to go beyond the limitations of everyday experience. Adults with **formal operations** can think scientifically. For example an adult can use formal logic to reason why a car won't start in the morning. The adult can formulate some hypotheses. Perhaps the car won't start because the fuel isn't getting to the engine; perhaps it won't start because there is insufficient air; perhaps there is an electrical fault: each hypothesis can be tested in turn until the problem is solved. Abstract thinking enables us to think up complicated ideas without having to see the concrete and practical issues at first hand.

> **Key concept**
>
> *Abstract thinking:* involves the ability to think about and solve problems in imagination without necessarily having concrete practical examples to work with. Abstract thinking involves an advanced ability to think using language.

An evaluation of Piaget's theory

Piaget's theory is very important because it reminds parents, teachers and care workers that children are likely to think differently from adults. Children will often need to experience practical demonstrations and examples in order to understand new ideas. Piaget's theory is also very important because it explains that we learn by building or constructing our own understanding of the world. We may remember things that we read or hear but developing an understanding involves a process of assimilation and accommodation – we have to develop our own personal store of knowledge and theory. So we learn ideas when we try to use the ideas to explain how the world works. Learning is not just about having information pumped into us.

There is a great deal of research evidence that suggests that intellectual development may not be as simple as Piaget's four stage theory suggests. A critique of some of his ideas follows.

The sensorimotor period – object permanence

Piaget believed that infants would be unlikely to understand object permanence until 18 months of

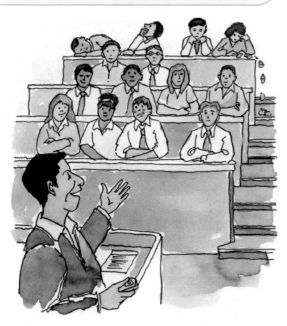 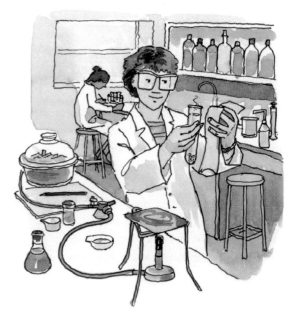

FIGURE 12.14 *Piaget identified the importance of actively using ideas in order to develop understanding – learning is more than just absorbing information*

age; but Berryman *et al* (1991) quote research by Bower (1982) that suggests that eight-month old infants can understand object permanence. Bower monitored the heartbeat of infants who were watching an object. A screen was then moved across so that the infant couldn't see the object for a short while. When the screen was removed, sometimes the object was still there and sometimes it had gone. Infants appeared to be more startled when the object disappeared. This suggests that these eight-month-old infants did expect objects to be permanent. Bower suggested that infants can begin to understand that their mothers are permanent from the age of five months. Berryman *et al* (1991) summarised the situation as follows: 'it seems that Piaget may well have under estimated the perceptual capabilities of the infant and that some sensorimotor developments take place at an earlier age than he suggested'.

The pre-operational period – conservation of number, mass and volume

Piaget believed that pre-operational children would not have developed the ability to understand the way the physical world worked. More recent research has argued that young children do have an understanding of conservation, but that they simply make bad judgments – perhaps dominated by the way things look – when they are pressured by adults. It may be the case that children will often try to please adults by giving the most obvious answer that they believe is wanted from them.

Bruner (1974) quoted a study about the conservation of volume (pouring water from one shaped glass into a differently shaped glass). But in this experiment, the experimenter used language and ideas that would be familiar to the child. The adult started with two full clear containers of water and got children to agree that there was the same water in each container. The adult then floated a small plastic duck on one container of water, making a story up about the water being the duck's water.

When the problem is presented as a story, children could conserve volume. Children said that the two final containers of water were the same – even though they looked different – because the duck had taken his water with him when he moved from one container to another. Children appeared to understand conservation when the situation became more playful and informal.

McGarrigle and Donaldson (1975) explored conservation of number using lines and piles of counters. But this time a 'naughty Teddy' soft toy was used to move the counters about creating an informal, playful atmosphere. In this situation young children were more likely to say that ten counters in a pile were indeed the same number as ten in a line. It may be that children as young as four do have some understanding of the way number mass and volume work, but that they rely on the way things look if they feel under pressure – and that this is something that older children and adults would not do.

Decentring

Pre-operational children were regarded as being egocentric to the point where they could not imagine that anyone could see or experience things differently from themselves. But Harris (1989) reports that children as young as three do understand emotion in other people and may try to comfort people who look distressed – even though they are not experiencing these emotions. Harris argues that even infants can recognise facial expressions for happiness, distress or anger and can respond to these emotions in other people. So why did children produce egocentric answers to the three mountains task that Piaget designed? It may be that the original three mountains task was just too complicated and difficult for the children. Hayes and Orrell (1993) quote research from Barke (carried out in 1975) and Hughes (also carried out in 1975) that suggests that young children could understand the views other people might see from different positions. In these studies the children worked in a relaxed, informal and playful context – and answered very simple questions. It may be that children are less capable of decentring in more formal test settings. It may not be true that all three- to seven-year-olds are incapable of imagining the emotions and experience of others.

Formal operations

Piaget believed that the ability to use abstract thinking developed soon after the age of the 11. Cohen (1981) quoted research by Watson and Johnson-Laird (1972) that suggested that 92 per cent of undergraduates did not apply formal operational thinking in order to solve a logical problem. There are also a number of cross-cultural studies suggesting that formal operational thinking is dependent on education and training rather than being some natural capability that simply unfolds in all humans.

These studies do not disprove Piaget's theory, but it does seem likely that many adults do not use abstract thinking and logical analysis to the extent that Piaget's theory would suggest. Table 12.3 lists the strengths and limitations of Piaget's theory.

STRENGTHS	LIMITATIONS
* Reminds adults that infants and children may not function in exactly the same way that adults do. Children are not miniature adults.	* Infants may understand object permanence much earlier than Piaget suggested.
* Explains learning as an active process that people undertake. Developing understanding is something you do – not something that is done to you.	* Young children may understand conservation – but fail to use their understanding in response to questions.
* Offers an outline for understanding intellectual development involving four stages.	* Young children may be able to decentre and may not be as egocentric as Piaget's theory suggests.
	* Adolescents and adults may not be as good at abstract and logical thinking as Piaget assumed – unless they have the education and training to apply these skills.
	* In real life, Piaget's four stages may not be as defined and clear-cut as the theory would imply.

TABLE 12.3 *Piaget's theory of cognitive development: evaluation summary*

Skinner's learning theory

Skinner (1904–1990) argued that behaviour is affected by the consequences that follow. This means that people learn to associate actions with the pleasure or discomfort that follows. For example, if a child puts some yoghurt in their mouth and it tastes nice, they will associate the yoghurt with pleasure. In future they will repeat the action of eating yoghurt. On the other hand if the yoghurt does not taste good they may avoid it in future.

Skinner developed some terms to explain learning by association. Behaviour operates on the environment to create outcomes. Pleasant outcomes are likely to reinforce the occurrence of the behaviours that created them. Behaviour operates on the world and so Skinner used the word 'operant' to describe behaviours which create learned outcomes. The term **operant conditioning** is used to describe learning through the consequences of action.

Key concept

Operant conditioning: learning to repeat actions which have a reinforcing or strengthening outcome. In other words, people learn to repeat actions which have previously felt good or are associated with 'feeling better'.

Reinforcement

Skinner used the idea of **reinforcement** to explain how behaviour is learned. Reinforcement means to make something stronger. For example, reinforced concrete is stronger than ordinary concrete. A reinforcer is anything that makes a behaviour stronger.

SCENARIO
Reinforcement at work

Amita is an infant who is eating while sitting in a highchair. Amita accidentally drops the spoon she is eating with. She reacts with surprise that the spoon has gone. Her mother picks the spoon up and gives it back to her, smiling and making eye contact as she does so. This makes Amita feel good. Amita's mother goes back to her own dinner and stops looking at Amita. By accident Amita drops the spoon again. Once again her mother gives Amita attention and the spoon is returned. Once again Amita feels good. Half a minute later Amita drops the spoon on purpose – dropping the spoon has become reinforced. The consequences or outcomes of dropping the spoon feel nice – it is followed by attention.

Without understanding human behaviour, parents might think that the child is being difficult, or that she is playing a game. What is happening is that Amita's behaviour of dropping the spoon is being 'reinforced' by her mother. Her mother is teaching her to drop the spoon, although she doesn't realise this. Reinforcement is happening because Amita is getting a 'nice feeling' each time she drops the spoon and her mother gives it back.

The theory of operant conditioning can help us to understand challenging behaviour.

Jason may be acting this way because of operant conditioning – he has learned this behaviour. The attention that he receives may be reinforcing (or strengthening) his behaviour of lying in the doorway; it may be that it feels nice to be the centre of attention. Alternatively Jason may feel bored; the attention received from lying in the doorway may relieve this boredom.

In order to change Jason's behaviour, Skinner would have argued that care workers should reinforce an alternative behaviour. If Jason looked bored staff might try to involve him in conversation. If Jason responds to conversation staff might try to be particularly attentive and supportive. Staff attention might act to reinforce conversational behaviour as an alternative to lying in the doorway. Staff might try to minimise the attention they give when he lies in the doorway but be very responsive and reinforcing towards any conversational activity.

Staff would not just ignore lying in the doorway because it would be unsafe to do this. Staff would not punish Jason – this would be unethical, but it would also fail to encourage an alternative behaviour. If Jason does not lie in the doorway – perhaps he will set the fire alarms off instead. Skinner's theory stressed the importance of reinforcing a new 'desirable' behaviour pattern to replace 'less desirable' behaviour.

Skinner argued that punishment was an inefficient way to influence behaviour.

It is important to remember that most conditioning happens without anyone planning or intending it. Reinforcement and punishment frequently take place in educational and social care settings. They can happen whether or not anyone intended reinforcement or punishment to happen.

The opposite of reinforcement is punishment; punishment has the result of blocking behaviour whilst reinforcement always strengthens it.

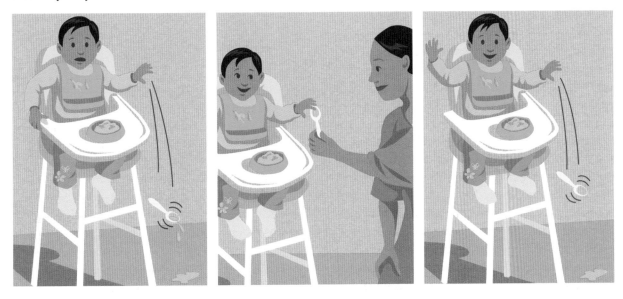

FIGURE 12.15 *Reinforcing behaviour*

Reinforcement: involves an outcome that strengthens behaviour. An outcome that creates pleasure or that results in a bad situation feeling better will strengthen your behaviour.

Punishment: unpleasant outcomes may inhibit or block a response. Punishment is the opposite of reinforcement; punishing outcomes will inhibit or weaken a behaviour. Your behaviour results in an outcome that is experienced as being unpleasant.

SCENARIO
Using reinforcement

Nia is a young person with learning difficulty who is used to being dependent on her carers. Nia does not attempt to put her own coat on or to do the buttons up – she leaves this to Ella who is her care worker. Nia likes Ella and trusts her. One day Nia points her finger to a button that has come undone. Ella guides Nia's fingers to push the button through the buttonhole. As soon as the button is done up, Ella smiles at Nia, and says thank you in a warm and friendly tone of voice. Nia smiles back and looks pleased.

In this instance Ella is trying to provide a good outcome that may become associated with the feeling of pushing a button through the buttonhole. Because Nia smiled back and looked pleased, Ella may have been successful in creating a reinforcing outcome. This one single incident is unlikely to be enough to teach the new behaviour of doing buttons up. Because Ella is conscious of operant conditioning theory, she will try and work with Nia on a number of occasions to reinforce the behaviour of pushing the buttons through the buttonholes. She might do this by guiding Nia's hands, but gradually reducing the guidance as Nia starts to push the buttons through on her own. Ella might smile and say thank you a lot in the early stages of teaching this skill, but she might reduce the amount of smiling and saying thanks as Nia gets better at the task. Skinner discovered that 'intermittent' (good outcome for only some of the time) reinforcement can be more effective than constant reinforcement (smiles and thanks in this instance) when trying to teach a new behaviour.

Reinforcement depends on outcome

Ella has to be very sensitive; smiling and saying thanks is only going to strengthen Nia's learning if Nia enjoys the response from Ella. If Nia gets bored with Ella's behaviour, then smiling and saying thanks will cease to have any effect. Reinforcement only happens if Nia experiences Ella's behaviour as a good outcome. The smiles and thanks are effective because Nia has a good relationship with Ella. Smiles and thanks from some other care workers would not be reinforcing because Nia does not like them so much.

Learning complex behaviours

Operant conditioning provides a way of teaching complex skills without needing to explain things using language. For someone like Nia, just putting a coat on will be a complex act. Her care workers might seek to increase her independence by teaching her how to put her own coat on. They would start by analysing the different steps involved in putting a coat on.

Try to identify how many small steps are involved in putting your coat on.

Remember to identify all the issues to do with getting the coat the right way round, finding the left and right arms, putting your arms into the sleeves and so on.

Care workers could analyse the task and then work one step at a time reinforcing each step until Nia could perform each step independently. The process of reinforcing one step and learning the step before teaching the next step is called chaining. Each link of the chain is completed (learned through reinforcement) before the next link is added. In theory, care workers might reinforce behaviours such as picking the coat up and then reinforce the step of putting the left arm through the left sleeve and so on.

Some tasks such as putting a coat on can be difficult to learn using forward chaining. This is partly because certain steps, such as getting your arm through the right hand sleeve after you have found the left sleeve, can be quite difficult – watch people at a restaurant after a meal. Care workers often use an approach called 'backward chaining'. In backward chaining the care worker does everything but the last step – such as doing up the coat buttons. The service user learns the steps involved in putting a coat on, starting with the last part of the process and working backwards. If they learn to do the buttons up independently, then they might move to the next but last step of pulling the coat around them. Once they have learned this step they learn the third from last step that might involve pulling the sleeves down and so on – until they have achieved independence. Many people learn to cook, make cups of tea, operate vending machines, etc., through teaching programmes that involve operant conditioning.

Reinforcement and language development

Skinner (1957) argued that children learn to develop speech and language through operant conditioning. He believed that the way in which adults responded to young children's verbal behaviour caused children to form appropriate words and later appropriate grammatical sentences.

Shaping language

Holly is an infant at the stage of 'babbling' – that is, she makes sounds such as 'da'. When her father looks at her she responds with 'da da'. Her father smiles at her and looks pleased and this reinforces Holly's response of 'da da'. Holly can also make 'ma' sounds. When Holly's mother looks at her she does not smile at 'da da' but becomes very pleased when Holly makes 'ma' sounds. Before long Holly has become operantly conditioned to respond with 'da da' to her father and 'ma ma' to her mother; and of course her parents think that she is saying 'daddy' and 'mummy'. What has happened is that Holly's babbling responses have been 'shaped' by the different reinforcement from the father and from the mother. Skinner believed that reinforcement could be used to explain the whole of language learning.

Critics of Skinner's theory of language acquisition

Very few language experts believe that children learn to speak or to understand other people because of reinforcement. Noam Chomsky (born 1928) argued that children are born with an inbuilt 'language acquisition device' (LAD) – the potential to recognise and speak a language. Chomsky (1959) believed that children simply needed to hear language in order to begin to develop language. The genetically inherited language acquisition device would enable them to understand the deep structure which all languages follow. Individual languages use different sounds and have special rules of grammar. Chomsky called these individual rules a surface structure, but all languages have the same underlying rules or

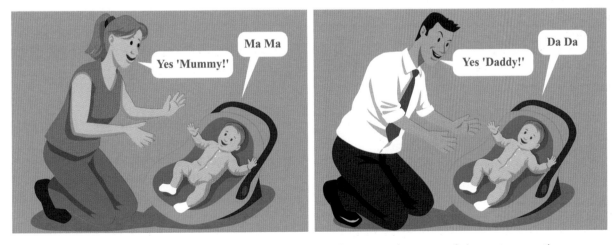

FIGURE 12.16 *Skinner believed that children learn to use language because of the outcomes they experienced*

deep structure, and we have a genetically inbuilt ability to use this deep structure. Chomsky argued that language could not result purely from reinforcement because:

* the majority of sentences that a person will speak or understand involve a new combination of words that may never have occurred before.

* there must be some sort of internal system for generating language and meaning, and this system is too complex to come into existence simply through operant conditioning.

Children develop the ability to speak and use language extremely rapidly. It is hard to believe that this ability could emerge so rapidly in most people if it depended on reinforcing responses from others. Pinker (1994) provides a detailed explanation of the way in which a genetically inherited ability to use language may work. We do not ask how bats learn to navigate in the dark; we accept that they are born with this special ability. Pinker argues that that we are born with a 'language instinct' – as our special human ability.

Another problem for reinforcement theory as an explanation for language comes from psychological research. Gross (1992), quotes research by Braine (carried out in 1971) and Tizard *et al* (carried out in 1972) that suggests trying to teach grammar to young children has little effect. Instead, there is evidence that trying to correct children's speech might actually slow down language development. Gross summarises some research as suggesting that children 'learn grammatical rules despite their parents'. It may not be a good idea to try to correct young children's grammar as they experience a genetically unfolding potential to understand and use language.

It may be that some of the words and phrases that we use are influenced by other people's responses and that the theory of reinforcement can be used to help explain some language behaviour. It is unlikely that your ability to make sense of this section has been learned purely as a result of operant conditioning.

Social learning theory

Social learning theories stress the importance of social expectations in influencing our behaviour. The

STRENGTHS	LIMITATIONS
* Skinner's theory identifies one way in which we can learn. * Operant conditioning provides a method for teaching skills and this method does not require language. * Operant conditioning provides a way of understanding challenging behaviour and responding to challenging behaviours in a positive and effective way. * We constantly affect other people and they affect us. The concept of reinforcement may help us to understand some of the ways in which we influence other people.	* Operant conditioning is not the only way in which we can learn. We also learn things in language – see Piaget's theory; and we learn by imitating other people – see Bandura's theory. * The theory of reinforcement can be made to look simple, but in practice there are a wide range of issues – including ethical issues – that need to be considered before the theory can be used to modify behaviour in health or social care settings. * There are limitations as to what the theory can effectively explain. Operant conditioning may influence our use of vocabulary but it cannot effectively account for the whole of human language behaviour.

TABLE 12.4 *Some strengths and limitations of Skinner's theory*

social learning perspective argues that it is important to understand the role of group expectations or norms when trying to understand human behaviour.

Tajfel (1981) argued that social identity plays a significant role in influencing what people do. Identity is learned through life experience. A range of social factors influences what we learn. These factors may be portrayed as layers of influence which affect the development of identity.

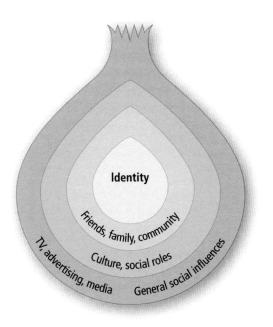

FIGURE 12.17 *Layers of influence – the onion theory*

Primary groups are small groups where you know each group member personally – such as your family. Secondary groups are large networks of people where you will not know everyone who belongs to the group – such as members of your gender or racial groups.

Try it out

Write down ten responses to the question 'I am…?'

You might tend to write things like caring, considerate, clever and so on. These might describe your personal identity. On the other hand you may have described aspects of your social group membership such as Woman, Black, Muslim.

People categorise themselves in terms of the groups that they identify with. Gender, religion, race, class, age group and social roles such as mother or sister signify groups that we may identify with. If we belong to a particular age group for example, we may categorise ourselves as being like other people who are the same age as us. People who are older may be seen as 'not like me'. It is possible to divide the world up into people 'who are like me' and people 'who are not like me'. An 'in-group' is a group that you identify with – people 'who are like me'. An 'out-group' means people who are different.

Tajfel (1981) argued that people develop social identities based on groups that they identify with. In some situations, personal identity will give way to social identity. For example, a thoughtful and caring individual may also be a football club supporter. When they join in with other supporters they may become abusive to supporters of other teams. Social identity takes over from the individual's 'personality' and behaviour conforms to the expectations of the group.

Social identity theory argues that a great deal of human behaviour can be understood as caused by an individual's conformity to the expectations of the social groups that they identify with. Social identity theory would argue that is wrong to try to explain everything in terms of individual personality.

Pro- and anti-social behaviour

Pro-social behaviour is behaviour that fits the norms and expectations of the broader society that we live in; encouraging social relationships amongst different groups of people. Anti-social behaviour can be understood as behaviour which deviates or is different from the norms and expectations of broader society. So being polite, holding doors open for others and so on may be seen as pro-social behaviour, whilst behaviours such as vandalism, littering and graffiti may be perceived as anti-social. But why do some people conform to social norms whilst others behave in an 'anti-social' manner?

One explanation comes from **social impact theory.** Social impact theory suggests that a lot of our actions are influenced, or even caused, by the people that surround us. But it is the actual people that we meet face-to-face that influence our behaviour rather than more general social norms. Put simply; humans often behave like sheep and simply copy what others around them are doing.

A lot of our actions are performed in order to conform to the expectation of other people that we mix with. If you need an explanation for why people tell racist jokes or commit acts of vandalism, there is no need to look inside their heads. Instead of looking for inner attitudes or motives, we might be better off looking at the social context that surrounds the person. For example, a person might vandalise a bus shelter because they are copying their friends – conforming to the expectations of their immediate social context. Such people may not be able to give a logical explanation of their actions – because their actions were not the result of some conscious plan or internal motive. Some people mix with groups that conform to broader social norms; some people mix with groups who do not identify with broader social norms.

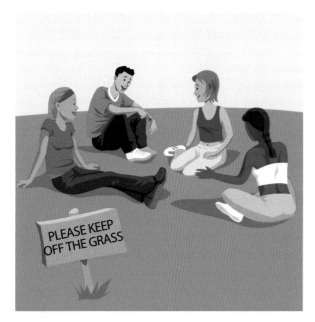

FIGURE 12.18 *Anti-social behaviour may often involve conforming to the expectations of others, and may help some individuals to identify themselves with a group*

Social impact theory developed from the work of Bibb Latané and John Darley who investigated 'bystander apathy' in the late 1960s. Their research discovered that when people are alone they will often come to the assistance of another person who has collapsed. When people are part of a group and that group generally ignores the person in need, then individuals will follow the lead of the group and not provide assistance to a person who has fallen down. The issue appears to be that many people are not directed by inner moral values – or even the wider social norms of

pro-social behaviour, but that they take their cue from what other people are doing. It is all right to do something if everybody else is doing it; that is ignoring someone in need. We respond to the 'social impact' of the people that surround us. We go with the crowd and seek to fit in with the social norms of others (Latané and Darley 1970).

What if?

Suppose you had a friend who said he was very concerned about the welfare of homeless people. One day you both walked through a crowded underpass and everyone including your friend ignored a homeless person who was begging. When you asked your friend why he ignored the homeless person he just looked embarrassed and couldn't explain.

How would social impact theory explain your friend's behaviour?

Gender roles

Other people's expectations may influence the way children learn gender roles. For example a boy might imagine himself as a person who is tough and who never cries if hurt. The act of being 'tough' may come about because the boy conforms to the expectations of other people that he mixes with. A girl living in the same neighbourhood may learn to behave in different ways in order to conform to social expectations about the way men and women should behave.

Think it over

In the past boys who did not appear tough and girls who were not gentle and caring may have been judged as not being ideal people.

Is this still the case today? What are the social expectations or norms associated with gender roles in your experience?

Bandura's theory

Albert Bandura (born 1925) argued that people's behaviour is often learned through imitating others. He argued that we often imitate or copy others without any reinforcement or conditioned learning taking place.

Bandura undertook a range of research that demonstrated that children would copy behaviours that they saw adults doing. One experiment in 1963 involved children watching adults behaving aggressively towards an object called a 'bobo doll.' A 'bobo doll' was a 1960s toy consisting of an inflatable plastic skittle shaped cylinder with some sand at the bottom to make the skittle stand upright if it was hit or knocked over. The dolls usually had cartoon character faces. Children who watched adults behaving aggressively towards the doll were more likely to get aggressive towards the doll when they had a chance to play with it than were children who had not seen the aggressive behaviour. This experiment confirmed that we are not just influenced by conditioning and reinforcement; we are also influenced by what we see in the media and what we see happening to other people (Bandura 1963).

It seems that people are more likely to imitate and copy another person's behaviour if:

* that person is rewarded for their behaviour

* that person is perceived as being generally liked and respected

* that person is perceived to have similarities with the observer

* the person's behaviour 'stands out' and is very noticeable

* the person's behaviour can be copied by the observer without too much difficulty

* the observer is rewarded in some way for watching the behaviour.

In a study in 1965 Bandura concluded that whilst children were more likely to imitate the behaviour of adults who had been rewarded for their behaviour, children learned and could later copy any behaviour that they had observed. So the key issue is that children can learn and imitate any behaviour they see – behaviour may not need to be rewarded in order for it to be remembered. It may be enough to see aggressive behaviour for it to have an impact on us (Bandura 1963).

Think it over

Suppose that some young children see Early Years care workers smoking outside a nursery building.

Children will not be able to obtain cigarettes in order to imitate the behaviour straight away, so does it make any difference to them if they watch an adult smoking?

Think it over

How might the following life experiences influence a person?

* seeing an elder brother or sister praised for school achievement

* seeing a friend being praised and looked up to because of violent behaviour

* seeing a neighbour do well from trading shares on the Internet

* seeing a person gain respect because they deal in drugs

* seeing a person being praised and thanked for caring for a relative.

Bandura's four-stage process

If we are going to model our behaviour on our observations of other people there appears to be four stages that are involved.

Attention

Your attention has to be drawn to behaviour – you have to notice it. You might not notice boring, everyday actions and habits that people around you perform. However, you may notice the mannerisms and actions of people that you see as being attractive or important. Equally, you may be more inclined to pay attention to people who are like yourself and are engaged with the kind of issues that you have to deal with. If you are a snooker player you might pay close attention to the moves of expert players. You might not pay attention if snooker doesn't interest you.

Retention

Retention means to retain or keep in memory. You have to be able to remember – sometimes to remember the picture of what you saw. If you are playing snooker you may have a clearer memory of what is involved in a particular shot than someone who doesn't understand the game.

Reproduction

You have to be able to turn your memories into actions – perhaps reproducing things you have seen as actions. If you play snooker you may be able to gradually 'fine tune' your actions to fit closely with expert performances you have observed. If you've never played snooker you probably won't be able to reproduce expert shots, even if you were able to pay attention and remember what was involved (and this might be unlikely).

Motivation

Why would you want to copy something you have seen someone else doing? Will it give you some sort of 'pay-off'? Can you imagine a good outcome? Have you seen other people like yourself receiving a reward for the behaviour? If you think you will receive praise, or indeed money, for being good at snooker you might be highly motivated to copy expert behaviour. On the other hand, if you cannot even imagine a pay-off, then why would you reproduce a particular skill or behaviour even if you were capable of doing this?

In Figure 12.19, the young male onlooker:

* pays attention to the skateboarder and his performance

* can remember or retain some of the detail of the performance

* has the physical ability to develop and reproduce the performance

* is motivated to imitate the behaviour because of the attention from the girls who are watching. There may be an imagined pay-off associated with imitating skateboarding.

So if the opportunity arises, this person might take up skateboarding and might be perceived as behaving in an anti-social way.

In Figure 12.19 the older woman:

* pays attention – but not to the detail of the actions; only to the perception that the activity is antisocial

* will probably not remember details of the skateboarding performance, she will only remember that the behaviour annoyed her

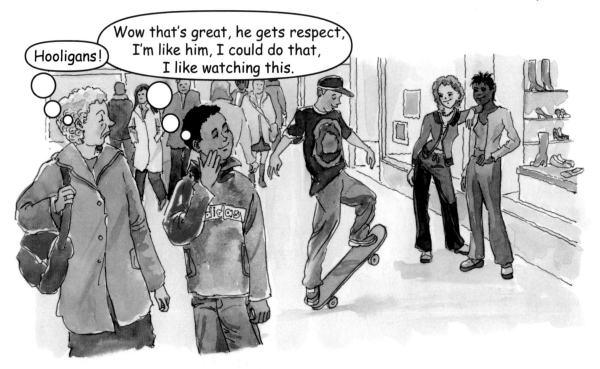

FIGURE 12.19 *People copy behaviours that are relevant to them*

* may not have the agility and co-ordination to reproduce the performance

* will not be motivated to copy the behaviour because there will be no pay-off, or imagined pay-off from others relevant to her social context.

Even if the older woman had an opportunity to try skateboarding, she will not imitate the perceived anti-social behaviour that she has seen. People do not spend their lives copying everything that they see anyone doing. We only copy behaviour that is relevant to us, that sticks in our mind, that we are capable of imitating and that we are motivated to imitate.

Think it over

Some films portray violent gun crime and people becoming rich and powerful as a result of violent behaviour.

Clearly most individuals do not imitate such behaviour, but do you think that certain people might model their behaviour on what they have observed in such films?

STRENGTHS	LIMITATIONS
* Identifies the importance of group and social context in influencing human behaviour. * Bandura's theory of observational learning explains how and why people copy the behaviour of others. * Identifies the importance of understanding an individual's immediate social context when seeking to explain behaviour.	* Like all the theories, social context theory should not be used on its own without reference to other possibilities. For example, a person may abuse alcohol, partly because they are imitating other people. But alcohol abuse may also involve a biochemical basis for dependency; together with cognitive and conditioning factors. It may be inappropriate to only use one theory to explain human behaviour.

TABLE 12.5 *Strengths and limitations of social learning theory*

Summary

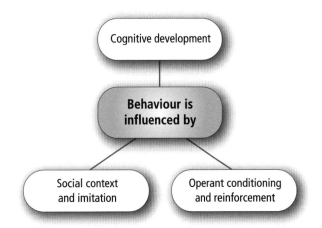

Consider this

Abbie

Abbie is a six-year-old child who has difficulties at school. Sometimes she will throw all her work, pencils etc. onto the floor and run round the classroom. Her class teacher cannot identify any specific issue that makes Abbie do this.

Using your knowledge of cognitive theory, can you identify what stage of cognitive development Abbie might be expected to be at?

If Abbie was being given lots of complicated verbal guidance she might have difficulty in understanding what was expected of her. Can you use Piaget's theory to explain why this might be so?

Using your knowledge of reinforcement theory, can you identify what might be happening if Abbie received a lot of attention from her friends when she threw her work on the floor?

Using your knowledge of operant conditioning and reinforcement theory, can you explain how the teacher might set about trying to reduce Abbie's disruptive behaviour?

One of Abbie's friends imitates her behaviour of throwing work on the floor. Using your knowledge of social learning theory, can you identify why her friend might copy Abbie's behaviour?

When the teacher asks Abbie's friend why she threw her work on the floor she cannot give an answer – because she doesn't understand her actions. Can you explain why it is that her friend does not understand her own actions?

12.3 Theories of personality development

People have different characters and react to events in different ways. For example, some people might respond to stressful situations calmly, whilst others might become depressed or angry. Many theorists would argue that personality differences cannot be explained purely in terms of imitation, conditioned learning or cognitive development, but that more complex processes of emotional development are involved.

Freud's theory

Sigmund Freud (1856–1939) developed a theory of the human mind that emphasised the interaction of biological drives with the social environment. Freud's theory emphasises the power of early experience to influence the adult personality.

Freud's theories are called **psychodynamic** theories. 'Psycho' means mind or spirit and 'dynamic' means energy or the expression of energy. Freud believed that people were born with a dynamic 'life energy' or 'libido' which initially motivates a baby to feed and grow, and later motivates sexual reproduction. Freud's theory explains that people are born with biological instincts in much the same way that animals such as dogs or cats are. Our instincts exist in the unconscious mind – we don't usually understand our unconscious. As we grow we have to learn to control our instincts in order to be accepted and fit in with other people. Society is only possible if people can 'control themselves'. If everybody just did whatever they felt like, life would be short and violent, and civilisation would not be possible. Because people have to learn to control their unconscious drives (or instincts), as children they go through stages of psychosexual development. These stages result in the development of a mature mind which contains the mechanisms that control adult personality and behaviour.

Freud's stages of psychosexual development

The oral stage

'Drive energy' motivates the infant to feed, and activities involving the lips, sucking and biting create pleasure for the baby. Weaning represents a difficult stage which may influence the future personality of the child.

The anal stage

Young children have to learn to control their muscles, and in particular their anal muscles. Toilet training represents the first time a child has to control their own body in order to meet the demands of society. The child's experiences during toilet training may influence later development.

The phallic stage

Freud shocked Europeans a century ago by insisting that children had sexual feelings towards their parents. Freud believed that girls were sexually attracted to their father and boys were sexually attracted to their mother. These attractions are called the Electra and Oedipus complexes, named after characters in ancient Greek mythology who experienced these attractions. As children develop they have to give up the opposite sex parent as a 'love object' and learn to identify with the same sex parent. Children's experience of 'letting go' of their first love may have permanent effects on their later personality.

Latency

After the age of five or six, most children have resolved the Electra and Oedipus complexes (Freud believed that this was usually stronger and more definite in boys, i.e. girls often continue with a sexual attachment to their father). Children are not yet biologically ready to reproduce so their sexuality is latent or waiting to express itself.

Genital stage

With the onset of puberty adolescents become fully sexual and 'life drive' is focused on sexual activity.

Think it over

Have you ever watched animals such as kittens develop? Freud's theories are often hard to accept in a society which is 'out of touch' with nature, but if you watch kittens they focus all their energy on getting milk from the mother cat – life energy seems almost visible. As kittens grow to young cats they will sometimes attempt to mate with parents. Freud's theories were based on the idea that people are animals – but animals that have to adapt their behaviour to the needs of society.

How far do you think we forget or even deny our inner 'drives'?

Mental mechanisms

Freud believed that we were born with an **'id'**. The 'id' is part of our unconscious mind that is hidden from conscious understanding. The 'id' is like a dynamo that generates mental energy. This energy motivates human action and behaviour.

When a young child learns to control their own body during toilet training the **'ego'** develops. The 'ego' is a mental system which contains personal learning about physical and social reality. The 'ego' has the job of deciding how to channel drive energy from the unconscious into behaviour which will produce satisfactory outcomes in the real world. The 'ego' is both unconscious (unknown to self) and conscious (a person can understand some of their own actions and motivation).

The 'super ego' develops from the ego when the child gives up their opposite-sex parent as a 'love object'. The 'super ego' contains the social and moral values of the parent that has been 'lost' as a potential partner.

The essence of psychodynamic theory is that people are controlled by inner forces, but that people do not understand and cannot explain what is happening to themselves. For example throughout adult life a person has to find a way to release 'drive energy' that is compatible with the demands of society and with the demands of the super ego. Sometimes people may feel sandwiched between the demands of their biology and social pressures. Typically today's world often creates

pressure to 'achieve a good career' and please parental values by 'doing well'. For some people the desire to enjoy their sexuality and perhaps have children may conflict with the pressure to achieve. The way people cope with these pressures will be strongly influenced by childhood experiences according to Freudian theory.

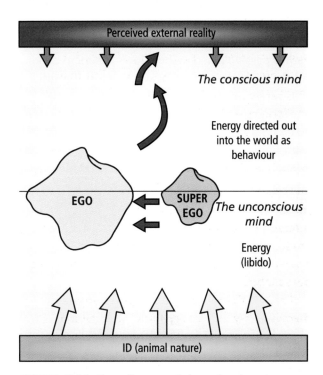

FIGURE 12.20 *Freudian mental mechanisms*

In order to understand an individual's behaviour, a therapist needs to be able to understand what is happening in that individual's unconscious mind. Therapists and counsellors cannot begin to understand the unconscious mind of an individual by asking direct questions. In order to understand how early experience has influenced the unconscious mind therapists might explore an individual's dreams. Alternatively, a therapist might ask a service user to make up a story about a picture (the Thematic Apperception Test) or ask them what they see in an ink blot (the Rorschach test).

These indirect conversations are a way of learning about another person's unconscious mind. Freud originally used the method of 'free association' to access the unconscious mind of his patients. This 'talking cure' involves getting the patient or client to relax on a couch and just explain whatever comes into their mind in response to words that the psychoanalyst says.

Psychosexual stages of development and personality

Freud believed that a person's experiences in the first three stages would influence their adult personality. An infant whose feeding needs were always anticipated and met might grow up to be a rather passive person who allows others to make all the decisions. An infant whose need for milk was rarely met might also become fixated with the struggle for food. Ideally, infants should learn to communicate their needs but also learn that communication will result in a good response. Many people do not experience ideal conditions in early life so it is possible for drive or life energy (Freud used the word 'libido' to describe this energy) to become focused or fixated on the early stages of development.

Personality characteristics associated with the oral stage

If life energy becomes fixated with the oral stage a person may tend to be passive, dependent on others and gullible. Such a person might also be attracted to oral pleasures such as eating, drinking or smoking. People who are extremely passive and perhaps manipulative might be understood as being fixated at the oral stage of development. Because of the way psychological defence mechanisms work, people with exactly the opposite personality, e.g. someone who is suspicious and avoids oral pleasure, might also be seen as reacting to an oral fixation. A well-

adjusted adult will have a personality that lies between these extremes.

Personality characteristics associated with the anal stage

A fixation of life energy at this stage of development might result in characteristics of:

* hoarding, or being mean with money
* being stubborn
* being obsessed with tidiness and cleanliness.

The term anal-retentive is sometimes used to describe people who are obsessed with tidiness, cleanliness and controlling their money.

Once again, a person who is extremely generous, extremely open to other people's suggestions and extremely untidy will be seen as reacting to a fixation with the anal stage. A well-adjusted adult will not be particularly mean or over generous; not particularly stubborn or over compliant; and not particularly tidy or untidy in his or her daily life.

Personality characteristics associated with the phallic stage

A fixation of life energy at this stage might result in extremes of personality involving:

* vanity and self-love
* recklessness
* obsession with sexual activity.

Again a person with exactly the opposite characteristics might be reacting to a fixation at this stage. So a timid adult who avoids all reference to sexuality might also be fixated at the phallic stage. A well-adjusted adult will not display extreme personality characteristics.

People do not become fixated with the latency period, and the genital stage represents adulthood.

Regression

When people experience extreme emotional stress it may be hard for their ego to maintain 'normal' age-appropriate behaviour. A person may feel pulled by unconscious desires to return to a safer time in life. An adult or adolescent might, for example, have a childish temper tantrum involving shouting and screaming over some minor annoyance. This behaviour could be interpreted as a regression to the oral stage. The person is behaving like a young child again because the ego has lost control of the flow of life energy. Life energy has regressed to an earlier stage of development.

Most people will react with some degree of emotional regression if they are stressed, but excessive amounts of childish behaviour might suggest a fixation of life energy with the early stages of development that makes it difficult for the ego to manage daily living.

Fixation means that the person's personality is strongly influenced – perhaps unbalanced – by experiences in the first three life stages. Regression means that a person is reliving some of their emotional experience from one or more of the first three stages of life.

Within Freudian theory, many people would be expected to experience some regression to and fixation with early stages of development.

Defence mechanisms

The ego is the decision-making part of our mind. The ego has to work out how to get on with other people whilst also coping with our unconscious animal instincts, and unconscious memories. The ego is under attack from the pressures of the real world and the pressures of the unconscious. If a person is to remain in good mental health their ego has to find a way of coping with all these pressures. Ego defences are ways in which people can make themselves feel safer and protect themselves from pressures.

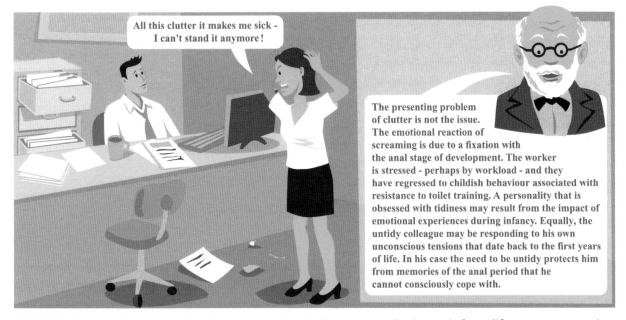

FIGURE 12.21 *An obsession with tidiness or untidy behaviour may both result from life energy regressing to the anal stage*

Examples of defence mechanisms include:

* *denial*: blocking threatening information or thoughts from awareness

* *repression*: forcing memories out of consciousness into the unconscious mind. Repression is a kind of motivated forgetting of unpleasant thoughts or memories

* *rationalisation*: reinterpreting events or memories in order to make them safer for the ego

* *displacement*: finding a different outlet for feelings such as transferring anger towards a parent to an 'out-group'

* *projection*: projecting forbidden emotions onto others, i.e. what we see in others is sometimes in ourselves

* *sublimation*: a change of state in the way mental energy is directed, e.g. sexual drive is directed away from partners and into activities such as collecting things

* *reaction formation*: changing an emotion into its overemphasised opposite, e.g. changing love to hatred or hatred into aggressively expressed praise.

SCENARIO

Defence mechanisms

What defence mechanisms might be involved in the behaviours described below?

Arnold lives alone in a three-bedroom house; he has filled all of the bedrooms, living rooms and corridor with old newspapers.

Arnold explains that he likes to collect newspapers because he is interested in recent history.

Andrea has chronic obstructive pulmonary disease which causes her distress and difficulty in breathing. She has a long medical history of illness. When asked about her health she claims that there is nothing wrong with her and that she is very well.

Andrea says that she has never experienced any serious illness in her life.

Andrea says that her carers are 'angels sent from God – the most wonderful people in the world and the kindest, cleverest people she has ever met in her life'.

Andrea says that the manager of the home is trying to poison her, and she knows this is true because he does not like her.

Possible defence mechanisms at work

Arnold may be using sublimation to redirect mental energy away from aspects of life which become threatening and into a much safer activity of collecting things.

Arnold may be using rationalisation to avoid recognising the real reasons for collecting so many old newspapers.

Andrea may be using denial to block out awareness of the seriousness of her illness.

Andrea may be repressing memory of past ill-health in order to make the situation feel safer for her.

Andrea may feel distressed and angry about the situation and about the care she is receiving, but she is using reaction formation in order to change her emotions into 'its over-emphasised opposite'. Reaction formation prevents her from being fully aware of her situation and feelings.

Andrea may be displacing her anger and distress onto the manager and defending her ego against full awareness of her motivation for doing this by using the defence of projection to claim that he dislikes her – it's his fault, he started it.

Strengths and limitations

Freudian theory provides a comprehensive system for interpreting the complexities of human behaviour. Freud emphasised that it was very important that only qualified therapists who had been through a process of self analysis should use psychodynamic theory to explain other people's behaviour. If used in an amateur way people will tend to use the theory to meet their own emotional needs. Another issue is that Freud's stages of development, his theory of mental mechanisms and the unconscious mind are not universally accepted. John Bowlby proposed a different emphasis for understanding the importance of early experience – see below.

Bowlby's theory of attachment

Like Freud, Bowlby believed that our early experiences in life can have a profound affect on our personality. But Bowlby did not believe in the importance of an 'oral stage,' where personality is influenced by the experience of obtaining food during breast-feeding. Bowlby believed that the most important issue during early life was making an attachment – a bond of love – between a caregiver and infant.

Bowlby developed his theory from experience of working with children and through observation of parent–child interaction. Bowlby was also influenced by studies of animal behaviour that showed dramatic evidence of attachment behaviours. Bowlby's studies of infants led him to the conclusion that there was a biological need for mothers and babies to be together, and that there was a sensitive or critical period for mothers and babies to form this attachment, which is known as bonding. Bowlby (1953) stated, 'The absolute need of infants and toddlers for the continuous care of their mothers will be borne in on all who read this book'.

If the bond of love between a baby and his or her mother was broken through separation, Bowlby believed, lasting psychological damage would be done to the child. If a mother left her child to go to work every day – or just once to go into hospital – there might be a risk of damage. Bowlby believed that children who suffered a lasting separation from their mother might grow up to be unable to love or show affection. Separated children might not care about other people. Separated children might also fail to learn properly at school, and might be more likely to turn to crime when they grew up. This theory, that children who are separated from their mother would grow up to be emotionally damaged, is known as maternal deprivation.

Bowlby's theory: an overview

An infant's experience in the first months and years of life will have long-lasting effects on their personality. We have an inbuilt need to form an attachment with a carer. Our experience

of attachment in infancy organises the way we understand social relationships – creating an internal working model of relationships in our minds.

If an infant does not make an attachment they may be incapable of loving and caring relationships in later life. If an infant is separated from his or her principal carer then they may be emotionally damaged by the experience of separation. Infants will seek to make a close attachment to one person – usually this will be their mother.

Key concept

Monotropic attachment: John Bowlby believed that every infant needed to attach to, or bond with just one principle caregiver. Usually this would be the child's mother. 'Mono' means one, and 'tropic' can be interpreted as 'attraction'. So Monotropic can be understood as 'seeking or being attracted to only one attachment'.

Key concept

Critical period/sensitive period: some animals, such as ducks and geese, display a 'critical period' in the first hours after hatching when they will attach to an adult figure. John Bowlby believed there was a sensitive period between six months and three years of age when infant humans needed to form an attachment. This 'sensitive period' might be similar to the 'critical period' identified in animal studies.

Separation

Bowlby observed that an infant who was separated from his or her mother would experience distress. Observations of short-term separations, such as that of a two-year-old going into hospital, suggested that children would respond with:

* *protest and anger:* to include behaviours such as crying, screaming, clinging to the mother

* *depression and sadness:* the child becomes withdrawn and does not seek comfort

* *normal behaviour that masks detachment:* the child responds normally to others but there is an unwillingness to share affection. If the mother returns the child may reject her and avoid her before the mother is accepted again.

Even a brief separation, for a few days, might result in a fear of being abandoned that will become absorbed into the assumptions that the child and later adult will make about other people.

Longer-term separations, such as the loss of a parent due to death or divorce, might result in separation anxiety – the fear that relationships will result in separation in the future. In such a situation the child may seek to become emotionally self-sufficient and detached in order to protect themselves from loss. A young child cannot understand what is happening if they are separated; and this may result in a deep unconscious fear that will influence or limit his or her ability to form an intimate loving relationship with an adult partner in later life.

Bowlby believed that each person develops an internal working model of the way social relationships work. An internal working model develops from our biological need to form attachments with carers during infancy. The way our carers behave will influence the development of our internal model of human relationships.

Ainsworth – anxious, avoidant and secure attachment

Mary Ainsworth undertook some research with infants using a 'strange situation' research approach. This approach involved mother and infant being in a playroom. A stranger would enter the room and talk to the mother. The mother would leave the room, and then return. The child's behaviour in these different strange situations and when the mother returns could be observed. Ainsworth (1978) categorised children's behaviour into four types (see Table 12.6).

The different types of attachment are thought to lead to different internal working models of relationship in adult life. Mary Main, quoted in McLeod (2003), undertook a range of research with adults. She concluded that people who had experienced secure attachment as a child were able to present a clear story of their past and of relationships – they appeared to develop an effective internal working model. This working model enabled them to think back and reflect on their life and evaluate the quality of emotional relationships. People who had experienced insecure attachment might be more likely to have confused or 'multiple' internal working models. It is possible that people who have not experienced secure attachment in early life may be less able to make sense of their relationships with other people.

Early experience may provide some people with a sense of security and confidence that enables them to feel confident with other people and naturally able to develop an intimate loving relationship. People who experience insecure attachment may be less automatically able to

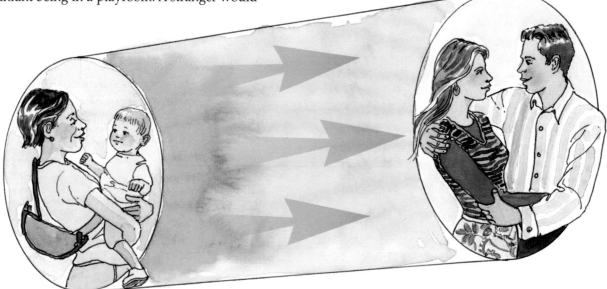

FIGURE 12.22 *The quality of early attachment experiences may influence adult emotional relationships*

BEHAVIOUR TYPE	DESCRIPTION
Secure attachment	Securely attached children are upset when the mother leaves but accept comfort and return to playing when the mother returns.
Insecure ambivalent (anxious) attachment	Insecure ambivalent children become upset and anxious but cannot be comforted when the mother returns. They may want to be comforted but resist the approaches of the mother.
Insecure avoidant attachment	Insecure avoidant children may ignore the mother on return, avoiding contact perhaps as a way of protecting themselves from emotional disappointment.
Insecurely attached – disorganised	These children appear confused when the mother returns and may show a range of contradictory behaviours.

TABLE 12.6 *Ainsworth's four types of attachment*

attach; there is also the possibility that insecure attachment may result in a lack of confidence and trust towards other people.

Marris (1996) believes that adult emotional security and quality of life depend on attachment. The quality of our early attachment influences our memory of love and our ability to feel secure. People who enjoy secure attachments are argued to have an advantage in life because they have the inner resources to cope with uncertainty in life. Life is full of transition and change. People who were securely attached as children are likely to have deep memories that enable them to cope emotionally. So success and happiness in life may be influenced by the degree to which you have experienced love during early childhood.

What if?

Suppose you heard a person say:

1. 'Well I guess I must just be very lucky – I never really had to think about relationships, I mean I met my partner when I was 17 and it just worked, I mean we're very happy. Sure we argue, but I never think about it, we just belong together, and we give and take and everything works out.'

2. 'I think if you've been with a person for more than three days then it's too long. I don't trust anyone – they always let you down in the end. The only person I can trust is me. I live for going out and meeting people, I enjoy sex, but I don't get involved with other people – it is always more trouble than it's worth.'

What kind of internal working model about attachments do you think each of these two people have developed? How do you think early experiences of secure or insecure attachment may have influenced each of these people?

Rutter (1981) found evidence that suggests that it is the quality of emotional attachment between a carer and the infant that matters. Not being able to make an attachment may damage a child emotionally. But it is the making of a bond of love between the baby and a carer that matters, not whether temporary separations happen.

There is research that suggests that babies can and do make bonds with their fathers and with their brothers, sisters, or other carers. In one study (Schaffer and Emerson 1964) almost a third of 18-month-old infants had made their main attachment to their fathers. It seems that babies give their love to the person or persons who give them the best quality affection and time. Rutter argued that research shows:

* Children can and do form important emotional attachments to fathers and to multiple members of the family. The theory that every infant seeks to make a monotropic attachment may not be true.

* Failure to make an attachment might cause lasting psychological damage, but there is evidence which suggests that children can and do recover from experiences of being separated.

It is important to make attachments during early life – but later life experience is also important. For example, disruption to family life or the loss of a parent after the age of three might also have damaging consequences; the loss of parents during adolescence may be closely associated with the development of adult depression. Rutter quotes research that suggests it might be a mistake to assume that only a critical or sensitive attachment period can influence development.

Strengths and limitations

Rutter's overview of research suggests that Bowlby's theory identifies some important issues but that it is important to understand human development as a very complex process. It may be wrong to assume that every adult problem can be traced back to the quality of attachment to a mother figure. It may be a serious mistake to assume that only the relationship between child and mother is important or that only the events during early childhood matter. It is also unlikely that mothers who go to work will inevitably deprive and damage their children. The quality of emotional contact between carers and children may be at least as important as the contact time available between carers and children.

Maslow's theory of human need

Abraham Maslow (1908–1970) developed a famous theory of human motivation. His theory is described as a humanistic theory because it shares assumptions with some other humanistic theories such as Carl Rogers' theory of personality (1902–1987). Humanistic theories stress the uniqueness of each person. Each individual builds their own system of belief and develops their own personal self concept. Humanistic theorists stress that it is important to understand the unique world of each person. Humanistic theorists argue that whilst genetics, conditioning, or early experience may influence people, individuals cannot be fully understood in terms of such general principles. In order to fully understand human behaviour we have to enter the unique thoughts of each individual person.

Maslow's theory also provides a way to understand human motivation and purpose. Existentialism explores the nature of human existence and what it is to be human. Maslow

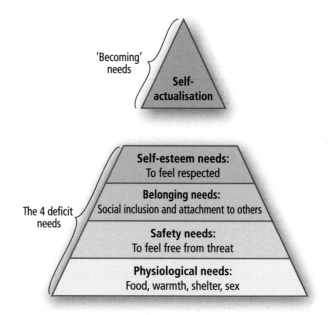

FIGURE 12.23 *Maslow's four deficit needs and the higher level need to self-actualise*

argues that fulfilling potential and going beyond self concept in order to 'transcend the self' represent the highest achievements of personal development. His humanistic–existential approach is explained below. Originally Maslow identified five basic needs. In 1943 he wrote: 'There are at least five sets of goals, which we may call basic needs. These are briefly physiological, safety, love (to belong), self-esteem, and self-actualisation.' These five levels of need form the basis of Maslow's theory.

Maslow identified four basic needs that he called deficit needs. Deficit needs have to be met before a person can fully develop their potential.

* *physiological needs:* food, warmth, shelter, sex, etc.

* *safety needs:* to feel physically and emotionally free from threat

* *belonging needs:* a need for social inclusion and attachment to others

* *self-esteem needs:* a need for respect and to develop a secure sense of self/self-concept.

Maslow argued that the majority of people in North American society spent their lives wrestling with deficit needs. Deficit needs limit and distort human development and the majority of people never achieve self-actualisation because they are unable to fulfil their deficit needs (see Figure 12.23).

Deficit needs: physical, safety, belonging and self-esteem needs are deficit needs. If you lack a sense of safety, or belonging with others, or self-esteem, then these deficits (things that you lack) will stop you from developing your potential and becoming what you are capable of becoming.

Becoming needs: when you have a secure sense of who you are and you feel content, safe, have appropriate relationships with others and have self-esteem then you can start to become what you are capable of becoming. Aesthetic, intellectual and self-actualisation are positive 'becoming needs'.

Self-actualisation: actualising self means that you fulfil your potential; you become everything that you are capable of becoming. Self-actualisation may involve developing a range of physical, artistic and intellectual abilities – because 'you have it in you' to achieve these things.

SCENARIO

Deficit needs

Michael is 22 years old and is homeless and drug dependent. He spends much of his time begging for money and much of his thoughts revolve around getting enough drugs to feel OK. Michael also thinks about food, warmth and having sex. Michael does not care about what other people think of him and he does not have a trusting relationship with any other person.

Emily is 22 years old and has had a large number of boyfriends although her relationships never work out. Emily says she intends to live alone when she can afford to buy her own house.

Olara is 22 years old and invests an immense amount of time and energy in physical training for sports competitions and in studying for qualifications. She says 'I want people to look up to me – I've got to become the best – I want people to see me as a winner'.

Identify the main deficit needs that each of these three people are likely to be struggling with.

Maslow argued that if you are hungry, tired and threatened your whole attention will be taken up in the struggle to survive. Other people spend much of their life looking for love or looking for a family or group that they feel they can belong with. More fortunate people will seek achievements and career goals that will help them to meet their self-esteem needs. Only a few people – usually people who are middle-aged – get to being fully satisfied in terms of self-esteem, belonging, safety and physical needs.

Maslow believed that there is a hierarchy with respect to the four deficit needs. This means that people will prioritise their survival and security before focusing attention on relationships. But physical, safety and belonging needs have to be at least partially fulfilled before people worry about what other people think of them. Concern about social status and self-esteem comes last among the deficit needs.

Self-actualisation

When a person has mostly met the deficit needs they have the potential to become self-actualising. A person who is not worried about physical needs, a person who feels secure, a person who has experienced loving emotional attachments and a person who has enjoyed a high level of self-esteem is free to go beyond the normal pressures of life.

Self-actualisation involves 'becoming needs.' When a person stops being controlled by deficit needs, he or she becomes free to explore their own creativity and potential. Self-actualisation is at the top of the pyramid, but it is not just another deficit need. Self-actualising people are free. They are free from the deficit pressures that restrict the lives of most people in Western society. Maslow once suggested that perhaps as few as 2 per cent of people in North American society would achieve full self-actualisation in their lifetime.

People who achieve self-actualisation might have special qualities, including:

* a more accurate perception of reality

* greater acceptance of self and others

* greater self-knowledge

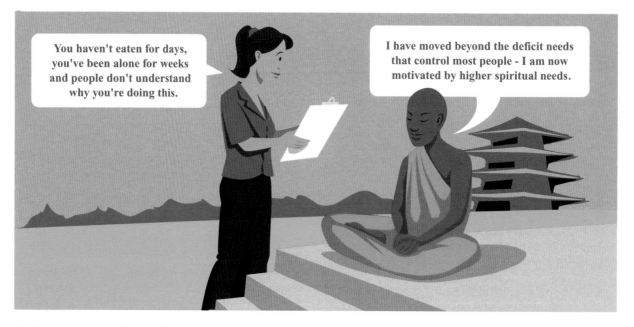

FIGURE 12.24 *A self-actualised person goes beyond the deficit needs that rule most people's lives*

* greater involvement with major projects in life
* greater independence
* creativity
* spiritual and artistic abilities.

So self-actualisation is the goal of living. People who self-actualise achieve a high degree of satisfaction from life. In a perfect world everyone would have the chance to self-actualise.

Maslow went on to develop his ideas about self-actualisation, and argued that many people experience becoming or 'growth' needs on the way to developing their full potential. These growth needs involve the need to understand and explore, and a need to explore artistic issues, such as beauty. People may develop their potential in stages. Maslow also went on to identify a spiritual stage of development that ventured beyond the fulfilment of potential – he called this stage 'transcendence'. Some textbooks therefore show Maslow's hierarchy as involving seven stages. Some websites show Maslow's hierarchy as involving eight stages with the ultimate stage of transcendence at the top.

Maslow's hierarchy and human development

Maslow did not specify age ranges in relationship to his theory of needs, but he did suggest that very few people would achieve self-actualisation during adolescence or early maturity. It is also reasonable to assume that the physical safety and belonging deficit needs are key issues during infancy and childhood, whilst self-esteem needs are likely to be centrally important to teenagers and young adults who are developing their self-concept and identity.

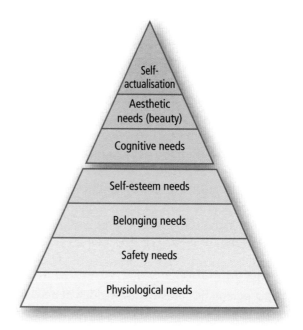

FIGURE 12.25 *Maslow's seven-stage hierarchy*

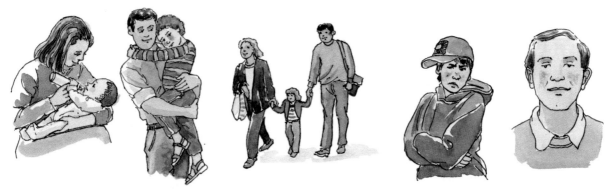

Physical needs	Safety needs	Love and belonging needs	Self-esteem needs	Self-actualisation
Demands on others: 'Feed me.'	Demands on others: 'Make it safe.'	Demands on others: 'Love me.'	Demands on others: 'Respect me!'	No demands on others: 'I'm taking care of myself now.'

FIGURE 12.26 *Some needs may be more important at different stages of development*

Strengths and limitations

Maslow's theory draws our attention to the manner in which human development involves physical, social, emotional (self-concept) and psychological needs. It is critically important that people who work in health and social care can understand that service users experience a full range of needs – and not just the need for physical well-being. Maslow also provides us with a theory that does not identify general stages of development, but focuses on the unique experiences of each individual. Maslow's theory is very critical of Western materialism. The purpose of life is the fulfilment of individual human potential – not the acquisition of financial wealth as such.

Maslow's theory offers us a general way of understanding key issues, but it might only offer limited insights into the explanation of our own or others' behaviours, and as with many other theorists described in this unit it may be inadvisable to only interpret human development using one theory.

Summary

These three approaches to understanding the development of human personality make different assumptions about the importance of life experience. It may be unwise to try to explain human development by relying on one single theory.

THEORY	DESCRIPTION
Freud's theory	Argues that people develop through a series of psychosexual stages during their early life and early experience has a powerful influence on personality.
Bowlby's theory	Argues that it is the quality of attachment in early life rather than psychosexual stages that influences personality.
Maslow's theory	Argues that there are four deficit and a range of becoming needs that will influence our personality and how we behave towards others.

TABLE 12.7 *Theories of personality development*

Joshua is an 18-month-old child. Joshua was taken into care at the age of ten months after being abandoned by his natural mother. When taken into care Joshua was seriously underweight due to a lack of feeding. Joshua's foster parents can no longer look after him because the foster mother is seriously ill in hospital.

Using your knowledge of Freudian theory can you identify some negative influences that Joshua might have been exposed to if he had been neglected during the first ten months of life?

Again, using your knowledge of Freudian theory, can you explain how poor quality experiences during the oral stage might be expected to influence an individual's personality in later life?

Using your knowledge of Bowlby's theory, can you identify some negative influences associated with neglectful or inconsistent early relationships?

Using your knowledge of Bowlby's theory, can you explain why consistent loving relationships are important during the early stages of a child's development?

Using your knowledge of Maslow's theory, can you identify the areas of unmet need that Joshua may have experienced during infancy?

Using your knowledge of Maslow's theory, can you explain why Joshua's experience might be considered a disadvantage in terms of the later development of self-esteem and self-actualisation?

UNIT 12 ASSESSMENT

How you will be assessed

This unit will be assessed through a two-hour written test. Some specimen questions relevant to this unit are set out below. They will give you an indication of what form the test will take and the maximum marks for each question (shown in brackets).

Test questions

Shevita is a skilled musician. Both her parents could play musical instruments and the school that Shevita went to provided interesting and exciting music lessons. When Shevita expressed an interest in learning to play a musical instrument, her parents paid for private tuition.

1. Explain some of the general factors that may have affected Shevita's development of musical skills. (6)

2. Explain what is meant by the term Phenotype. (3)

3. Mitesh lives in a flat within a low income housing estate. Olara lives in a detached house in a wealthy area. Describe three likely socio-economic factors that are likely to be different for Mitesh and Olara. (6)

Some children are watching a teacher performing an experiment using two identical glass tumblers and a glass bowl. The teacher fills the two glasses to the same level. The children all agree that there is the same amount of water in each glass. The teacher then pours one glass of water into the glass bowl. The children agree that all the water has gone into the bowl. The teacher then asks the children if they think there is more water in the first tumbler or in the bowl, or the same amount of water in both.

Some children think that there is more water in the tumbler; others say more water in the bowl. A few children are very clear that the must be the same water in the tumbler and the bowl.

4. Using your knowledge of Piaget's theory explain what aspect of cognitive development is being tested here. (4)

5. Using your knowledge of Piaget's theory explain why some children might be able to give the right answer whilst other children give wrong answers about the volume of water. (6)

6. Within Piaget's theory explain what is meant by object permanence. (4)

7. Within Piaget's theory children in the 'pre-operational period' of development may have difficulty decentring. Explain what is meant by decentring. (4)

8. Identify any two limitations of Piaget's theory of developmental stages. (6)

Ross is a five-year-old boy who has difficulty in attending to school work. Ross will often leave his seat to look for things on the floor or to talk to other children.

9. Explain how the theory of reinforcement might be used in order to explain why Ross often gets out of his seat. Explain how a classroom assistant might use the theory of reinforcement in order to encourage Ross to concentrate on his schoolwork. (6)

10. Mark watches an aggressive argument between a male parent and a teacher in class. Later Mark acts out shouting and aggressive behaviour while playing with other children. Sarah also watched the argument but did not copy any of the behaviour. Explain Bandura's theory of observational learning. Using Bandura's theory Identify why Mark may have been aggressive. With reference to Bandura's theory explain why Sarah did not act out the aggression, yet Mark did. (6)

11. Explain what is meant by the terms Id, Ego and Superego within Freudian theory. (6)

Read the following statements made by Tom:

'I may be 75 but there are a lot of things I want to do with my life. I think that life is what you make it, isn't it? I learned to stop worrying about trivial things like money and jobs a long time ago. I enjoy my life and I think positively about every opportunity I get. I've always been a craftsperson, I make wooden furniture – it might not be your thing, but I get a nice feeling out of designing and creating things. Many years ago, I worked as a cabinet maker for a furniture company, but in the end it got me down. I was told to do things cheaply rather than do them properly, so I left. I think if you're not enjoying your work then something is wrong. What really matters in life is being able to look back on life and feel proud and pleased with what I've done. There is no one else I would have liked to have been. I've lived my life as I wanted.'

12. With reference to Maslow's theory explain what level of need Tom might be experiencing. Explain what is meant by 'deficit needs' and 'becoming needs'. (6)

Modern health facilities for children are usually very concerned to prevent children being separated from their parents.

13. With reference to Bowlby's theory of attachment explain some of the possible harmful effects that might arise from separation. (6)

14. Explain what is meant by 'monotropic attachment.' Explain Michael Rutter's conclusions with respect to Bowlby's theory of monotropic attachment. (6)

References and further reading

Acheson, D. (1998) *Independent Inquiry into Inequalities in Health* London: HMSO

Ainsworth, M. D. S., Blehar, M. C., Water, E. and Wall, S. (1978) *Patterns of attachment: A psychological study of the strange situation.* Hillsdale, New Jersey: Lawrence Erlbaum Associates Inc.

Bandura, A., Ross, D. and Ross, S. A. (1963) Imitation of film-mediated aggressive models *Journal of Abnormal and Social Psychology,* 66, 3–11

Bandura, A. (1965) Influence of model's reinforcement contingencies on the acquisition of imitative responses *Journal of Personality and Social Psychology,* 1, 589–95

Berryman, J. C., Hargreaves D., Herbert, M. and Taylor, A. (1991) *Developmental Psychology and You* London: Routledge

Bower, T.G.R. (1982) *Development in Infancy* Second ed. San Francisco: WH Freeman

Bowlby, J. (1953) *Child Care and the Growth of Love* Harmondsworth: Penguin.

Brown, H. (1996) Classic studies of conformity. In Wetherell, M. *Identities Groups and Social Issues* London: Sage Publications

Bruner, J. S. (1974) *Beyond the information given* London: George Allen & Unwin

Chomsky, N. (1959) Review of Skinner's Verbal Behaviour *Language,* 35, 26–58

Cohen, D. (1981) *Piaget: Critique and Reassessment* London & Sydney: Croom Helm

Gross, R. (1992) *Psychology* Second ed. London: Hodder and Stoughton

Harris, P. (1989) *Children and Emotion* Oxford: Basil Blackwell

Hayes, N. and Orrell, S. (1993) *Psychology an Introduction* Second ed. Harlow: Longman.

HM Government (2000) *The NHS Plan* London: HMSO

Latané, B. and Darley, J. M. (1970) *The Unresponsive Bystander: Why Does He Not Help?* New York: Appleton-Century-Croft

Marris, P. (1996) *The Politics of Uncertainty* London: Routledge

Maslow, A. H. (1943) A Theory of Human Motivation *Psychological Review,* 50, 370–96

McGarrigle, J. and Donaldson, M. (1975) Conservation Accidents *Cognition,* 3, 341–50

Paxton, W. and Dixon, M, (2004) *The State of the Nation – an Audit of Injustice in the UK* London: Institute for Policy Research

Pinker, S. (1994) *The Language Instinct* London: Penguin Books

Rutter, M. (1981) *Maternal Deprivation Reassessed* Second ed. Harmondsworth: Penguin

Schaffer, H. R. and Emerson, P. E. (1964) The development of social attainments in infancy *Monographs of Social Research in Child Development* 29 (94)

Skinner, B. F. (1957) *Verbal Behaviour* New York: Appleton-Century-Croft

Social Exclusion Unit (1999) *Opportunity for All* London: HMSO

Social Trends Vol. 34 (2004) London: HMSO

Social Trends Vol. 35 (2005) London: HMSO

Tajfel, H. (ed.) (1978) *Differentiation Between Social Groups: Studies in the Social Psychology of Intergroup Relations* London: Academic Press

Tajfel, H. (1981) *Human Groups and Social Categories* Cambridge: Cambridge University Press

Watson, P. and Johnson – Laird N.J. (1972) *Psychology of Reasoning: Structure and Content* London: Batsford

Useful websites

www.ippr.org
Institute for Policy Research

The role of exercise in maintaining health and well-being

Unit 13

This unit covers the following sections

13.1 Exercise-related fitness

13.2 Physical, social and psychological benefits of regular exercise

13.3 Standard monitoring methods and tables

13.4 Safety in physical activity

13.5 Barriers to participation in regular exercise

13.6 Exercise and disease prevention

13.7 Exercise programmes for different clients

This unit aims to develop your understanding of a range of different aspects of exercise which help maintain health and well-being. You will learn about the fundamentals of exercise-related fitness which enable the body to function with maximum physical efficiency. You will explore the physical, social and psychological benefits of regular exercise, as well as barriers to participation, and become informed about exercise programming for different clients.

Good nutrition and exercise work together to support our health and well-being, whilst health can be considered as an integrated method of functioning that is orientated towards achieving our maximum potential, and wellness as our approach to personal health. Regular exercise and physical activity make us feel fitter, look better and provide us with more vitality and energy to go about our daily tasks with ease. Numerous health benefits are afforded by regular exercise participation, such as weight management, a reduced risk of coronary heart disease, diabetes and osteoporosis, maintenance of physical work capacity as the body ages, and reduced feelings of depression and anxiety. Hence the importance of regular exercise and physical activity in promoting good health is a common feature in policy initiatives to improve the nation's health and well-being, but the lack of exercise and physical activity participation within the population remains a serious public health concern, with most of our population deemed to be sedentary or irregularly active.

Unit assessment

This unit will be assessed by a two-hour written examination. A more detailed guide to the assessment is given at the end of the unit.

13.1 Exercise-related fitness

You should understand that there are many different kinds of exercise-related fitness, often referred to as health-related fitness, that enable your body to function with maximum physical efficiency to cope with the demands placed on your body by daily life. Exercise-related fitness has several components and you require a minimum level of fitness in each of these individual components to cope with everyday living with ease. Athletes, however, require higher levels of fitness in these components and different sporting activities will require the development of different aspects of exercise-related fitness.

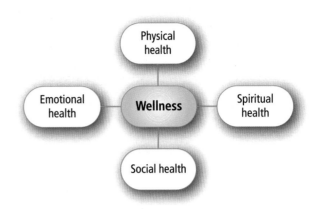

FIGURE 13.1 *The components of wellness*

> **Get set introductory activity**
> You should undertake the following activity before reading this unit, but for your safety before you get started you need to check your suitability to undertake the practical activities throughout this unit using the **health status questionnaire** described at the end of the unit on page 135. Complete this questionnaire before you read on any further.

Key concepts

Health: as defined by the World Health Organisation (WHO), is a state of complete physical, mental and social well-being and not merely the absence of disease and infirmity.

Wellness: can be viewed as our approach to personal health that emphasises individual responsibility for well-being through the practice of health-promoting lifestyle behaviours.

These behaviours include regular physical activity, a healthy diet and the maintenance of good emotional and spiritual health. There are strong interactions between the different components of wellness; none of these work in isolation. Total wellness is achieved by balancing physical, social, emotional and spiritual health.

Whether you normally exercise alone, or as part of a sports team you will have already

recognised some of the changes and adaptations that occur within your body in response to exercise. After you have worked through this unit you can return to this activity to assess what you have learned. Choose your favourite individual sporting or fitness activity such as aerobics, running, cycling, rollerblading or swimming.

Take five to six minutes to warm-up and then undertake your favourite activity at a relatively high intensity for about 15 to 20 minutes. At the end of this fitness session, be sure you finish with a minimum five-minute warm-down. At each stage of the fitness session you should pay close attention to how the different parts of your body respond and adapt to the activity you have chosen to undertake.

Think it over

Identify the components of wellness and consider their importance to the maintenance of health.

Try it out

On a separate piece of paper list the body changes that you have experienced. How did your body adapt to the different stages of the workout?

You will have an opportunity to assess your fitness level during this unit.

Poor health is a serious drain on national resources and increases the expenditure required on health care by the government.

As individuals we may encounter many difficulties in attaining wellness. Our age, ethnicity and socio-economic status may present challenges to achieving wellness, and these and other potential barriers will be discussed further later in the unit.

Let's take a closer look at the components of fitness

Aerobic fitness

Also referred to as cardiorespiratory fitness or cardiorespiratory endurance, this relates to the efficiency of the heart, lungs and circulatory system. It is essentially a measure of the heart's ability to pump blood rich with oxygen to the working muscles, and the ability of the muscles to take up and utilise this oxygen to produce the energy required for the muscles to continue contracting. In simple terms, aerobic fitness is the ability to perform endurance-type activities such as swimming, cycling, running and walking. Essentially, individuals with high levels of aerobic fitness will be able to undertake these types of activities more vigorously and for longer without undue fatigue. Many high intensity intermittent team sports, such as football and hockey, require a good level of aerobic fitness. In aerobic work, oxygen obtained from the air is used to burn fat and carbohydrate to produce the energy necessary to perform the work.

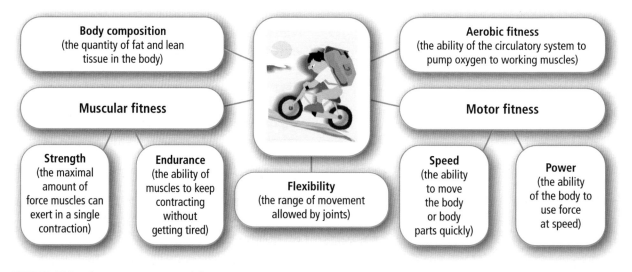

FIGURE 13.2 *The components of fitness*

The most accurate measure of aerobic fitness is the laboratory assessment of maximal oxygen consumption known as the **VO₂ max test**. This test measures the highest oxygen consumption achievable during exercise. The test usually consists of walking or running on a treadmill, or cycling on a cycle ergometer for approximately 15 minutes with increasing loads with maximal effort. The oxygen used during the maximal effort is the maximal oxygen uptake. The higher the VO_2 max score the fitter the individual.

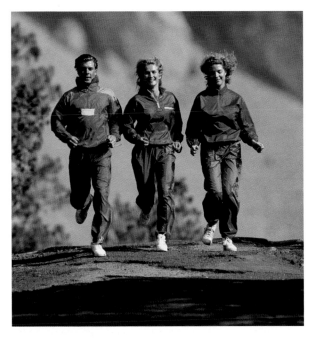

Running helps maintain health and well-being

Rockport 1-mile walk test

This is a simple weight bearing field test to determine cardiorespiratory fitness, which is particularly useful for sedentary subjects or those about to embark on a training programme. The objective of the test is to complete the mile walk in as fast a time as possible. It involves a timed 1 mile walk on a smooth level surface, preferably a running track, in good weather conditions with the subject aiming to maintain a steady even pace throughout. The test procedure is as follows:

* prior to commencing the test the subject should undertake a 5–10 minute warm-up

* the subject should be informed that the test requires maximum effort, but that if any distress is suffered during the test he or she should slow the pace, inform the researcher and seek medical advice as soon as possible

* activate the stop watch at the start of the measured mile and on completion of the test record the time taken

* the subject should then undertake a 5–10 minute warm-down.

Cooper's 1.5-mile run test

This is another simple-to-perform weight-bearing field test designed to evaluate cardiorespiratory endurance which can be more readily applied to physically active subjects. Again, the objective of the test is to complete the distance in the shortest time possible. It involves a timed 1.5 mile run on a smooth level surface, preferably a running track in good weather conditions. Again a useful strategy is to aim to maintain a steady even pace throughout. The test procedure is as follows:

* prior to commencing the test the subject should undertake a 5–10 minute warm-up

* the subject should be informed that the test requires maximum effort, but that if any distress is suffered during the test he or

she should slow the pace, inform the researcher and seek medical advice as soon as possible

* activate the stopwatch at the start of the measured 1.5 mile and on completion of the test record the time taken

* the subject should then undertake a 5–10 minute warm-down.

Try it out

Using the Internet and sources identified at the end of this unit, identify the fitness scores and classifications for the Cooper's running test.

The 3-minute step test

The 3-minute step test is another submaximal test to determine aerobic fitness. The basic principle of this test is that subjects with a higher level of aerobic fitness will recover more rapidly and have a lower heart rate during recovery from a three-minute standardised bench stepping test. One of the additional advantages of this test is that it can be performed indoors. The standardised height of the step is 45 cm (18 inches) and cadence 60 beats per minute (bpm) for both male and female subjects. Thirty complete steps in a four beat cycle (up, up, down, down) should be completed during each minute of the test. The test procedure is as follows:

* prior to commencing the test the subject should undertake a 5–10 minute warm-up

* the subject should be informed that the test requires maximum effort, but that if any distress is suffered during the test he or she should slow the pace, inform the researcher and seek medical advice as soon as possible

* set the metronome to 60 bpm

* the subject starts stepping ensuring that the knee is straightened during the up phase of the step

* on completing the test the subject sits on the bench and the pulse is located and counted for a 30 second period during three separate recovery times: 1–1.5 minutes, 2–2.5 minutes and 3–3.5 minutes post exercise

* the subject's fitness category is determined by adding the three values obtained for the 30 second heart rates during recovery and referring to Table 13.1.

* the subject should then undertake a 5–10 minute warm-down.

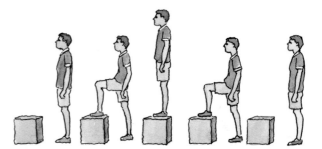

FIGURE 13.3 *The 3-minute step test*

FITNESS CATEGORY	MEN	WOMEN
Very poor	194+	206+
Poor	167–193	176–205
Average	144–166	155–175
Good	134–146	137–154
Excellent	119–133	122–136
Superior	<118	>121

TABLE 13.1 *Fitness classifications for the sum of heart rate recovery values for the 3-minute step test expressed in beats per minute*

Try it out

Working in pairs, taking roles as subject and researcher, undertake one of the test protocols for establishing aerobic fitness and determine each other's fitness scores.

Remember this test should only be attempted if you have met the medical clearance criteria as outlined at the end of this unit on page 135.

Women have lower $\dot{V}O_2$ max values than men. This is, in part, due to their smaller total muscle mass and higher body fat content.

Muscular fitness

Muscular fitness has two components:

* muscular strength
* muscular endurance.

Muscular strength is defined as the maximal amount of force a muscle can exert to overcome a resistance in a single contraction. It is an important characteristic of many sports, such as football, rugby, several athletic events and gymnastics. Females have only about two-thirds of the muscular strength of males, due to differences in hormones and muscle mass. Maximum strength is usually reached in our twenties and then declines with advancing age. However, regardless of age, strength can be improved. In order to improve muscular strength, exercises requiring relatively short intense work periods are required.

Muscular endurance, on the other hand, is the ability of the skeletal muscles to generate force for extended periods of time without becoming fatigued. Although muscular strength and muscular endurance are related, it is important to note that they are not the same. Any activity where movement patterns are repeated over and over again will require high degrees of muscular endurance, for example the squash player who needs to repeatedly swing their racquet during a match, or the athlete rowing on a rowing machine in the gym.

Flexibility

Flexibility is the ability to work a joint and its associated soft tissue structures freely through its

full range of movement. In the absence of routine stretching, muscles and tendons shorten becoming tight and impairing the range of movement around their joints. Individual requirements for flexibility vary and in a sporting context some sports such as gymnastics and diving require much greater degrees of flexibility. In a health context adequate flexibility could mean the difference between being able to tie your own shoe laces or not, or do up the zip on a dress.

Motor fitness

Motor fitness is a general term that refers to many factors such as agility, balance, reaction time, co-ordination, power and speed. These are sometimes referred to as performance-related components of fitness, but many have great relevance to maintaining health-related fitness and well-being. Maintenance of some of the above aspects of motor fitness are important in the co-ordination of muscle movement, so that movements can be performed accurately while still maintaining the desired posture, and potentially lead to less energy expenditure.

Body composition

Body composition is not the same as body weight. It is a technical term that refers to the quantification of the various components of the body, namely fat and lean body mass, the muscles, organs and bone. This measure plays an important role in both health and sport. Excess body fat, for example, may lead to obesity and increase the risk of chronic disease in the context of health, and in some sports excess body fat may hinder performance, requiring additional energy to move around.

Undertake your own research to investigate the relative merits of these measures of body composition when applied to the sedentary and sporting individual.

Body responses and adaptations to exercise

Exercise produces a stress on the body. The body responds to the stress of exercise or physical activity in a variety of ways. Some of these responses are immediate and are often referred to as the 'acute responses' to exercise, such as an increase in body temperature and heart rate. These are the body's immediate responses to a single bout of exercise. Others are long term, often referred to as 'chronic responses' or adaptations that contribute to improved fitness for sports participation and reduced health risk. Chronic adaptations are the body's response over an extended period to the stress of repeated frequent bouts of exercise.

When exercise is performed over a period of weeks or months, the body adapts. The physiological changes that occur with repeated exposure to exercise improve the body's exercise capacity and efficiency. With aerobic training, such as running and cycling, the heart and lungs become more efficient and endurance capacity increases, while the muscles become stronger with resistance modes of training, such as weight training. Adaptations derived from training are highly specific to the type of exercise training undertaken. To understand the responses and adaptation observed as a result of training it is necessary to understand the basic principles of training and exercise prescription, some of which can be applied to all forms of exercise training. This will be covered later in the unit.

Aerobic system responses to exercise

During exercise the contracting muscles require a continual supply of nutrients and oxygen to support energy production (**aerobic** training). These requirements are over and above those required to support normal activities at work or rest. As a result the heart has to beat harder and faster to meet these increased demands. If these demands are repeated frequently as a result of a systematic training programme, over time the heart becomes stronger. The heart and blood vessels of the circulatory system adapt to repeated bouts of exercise.

* The heart increases in its size and blood volume. The wall of the left ventricle thickens increasing the strength potential of its contractions.

* It pumps more blood per beat, increasing stroke volume. Stroke volume at rest has been shown to be significantly higher after a prolonged endurance training programme.

* It can therefore pump more blood per minute increasing cardiac output during maximal levels of exercise.

* Blood flow increases as a consequence of an increase in blood vessel size and number. This allows for more efficient delivery of oxygen and nutrients.

* Resting heart rate falls, reducing the workload on the heart and the heart rate returns to normal after exercise more quickly.

However, it would not matter how efficient the circulatory system was at supplying blood to the tissues during exercise if the respiratory system, could not keep pace with the demand for oxygen. In common with the cardiovascular system, the respiratory system undergoes specific adaptations in response to a systematic training programme, which help to maximise its efficiency. The respiratory system adapts to repeated bouts of exercise in the following ways:

* an increase in the rate and depth of breathing – the muscles demand more oxygen and the corresponding increase in carbon dioxide production stimulates faster and deeper breathing

* the muscles of the diaphragm and intercostals increase in strength, allowing for greater expansion of the chest cavity

* the capillary network surrounding the alveoli expands, increasing blood flow to the lungs and pulmonary diffusion.

Key concepts

Muscle strength and size increases with high intensity resistance training, while *muscle endurance* increases with repetitive low intensity training.

Muscular system responses to exercise

Muscle tissue response to exercise is dependent on the type of training undertaken and the degree of overload achieved. Muscle strength and size increases with high intensity resistance training, while muscle endurance increases with repetitive low intensity training. In addition, stretching exercises will improve flexibility and the range of motion around joints. Increases in muscle size and bulk, **hypertrophy**, are the result of increases in the volume of contractile proteins within the muscle cells so that they can contract with greater force. In general, males have a greater potential to achieve increases in muscle bulk and size due to higher levels of the hormone testosterone.

Key concept

To achieve a higher level of fitness it is necessary to stress the body systems and place it in a state of *overload*, a point that reaches above and beyond that which is usually achieved.

Ligaments and tendons, the connective tissue structures around the joint, will increase in flexibility and strength with regular exercise. Cartilage also becomes thicker. Bones are strengthened as a result of the stress exercise imposes on them, with greater quantities of calcium and collagen being deposited within them.

Anaerobic training, the capacity to undertake all-out exercise for periods up to around 90 seconds, stimulates the muscles to become better able to tolerate lactic acid, and clear it away more efficiently. With endurance training the capillary network around the muscle extends, allowing greater volumes of blood to reach the muscle to supply oxygen and nutrients. The muscles are able to use more fat as a fuel source, and be more efficient at using oxygen, increasing the body's ability to work harder for longer without fatiguing. The net result is an increase in the body's maximal oxygen consumption.

Exercise also increases the body's metabolic rate, the rate at which it uses up energy. Carbohydrate stored in the muscles as glycogen is the main source of energy for high intensity activities, whilst fat is the main fuel source for activities of low to moderate intensity.

Key concepts

Aerobic: means 'with oxygen'– this relates to energy processes that occur in the presence of oxygen.

Anaerobic: means 'without oxygen'– this relates to energy processes that occur in the absence of oxygen.

Summary

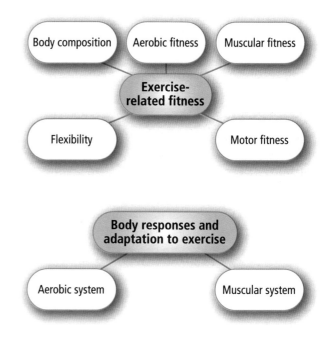

Ian is a 40-year-old white male maintenance worker who was screened at his company's occupational health centre and found to have a high percentage of body fat. The occupational health nurse has told him he needs to lose some weight and begin a programme of exercise. He was a 40-per-day smoker up until three years ago when he quit, but since giving up smoking he has gained weight progressively.

Ian admits to a sedentary lifestyle away from work, preferring to watch sport from the comfort of his armchair. He was a competitive athlete in his early youth, but can't seem to get motivated to do any exercise at present. He has thought about joining his local health club, but is sensitive about his current size and poor level of fitness.

Ian's current measurements:
Height – 1.80 m
Weight – 96 kg

1. What benefits would a regular programme of physical activity or exercise bring for Ian?

2. How long would you expect it to take before Ian would notice any benefits to participation in a regular programme of physical activity or exercise?

3. What do you think would be the most appropriate types of exercise to include in a regular programme of physical activity or exercise at this stage?

4. What field tests of aerobic fitness could you use to assess Ian's level of aerobic fitness before he commences his programme?

5. What strategies could you use to overcome his current barriers to participation in a regular programme of physical activity or exercise and get him motivated to start?

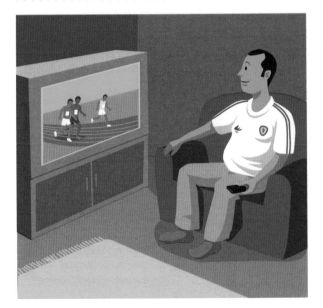

FIGURE 13.4 *Ian has a sedentary lifestyle*

13.2 Physical, social and psychological benefits of regular exercise

Science has confirmed, with overwhelming evidence, that individuals who lead active lives are less likely to die early, or suffer from chronic disease such as coronary heart disease and diabetes.

Physical activity: any activity that increases energy expenditure above resting level. Physical activity undertaken for health benefits would be targeted at avoiding disease and delaying death.

Exercise: physical activity that is structured and undertaken usually for fitness gains. Exercise undertaken for fitness benefits would be targeted at improving one or more components of health-related fitness.

1. Before you read on further in this section of the unit take a few minutes to consider all the benefits a regular programme of physical activity and exercise can bring. Record your thoughts in your notebook for discussion with your tutor.

2. Are you able to group the benefits you have identified into the following categories?

   * physical
   * social
   * psychological
   * economic
   * environmental.

In the 1950s researchers studying workers on London's double-decker buses found that 30 per cent fewer conductors had heart disease compared to their fellow bus drivers. The proposed argument for this was that the conductors were much more active in their job role, moving between the decks to collect fares and issue tickets. In addition to this, American studies in the early 1980s showed that men who expended more than 2000 calories a week by regular walking also had a much lower risk of heart disease. These early studies, and many more since, have demonstrated numerous health benefits of physical activity and exercise. With the boom in the private health and fitness industry it would be easy for people to think that exercising for health and well-being requires a considerable amount of special equipment, clothing and money. However, this is not necessarily the case; there are many types of exercise accessible to those on a limited budget, walking being an excellent example. It is also important to remember that whatever your age, regular exercise offers many health benefits, both short and long term.

The wider benefits of physical activity and exercise for society

Physical activity can benefit not only individuals but the whole of society. Table 13.2 summarises some of the main benefits for society.

SOCIAL	ECONOMIC
* encourages connectedness and social interaction	* reduces health costs
* improves social skills	* creates employment
* reduces isolation	* supports local business
* enhances self-esteem and confidence	* reduces absenteeism
	* enhanced productivity

TABLE 13.2 *The benefits of exercise for society*

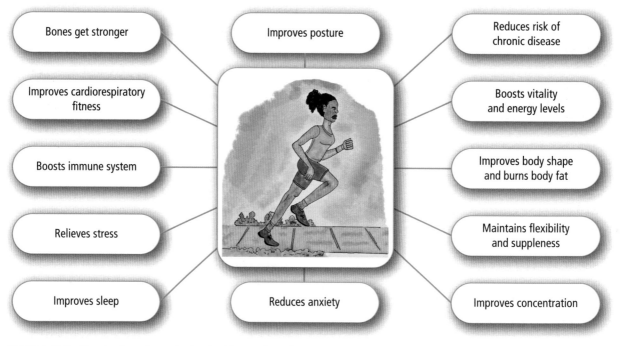

FIGURE 13.5 *Physical and psychological benefits of exercise*

Active transport

Active transport, such as walking and cycling, provides great opportunities for increasing physical activity in the sedentary population, and presents low risks in terms of injury. There is an added environmental benefit for society, since travelling on foot or by bicycle means fewer cars on the road.

Benefits of physical activity and exercise for the individual

As we have seen, an active lifestyle can have social, environmental and economic benefits for society. At an individual level, let's take a closer look at the short- and long-term benefits of exercise in maintaining health and well-being. Some of the main benefits for individuals are that it:

* provides an opportunity for fun and enjoyment

* relaxes and revitalises the body, reducing muscular and mental tension

* boosts self-esteem and confidence

* clears the head and improves concentration

* reduces anxiety and feelings of stress that may be associated with an increased risk of high blood pressure

* lowers the risk of heart disease and stroke.

Exercise not only strengthens the heart muscle, it also reduces some of the 'risk factors' associated with heart disease and stroke, such as high blood pressure and cholesterol, as well as overweight and obesity. Exercise lowers blood pressure and has a favourable effect on blood lipid profiles, improving blood flow. It also lowers body weight and body fat, assisting in the maintenance of optimal body weight and composition. A programme of regular exercise combined with a healthy diet is the best way to lose excess weight, and maintaining a regular programme of exercise provides the best opportunity for maintaining weight loss. Physical activity and exercise facilitates the development and maintenance of muscle mass thereby improving the body's ability to burn calories.

Exercise also:

* lowers the risk of Type 2 diabetes and increases the uptake of glucose in those who are already sufferers, primarily by reducing body fatness

* lowers the risk of certain types of cancer, such as cancer of the breast and colon

* lowers the risk of osteoporosis as regular exercise promotes bone density by the pulling and tugging on the bones by muscles during exercise, stimulating the bone-making cells

* alleviates the symptoms of arthritic pain by keeping joints flexible and maintaining the strength of muscles surrounding joints

* combats ageing by maintaining the effectiveness of body systems, such as the respiratory, circulatory and musculo-skeletal systems. As we age several structural and functional changes occur that result in a decline in 'optimum' physical capacity. Factors such as breathing capacity, heart function and muscular strength are greatly influenced by fitness level, while other age-related changes such as changes in skin, vision and hearing occur irrespective of fitness level

* improved digestion as exercise and activity support the proper functioning of the gut

and reduce the risk of indigestion and constipation

* improved cognitive capabilities, particularly in older adults. Aerobic exercise, such as walking, has been shown to sharpen focus and improve decision making

* promotes the 'feel good factor' by the production of endorphins, chemicals produced in the brain that provide relief from stress and pain.

The role of exercise in weight loss and maintenance

The highly mechanised environment that we live in today has significantly reduced the number of opportunities open to us to incorporate moderate intensity physical activity into our daily living, but exercise has a crucial role to play in weight loss and weight maintenance. Firstly, increased physical activity elevates total daily energy expenditure, helping to maintain a higher energy output. In the case of initiating weight loss, increased physical activity can assist in achieving a negative energy balance. Regular endurance-type exercise improves the ability of our muscles to burn fat as a fuel, while regular resistance-type exercise can help to combat the loss of lean body mass that often occurs as a result of dieting. Gains in lean body mass, contributing to an increase in resting metabolic rate, can further aid weight loss and maintenance by increasing energy requirements even at rest. The best approach is to undertake a combined programme of progressive aerobic and resistance training in which training sessions should aim to expend at least 250 kilocalories. A lifelong commitment to regular exercise is essential to facilitate weight maintenance.

Despite the very strong case presented for keeping active, many individuals find it extremely difficult to incorporate physical activity or structured exercise in to their daily lives. We will explore why this might be in the section on barriers to participation in regular exercise, but before we do, try out the activity outlined below.

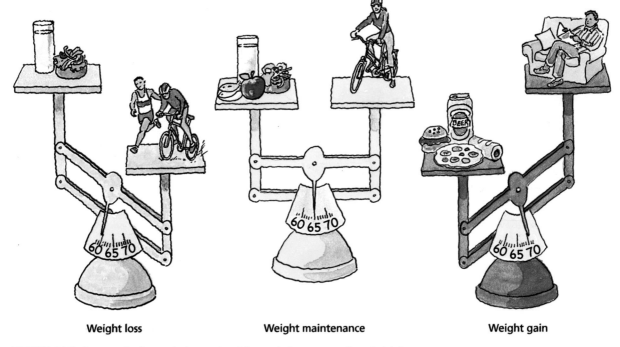

Weight loss   **Weight maintenance**   **Weight gain**

FIGURE 13.6 *Energy balance is important in maintenance of weight loss*

Try it out

Working in small groups, undertake a short survey within your college that aims to establish the level of physical activity and exercise participation of staff and students.

You should:

* consider how you are going to undertake your survey and what information you want to obtain

* assess for knowledge of current physical activity and exercise guidelines aimed at promoting health and well-being

* consider how you are going to collect, analyse and present your data

* disseminate your findings in an appropriate media (poster, flyer, article on college intranet).

Consider this

While low levels of physical activity can afford us some health benefits, moderate to high levels are required to deliver major benefits to our health and well-being. Undertake your own research of scientific journals and key authoritative sources on physical activity participation, such as the American College of Sport Medicine (ACSM) and British Association for Sport and Exercise Sciences (BASES), to investigate the scientific bases for this statement.

Summary

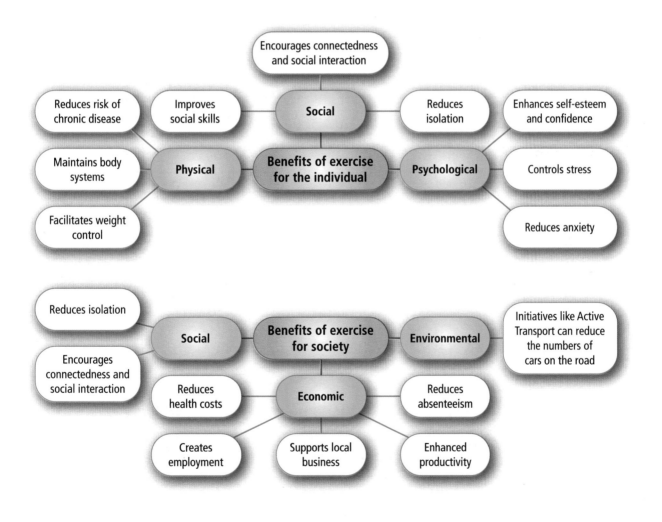

13.3 Standard monitoring methods and tables

Periodic objective evaluation of your fitness is important in maintaining interest and motivation to sustain physical activity or exercise programmes. Monitoring fitness goals and outcomes can provide useful information in the design and progression of physical activity and exercise programmes. Methods of monitoring can be sophisticated and complex, such as the direct measurement of VO_2 max (see page 95), or simple measures of body weight and composition.

Body weight and composition

A variety of methods can be used for assessing weight and body composition. These include:

* height and weight charts
* waist circumference
* body mass index.

Body weight

Height and weight charts

Height and weight charts represent one of the most widely used methods of assessing an individual's body weight and composition, presenting a crude assessment of the individual's weight in relation to his or her height (see Figure 13.7).

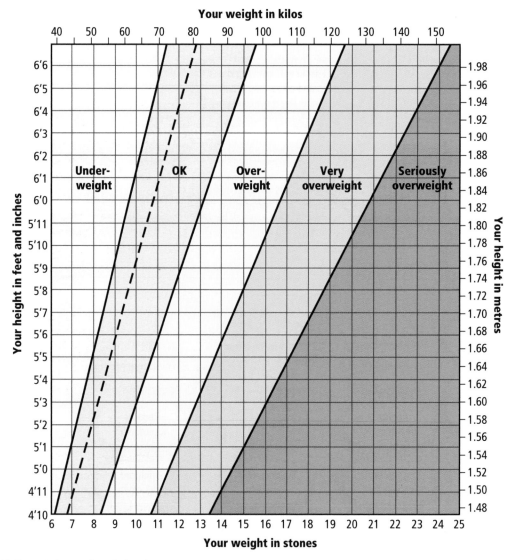

FIGURE 13.7 *Height and weight charts*

These charts suggest acceptable weight ranges for a given height, but do not take in to account body fat or body type. In relation to health, it is actually fat weight, not total body weight, which is more important in determining our health risk. Total body weight alone is of little importance, particularly when working with sports people, but too many people base their weight loss regimes on what they see on the bathroom scales. Although weight is a useful measurement in some respects, body composition has become a more important health indicator. Sportspeople and those actively engaged in fitness regimes are often concerned about their weight, whether for performance or health reasons. Unlike your basic body type, it is possible to alter your body composition, with exercise generally having the effect of increasing lean body mass and decreasing body fat. On the whole, women tend to have a greater percentage of their total body weight as fat. Average figures are around 25 per cent of total body weight as fat for adult women, and about 15 per cent for adult men.

Try it out

To find out if your weight falls within the acceptable range for your height, locate your height on the y-axis of the height and weight chart in Figure 13.5, and move across the row to find your weight until the lines cross. If you fall in the overweight, very overweight or seriously overweight categories you are more likely to suffer health problems.

Body mass index (BMI)

The body mass index is an index of body fatness. BMI is the sum of the ratio of body mass expressed in kilograms to the square of height in metres.

$$BMI = \text{body mass in kg} \div (\text{height in m})^2$$

BMI assumes that there is no single weight for a person of a specific height, but that there is a healthy weight range for any given height. BMI can be used to classify different grades of weight. A ratio between 20 and 24.9 is deemed desirable for both men and women. Values above this level are associated with increased risk of disease. Extremely muscular individuals, such

as sportspeople, particularly those involved in strength sports, may present with values that are high but these will not reflect the same degree of risk as those of a sedentary individual with the same BMI.

BMI classifications
<20	underweight
20–24.9	healthy, desirable weight
25–29.9	overweight
30–40	moderately obese
40+	severely obese

Try it out

Using your weight and height calculate your BMI and determine your BMI classification.

What limitations do you think there might be to using BMI and its classifications?

Waist circumference

More recently this measure of fatness has become a common index for determining health risk, particularly of coronary heart disease (CHD). The theory behind this measure is that a high percentage of body fat, particularly in the abdominal region, is associated with an increase in risk of CHD. A waist circumference of more than 94 cm in men and 80 cm in women is suggestive of central obesity.

Body composition

Our bodies are composed of a perplexing number of cells, tissues, organs and systems but the components of most interest to exercise scientists and nutritionists are muscle, bone and fat. Body composition simply refers to the amount of lean body mass and body fat that makes up our total body weight. Lean body mass includes the bones, muscle, water, connective and organ tissues. Body fat includes both essential and non-essential fat stores. As mentioned above, in relation to health and well-being, it is actually fat weight not total body weight that is more important in determining our health risk. Although weight is useful in some respects, body composition has become a more

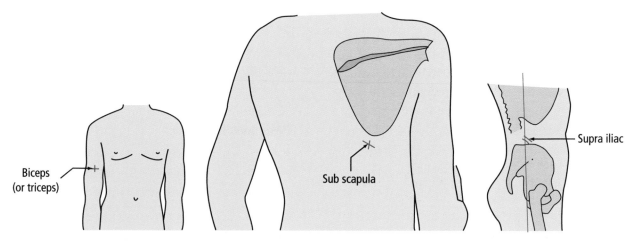

FIGURE 13.8 *Sites for measurement of skinfold thickness*

important health indicator. Methods of assessing body composition include:

* skinfold thickness
* underwater or hydrostatic weighing
* body impedance analysis
* near infrared interactance
* body plethysmography.

Skinfold thickness

With this technique, callipers are used to measure the thickness of skinfolds at various sites, with the biceps, triceps, sub scapula and supra iliac crest being the most common anatomical sites of measurement (see Figure 13.8). The sum of these measurements is then used to calculate the percentage of body fat, using a calculation that takes into account the age and sex of the individual from equations or tables. This is a relatively cheap and convenient method, but does require a high degree of skill. This method is thought to be generally reliable if performed correctly, but has been shown to have an error margin of ± 3–4 per cent and may not be effective for the use on very fat or very thin individuals.

Underwater or hydrostatic weighing

This is considered to be one of the most accurate methods of assessment of body composition. However, it is expensive and time consuming to perform and can be potentially stressful to the individual, requiring total submersion in water. The technique measures body density which can be translated mathematically into percentage body fat, and relies on Archimedes' principle of water displacement to estimate body density. As muscle and bone weigh more in water, an individual with more lean tissue for the same body mass will weigh more in water, while an individual with more fat will weigh less. The first individual will have a higher body density and a lower body fat reading, while the second will have a lower body density and a higher body fat reading. As a technique it is rarely used due to expense.

Did you know?

Archimedes' Principle states that when a body or object is immersed in water it is buoyed up by a force that is equal to the weight or volume of fluid displaced.

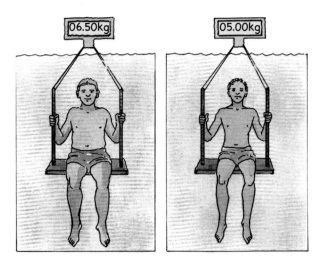

FIGURE 13.9 *Measurement of body composition by hydrostatic weighing*

Body impedance analysis (BIA)

BIA is fast becoming the standard technique for the assessment of body composition, particularly in the health and fitness sector. BIA machines have an advantage over callipers in providing a quick, easy and non-invasive method of estimating percentage body fat, requiring the individual to either fix electrodes to the body, stand on a plate, or grip handles.

BIA measures the resistance to the flow of an electrical current through the body utilising the fact that different body tissues display different impedance to the flow of the current. Tissues that contain a large amount of water, such as lean tissue, provide lower impedance than tissues such as bone and fat.

When using BIA techniques a number of assumptions have to be made, and equations applied, to obtain a body fat percentage figure. One potential drawback to this method is that impedance measurements are related to the water content of tissues. This means that for accurate results, subjects must be fully hydrated and are required to abstain from exercise and substances which exert a diuretic effect, such as alcohol or caffeine, for a period of at least 24 hours prior to the test. Invalid results may also be obtained for women if measured immediately before or during menstruation, when the body water content may be higher than normal.

Many household bathroom scales now use the principle of body impedance, but as with traditional scales daily fluctuations in hydration status can influence the accuracy of body fat readings, so overuse is not recommended.

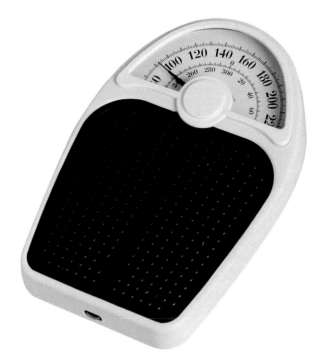

FIGURE 13.11 *Some bathroom scales now use the principle of body impedance*

Near infrared

In this method a wand emitting infrared light is placed against, most commonly, the biceps muscle of the upper arm. The infrared beam contains two specially selected frequencies which interact with chemical bonds found in high concentrations in fatty tissue, but which do not interact with those found in lean tissue. The fattier the tissue the less infrared light is reflected back to the wand. An equation built into the device is then used to calculate percentage body fat taking into account weight, height, gender and exercise frequency, intensity and time.

Body plethysmography

This is a relatively new and expensive method of assessing body composition that applies the gas law to determine body volume. It requires the individual to sit in a structure resembling a pod, hence the name 'Bod Pod', which comprises two chambers, both of a known volume. Changes in pressure between the two chambers are recorded and various equations are applied to compute percent body fat.

All of the methods outlined here have some merits in measuring changes in body composition over time rather than absolute values. When attempting to assess body composition a number of steps can be taken to minimise potential errors

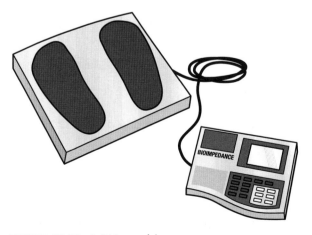

FIGURE 13.10 *A BIA machine*

in measuring changes in body composition over time:

* always use the same method
* ensure the subject is always assessed by the same person
* ensure repeat measurements are always taken at the same time of day.

Lung function

Your respiratory rate refers to the amount of air breathed in one minute. For a typical 18-year-old this represents about 12 breaths per minute at rest, during which time about 6 litres of air will pass through the lungs. Respiratory rate can increase significantly during exercise by as much as 30–40 breaths per minute.

Tidal volume is the term used to represent the amount of air you breathe in and out with each breath, and on average tidal volume at rest represents about 0.5 litres of air. During exercise our tidal volume increases to allow more air to pass through the lungs. The volume of air passing through the lungs each minute is known as the minute volume and is calculated by multiplying your breathing rate by the amount of air taken in with each breath. When we exercise, our breathing rate increases in order to take in more oxygen and expel greater levels of carbon dioxide.

Key concept

Minute volume = Tidal volume x Respiratory rate

Your total lung capacity after you have inhaled as deeply and as maximally as you can is normally around 5 litres of air. Your lungs are never fully emptied of air; otherwise they would collapse. The air that remains in the lungs is referred to as the residual volume and is the amount of air

remaining in the lungs after you have breathed out as hard as you can. This usually represents around 1–1.5 litres of air. Residual volume decreases in response to increased fitness through training.

The maximum amount of air that can be exhaled when you breathe out as hard and as deeply as you can is referred to as your vital capacity. This usually represents around 4.5–5 litres of air. Vital capacity increases in response to physical training to provide an increased and more efficient supply of oxygen to our working muscles. During strenuous exercise oxygen diffusion may increase by as much as threefold above the resting level.

When it comes to sport and exercise it appears that the efficiency of the exchange of oxygen and carbon dioxide between the lungs and the blood, and between the blood and muscle fibres, is more important in determining performance than the total lung volume.

Lung function can be measured using a technique known as spirometry. This measures how efficiently the lungs work and determines how much air the lungs can hold and how efficiently they transfer oxygen in the blood. For this test you need to breathe into a mouthpiece attached to a recording device, where the information collected is printed out on to a chart known as a spirogram.

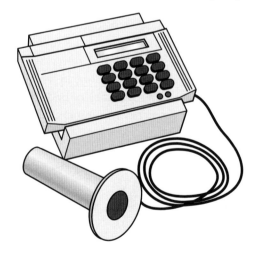

FIGURE 13.12 *Measurement of lung function by spirometry*

A more common measure of lung function is the measurement of peak flow. This is a simple measurement of how much air can be pushed out of the lungs in one fast blast using a portable, inexpensive hand-held meter.

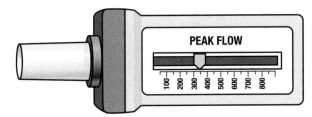

FIGURE 13.13 *Peak-flow meter*

When measuring peak flow it is important to use the correct procedures:

* attach a mouthpiece to the meter and make sure it is set to zero

* if possible, the individual should stand

* the individual takes a deep breath and places his or her lips tightly around the mouthpiece

* the individual breathes out as hard and as long as he or she can

* the process is repeated a maximum of three times taking the highest value attained.

Peak flow scores are dependent on age, height and sex, for example, a young boy who is 1.50 m tall should have a peak flow of approximately 350 litres per minute, while a 50-year-old who is 1.75 m should have a peak flow of approximately 600 litres per minute. Scores should always be evaluated in line with previous test scores.

Try it out

Using your own research, what peak flow test scores would you expect for a healthy adult female aged 35 years and 1.70 m tall?

How might you expect this score to differ if she was an asthma sufferer (see Unit 19 for more details on lung function)?

Monitoring exercise intensity

The best way to monitor intensity during exercise is to use a combination of heart rate measures and ratings of perceived exertion, or RPE. Heart rates can be taken manually, or by wearing a heart rate monitor. RPE is a ten-point scale that focuses on tuning body function into physical cues for recognising intensity of effort, such as a quickened breathing rate, breathlessness or flat out effort. The RPE scale provides a way of quantifying subjective exercise intensity, but has been shown to correlate well with heart rate and oxygen uptake.

Modified rate of perceived exertion (RPE) chart

0	Nothing at all
1	Very weak
2	Weak
3	Moderate
4	Somewhat hard
5	Hard
6	Moderately hard
7	Very hard
8	Very, very hard
9	Near maximal
10	Extremely hard or maximal

Did you know?

Borg's original RPE scale was a scale from 6–20, with 6 representing complete rest and 20 exhaustion. The reason for this odd numbering is reflected in the individuals he used in his original exertion studies. These were all fit and had heart rates that corresponded to around 60 bpm at rest and a maximum heart rate of 200 bpm.

Pulse taking

Coinciding with every heartbeat, a pulse can be felt wherever an artery can be compressed gently against a bone. It is possible to feel this movement of the blood through the arteries by placing two or three fingers over the artery. Common sites for measurement of the pulse are the wrist (radial artery), the neck (carotid artery) or the elbow (brachial artery). Counting the 'pulse' of the blood at these points is a simple method that is often used to estimate heart rate. It can provide a useful estimate for training purposes, but it is important to note that the true maximum heart rate can vary by plus or minus 15 beats per minute. The average range of pulse in healthy adults is between 60–80 beats per minute. Increases in temperature, exercise and intense emotion can all raise pulse rate.

Record your pulse at various points throughout the day and produce a chart or table showing how your pulse responds to different activities and situations including:

✴ on waking

✴ after eating and drinking

✴ after walking to college

✴ during participation in sport and exercise

✴ after sport and exercise

✴ sitting watching television

✴ after a bath or shower.

Record your pulse rate for 60 seconds to give beats per minute.

What have you observed?

Using a heart rate monitor

The use of heart rate monitors provides immediate and potentially more accurate measures of heart rate before, during and after exercise and is less time consuming than manual measures. If working accurately, heart rate monitors transmit the electrical activity of the heart through an electrode harness or strap worn around the chest. This sends information about the heart's electrical activity to a watch-like receiver worn on the wrist that calculates heart rate. Erroneous readings can occur, so it is a good idea to use heart rate monitors alongside RPE.

The best way to monitor intensity during exercise is to use a combination of heart rate measures and ratings of perceived exertion or RPE.

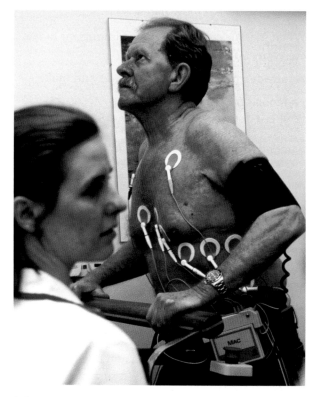

FIGURE 13.14 *Monitoring heart rate during exercise*

Summary

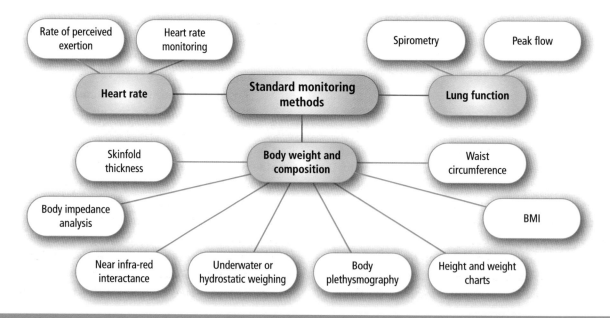

- Rate of perceived exertion
- Heart rate monitoring
- **Heart rate**
- **Standard monitoring methods**
- Spirometry
- Peak flow
- **Lung function**
- Skinfold thickness
- **Body weight and composition**
- Waist circumference
- Body impedance analysis
- BMI
- Near infra-red interactance
- Underwater or hydrostatic weighing
- Body plethysmography
- Height and weight charts

Let's take another look at Ian, the 40-year-old white male maintenance worker who was screened at his company's occupational health centre and found to have a high percentage of body fat. Reread the information about him on page 101 to remind yourself.

Ian's current measurements:
Height – 1.80 m
Weight – 96 kg

You were asked to consider the benefits of a regular programme of physical activity and exercise for Ian and the most appropriate types of exercise and activity to include as he embarks on a new path to improved health and wellness.

Now consider:

1. What assessment do you make of Ian's current weight for height?

2. Calculate his BMI and consider the score in line with your assessment of his weight for height.

3. What might be the most appropriate measure of body composition to use with Ian?

4. Bearing in mind Ian's lifestyle history, other than weight and body composition, what might you want to assess?

5. As he embarks on his programme of increased physical activity and exercise, consider how you are going to monitor Ian's progress.

13.4 Safety in physical activity

For many individuals, the mere notion of physical activity or exercise conjures up unpleasant thoughts or images of boring exercise classes or programmes, or rough competitive sports where the risk of injury would be a real turn-off. Equally, the risks associated with participation in a regular programme of physical activity or exercise are commonly less than the risks associated with that of living a sedentary lifestyle, but the potential benefits of exercise must outweigh the potential risks to the participant. Those who have never exercised before, or are in poor shape, should not expect to see immediate results. Achieving physical fitness requires time and consistency.

Risks: those associated with participation in a regular programme of physical activity or exercise are commonly less than the risks associated with that of living a sedentary lifestyle.

Health and lifestyle screening

It is very important to assess health status before starting a physical activity or exercise programme. An objective evaluation of current health status will give information on the participant's fitness, strengths and weaknesses, providing the basis for establishing realistic fitness goals and avoiding injury. In addition to health and lifestyle screening, testing initial fitness levels provides a useful benchmark to measure progress against, with periodic fitness testing providing the potential for motivating feedback as the exercise programme progresses.

It is essential that health and lifestyle screening occurs before fitness testing and exercise prescription, preferably by a medical or fitness practitioner, with all who are contemplating starting an exercise programme. Health and lifestyle screening is usually carried out in the form of an interview or questionnaire. Comprehensive lifestyle and pre-exercise screening will help to identify any medical conditions that may prevent the participant from exercising safely. It will also highlight the participant's objectives and ensure that the exercise prescription fulfils their needs.

Pre-exercise health screening questionnaires can be self- or practitioner-administered, such as the Canadian PAR-Q (Physical Activity Readiness Questionnaire), which is available from the Canadian Society for Exercise Physiology (www.csep.ca). This questionnaire is designed for use by individuals between the ages of 15 and 69, and aims to identify the small number of individuals for whom physical activity might be inappropriate, or those that would require medical advice before embarking on a programme or supervision during physical activity or exercise participation.

For some, pre-exercise screening may involve a complete medical examination by a medical practitioner. The choice of method will depend on a number of factors, such as age and health status, previous training history and resources.

Fitness testing

This is used to measure and evaluate components of fitness, such as aerobic fitness, strength, or body composition; it can be a useful addition to the health and lifestyle screening process in identifying individual fitness, strengths and weaknesses.

IMPORTANT
When in any doubt about an individual's suitability or readiness to exercise, make sure they consult their doctor.

It is important that any information obtained from health and lifestyle screening is stored in a secure place for reasons of confidentiality, and that the information is only accessed by authorised personnel. A good health, lifestyle and fitness screening protocol includes:

* participant's past and current medical history
* family medical history
* recording blood pressure
* measuring body composition
* measuring current fitness status
* considering participants' fitness goals.

Once readiness to participate is assessed and evaluated, consideration can be given to the exercise prescription. Whatever the exercise prescription, some basic rules apply to maintaining safety and reducing the risk of injury. These are outlined in the following basic structure of an exercise programme.

The basic structure of an exercise programme

All fitness programmes should follow this structure.

Warm-up
Activities to mobilise the joints, gradually raise the pulse and slowly stretch the muscles to be used in the activity.

Main activity
This is sometimes referred to as the conditioning phase. Exercises to emphasise the components of fitness should be specific to the training requirements of the individual or group.These activities will usually promote aerobic fitness, muscular strength and endurance and flexibility.

Warm-down
Warm-down activities to decrease the pulse rate and stretch muscles.

The warm-up

This should be included at the beginning of **all** exercise programmes to achieve the following objectives:

* prepare the body for exercise
* maximise performance
* prevent injury.

Physiological changes occur in the body during the warm up. These include:

* increase in body temperature
* increase in gaseous exchange from the blood to the tissues
* dilation of blood vessels as blood flow increases
* redistribution of blood from relatively inactive tissues, such as the digestive system and kidneys, to the working muscles
* increase in heart rate and stroke volume
* increase in respiration and metabolic rate
* increase in supply of synovial fluid to the joints
* increase in muscle temperature and greater pliability of muscle fibres, ligaments, tendons and connective tissue.

If the exercises undertaken during the warm-up are related to the main component or activity of the exercise programme to follow, the individual or group will have the opportunity to rehearse the relevant movements, and incorporate neuromuscular response patterns, leading to better co-ordination.

Key concepts

Cardiac output and stroke volume: the rate at which blood leaves the heart is referred to as *cardiac output.* This is the amount of blood the heart pumps in one minute. Cardiac output is the sum of the *heart rate* (the number of times the heart beats in each minute) multiplied by the *stroke volume* (the volume of blood that leaves the heart with each beat).

Heart rates are dependent on age, with children having relatively higher rates than adults. When the body is in action cardiac output can increase five to seven times in order to accelerate the delivery of blood to exercising muscles, and to meet their demand for increased oxygen.

During participation in sport and exercise, cardiac output will be increased as a result of increases in either heart rate, stroke volume or both. Stroke volume does not increase significantly beyond the light work rates of low intensity exercise, therefore the increases in cardiac output required for moderate- to high-intensity work rates are achieved by increases in heart rate. Maximal attainable cardiac output decreases with increasing age, largely as a result of a decrease in maximum heart rate. A warm-up should always include:

* exercises to gradually elevate the heart rate and body temperature
* mobilising exercises incorporating gentle rhythmical movements to promote the production of synovial fluid
* stretches of an easy static nature based around the muscle groups to be used in the main component or activity
* activities to re-warm the body to bring the heart rate up to the work out level.

The stretching of the appropriate muscle groups should only be undertaken when the body temperature has been raised and the joints taken through their full range of movement.

Guidelines for warming-up

* intensity should be low, raising the heart rate to 50–65 per cent of maximum heart rate (MHR)
* progressive movements, starting with the basic move and building up to more demanding movements, should be used
* movements should be rhythmic and continuous, involving the large muscle groups
* the exercises chosen should be appropriate to the level of fitness of the individual or group.

There are no set guidelines for the length of a warm-up. However, timings should take into account the fitness level of the individual or group participating in the exercise session. Beginners require a longer warm-up period to gradually lead them into the more strenuous component of the exercise programme. The temperature of the environment in which the exercise takes place is also an important factor. Colder conditions require a longer warm up period.

> **IMPORTANT**
> Failure to warm-up properly can result in injury and sub-maximal performance during exercise.

The warm-down

This should be included at the end of **all** exercise programmes to achieve the following objectives:

* return the body to the pre-exercise state
* relax the body and reduce tension
* re-align muscle fibres and prevent muscle soreness injury
* promote circulation and motor fitness.

A warm-down should always include:

* activities to gradually lower the heart rate
* stretches to promote flexibility and mobility.

By the controlled lowering of the exercise intensity the circulatory system:

* maintains adequate venous return and cardiac output, thus avoiding blood pooling, preventing dizziness and fainting
* assists in the removal of lactic acid and other by-products from the muscles, which might otherwise cause stiffness and soreness
* reduces tension and promotes flexibility.

Guidelines for warming-down

* the choice of exercises will be determined by the preceding activities and the fitness level of the individual or group
* activities chosen should be mild and rhythmic, gradually decreasing in intensity of effort enabling the heart rate to be lowered towards resting levels
* encourage participants to replace clothing to retain body heat.

There are no clear guidelines on the duration of the warm-down, however similar considerations as to the length of the warm-up should be applied in respect of the individual and the environment.

> **IMPORTANT**
> Exercisers are advised not to take hot showers, baths or saunas immediately after exercise, due to the effects of vasodilation (dilation of the veins). This can lead to hypotension (low blood pressure), irregular heart beat, dizziness and fainting. The use of saunas can also lead to dehydration as a result of increased fluid losses from the body.
>
> If participants feel dizziness, any pain or shortness of breath, or excessive fatigue during exercise they should cease the activity immediately and seek the advice of their doctor before exercising again.

General health and safety guidelines for exercise participation

Beyond the structure of the exercise session or programme, whatever the exercise there are certain health and safety issues that should always be considered.

* Clothing and footwear should be appropriate for the specific activity or exercise to be undertaken. This will minimise the risk of injury or illness, help the participant perform better and facilitate the enjoyment of the activity or exercise.

* Adequate hydration should be maintained by drinking plenty of fluids before, during and after the activity or exercise. Exact amounts will depend on factors such as the length of the activity or exercise, temperature and humidity.

* Interactions between medication and exercise should be monitored carefully, such as medications to control diabetes.

* If the exercise requires the use of equipment this should only be used in the appropriate manner for which it was designed and be well maintained.

In order to maximise efficiency, maintain comfort and reduce the risk of injury it is essential that the participant invests in the correct equipment and clothing for their chosen activity. Some activities will require minimal equipment, whilst others much more specialised elements. Complete Table 13.3 by identifying the most essential elements of equipment and clothing required to ensure the above can occur. The first column has been completed for you.

Monitoring fitness progress

Monitoring progress in attaining and maintaining physical fitness is a vital factor in providing motivation to maintain an exercise regime. Progress can be monitored by keeping training logs or diaries which record, for example, the distance walked or run, or the amount of weight lifted. Another means of monitoring fitness progress is by fitness testing. Fitness testing can provide very strong positive feedback when fitness levels are improving, but may be demotivating when they are not.

IMPORTANT

When using monitoring equipment during the screening process, or during periodic fitness testing throughout an exercise programme, it is very important to understand how the monitoring equipment works and ensure it is always used according to the instructions.

What do you think are the key factors in terms of maintaining client safety in adopting any of the monitoring equipment and techniques identified in this section of the unit? (See Unit 19 for more information on this subject.)

Good practice guide to physical activity safety

* have a plan
* get a fitness check up
* attain and monitor fitness goals
* start and progress slowly
* warm-up and warm-down.

Things to avoid during exercise

* performing exercises too fast and without control
* too many repetitions
* jerky, bouncy movements
* forcing a movement
* over-exertion if overweight, unfit, have high blood pressure or heart trouble
* weight-bearing exercises if joints are stiff or damaged.

WALKING	RUNNING	GYM TRAINING	RACQUET SPORTS	A SPORT OF YOUR CHOICE
* A sturdy pair of walking shoes * Any loose comfortable clothing * Reflective clothing if walking at night				

TABLE 13.3 *Essential equipment and clothing for exercise*

Summary

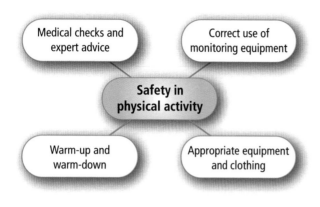

Safety in physical activity

- Medical checks and expert advice
- Correct use of monitoring equipment
- Warm-up and warm-down
- Appropriate equipment and clothing

13.5 Barriers to participation in regular exercise

As mentioned previously, poor health is a serious drain on national resources and increases expenditure on health care by the government. As individuals we may encounter many difficulties in attaining wellness. Our age, ethnicity and socio-economic status may present challenges to achieving wellness. Beyond these factors there may be many more barriers to adopting a regular exercise programme:

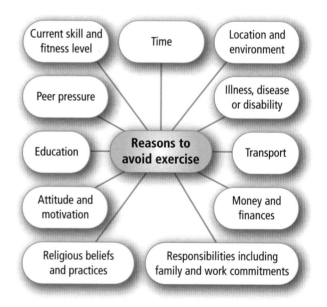

Reasons to avoid exercise

- Current skill and fitness level
- Time
- Location and environment
- Peer pressure
- Illness, disease or disability
- Education
- Transport
- Attitude and motivation
- Money and finances
- Religious beliefs and practices
- Responsibilities including family and work commitments

FIGURE 13.15 *There are many reasons that may stop or prevent us from exercising*

Overcoming barriers

Location and environment

The easier it is to get to a sporting facility, or the safer the streets are to walk or run in, the easier it may be to take exercise. Think about how you could adapt your exercise plans to suit your location. For example:

* if you live near the sea or a lake you might take up rowing or windsurfing

* if your neighbourhood has a high crime rate you may not want to walk or run in the streets, but you could exercise indoors, or cycle, drive or take public transport to a sports centre.

Education

If your school has a strong tradition of sport and exercise, and you enjoy these at school, you are more likely to continue participation later in life. If, through education, you become aware of the benefits of regular participation to health and well-being you are also more likely to remain physically active. If your education has not introduced you to exercise in an enjoyable way, it is not too late to learn to exercise as an adult. There are many sports classes and social activities which can introduce young people and adults to sporting activities, or you could take up a simple form of exercise which doesn't need to be taught formally, such as walking, running or cycling.

Work and family commitments

Responsibilities including work and family commitments can make you feel that you have no time to exercise. There are various ways of making time for exercise, even in a crowded schedule, for example, swimming or walking in your lunch hour or before work; getting help with childcare to allow attendance at an exercise class; cycling or walking to work instead of driving, etc.

Cost

Some activities such as playing golf or joining a gym can be quite expensive, but not all activities require hefty budgets to support them, for example walking or running.

Skill and fitness level

Obviously some activities require higher degrees of skill and fitness, such as gymnastics and many athletic events, but again walking or running require limited levels of skill and can be undertaken almost anywhere that is safe.

Try it out

Take a closer look at the barriers previously identified and consider any additional ways that they might be overcome in order to promote physical activity and exercise participation.

What about other barriers such as:

* peer pressure, where friends put on pressure to take part in activities that don't involve exercise

* finances, where a person may feel they don't have enough money to take part in exercise

* transport, where a person does not have access to a car and would find it difficult to reach the sports centre by public transport

* motivation, where a person may feel that he or she has never enjoyed sports and therefore doesn't feel positive about exercise.

How might these be overcome in order to promote physical activity and exercise participation?

The role of local and national government in exercise promotion

The promotion and maintenance of physical activity and exercise requires intensive efforts from several agencies to support individuals to reduce sedentary behaviours and become more active more often, and to promote the environment necessary to encourage people to become more active. This requires co-operative working by national, regional and local governments in the consideration of healthy transport, schools and work places that promote activities such as walking, cycling and other active leisure pursuits, but at the same time the individual must take responsibility for assessing their physical activity patterns.

Keeping the exercise habit

The following are useful tips to assist people to start and stick to an exercise programme:

* choose an activity you like
* find a partner
* vary your routine and activities
* make it fun
* keep a diary.

Summary

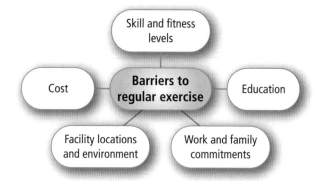

Consider this

Pamela's current measurements:

Age	–	37 years
Height	–	1.63 m
Weight	–	130.0 kg

Weight history
Pamela was moderately overweight as a child. Her weight has steadily increased over the last ten years, with her lowest adult weight being 74.0 kg. Over the years she has generally been concerned about the weight around her thighs, but recent weight gain appears to be on the upper body, particularly around her waist.

Occupation
She is an account manager who has worked in sales for 12 years, working her way up to her current position. She is considering working freelance due to the high levels of stress associated with her current position.

Social history
She lives with her partner who is also overweight. She has no children and enjoys eating out, fine wines and foreign holidays.

Personal medical history
She suffers from low back pain which impacts on her ability to be physically active.

Family medical history
She has a family history of heart disease.

Relevant measurements
Resting heart rate: 90–96 bpm.

These measurements were obtained from a recent fitness test undertaken at a private sector Health & Fitness Club which she joined about a month ago but has found little time to attend since.

Physical activity and exercise
As mentioned above, Pamela has recently joined a local health and fitness club that has extensive and excellent facilities but she has found little time to attend since joining. In addition, she is concerned about her appearance and does not feel confident in the exercise environment. In the past she did enjoy going for the occasional swim at the ladies only sessions at the local swimming pool.

1. How would you summarise Pamela's lifestyle and exercise habits?

2. What potential barriers do you think there are to Pamela engaging in a regular programme of physical activity and exercise?

3. How might she overcome some of these barriers?

4. What physical activity and exercise recommendations would you make?

5. Are there any safety aspects that require consideration in this case?

13.6 Exercise and disease prevention

The diseases that can be prevented or treated by physical activity and exercise participation can be thought of as chronic or persistent. Physical activity must be consistent if it is to have optimal benefits for the management and treatment of these diseases.

Did you know?

The World Health Organisation (WHO) has reported that physical inactivity is one of the ten leading causes of death in the developed world.

Try it out

Visit the Department of Health website (www.dh.gov.uk) to view the Chief Medical Officer's Report on *At least 5 a week: evidence on the impact of physical activity and its relationship to health* (2004). This report sets out the latest research evidence on the benefits of exercise and physical activity for health and here you will find more supporting evidence for the role of physical activity and exercise in the prevention and management of disease.

You could also take a look at the *National Service Frameworks for Coronary Heart Disease, Diabetes, Mental Health and Older People* available from the Department of Health website (www.dh.gov.uk). These frameworks set out long-term strategies for improving prevention and treatment, and identify the role that increased participation in physical activity can play in improving the health of the nation.

Obesity

Obesity is now clearly recognised as a disease in its own right, one which is now thought to be largely preventable through lifestyle changes, particularly to diet and activity patterns. In spite of high levels of dieting among particular groups of the population, obesity continues to be a growing problem and is increasingly becoming a major public health concern. Undeniable evidence suggests that fitness and fatness can have a profound effect on our health, but the fitness and nutrition boom of the 1980s in response to the emergence of healthy eating principles appears to have had little impact on the increasing rates of overweight and obesity that now face our nation, with 25 per cent of the adult population predicted to be obese by the year 2010.

Levels of physical inactivity in the UK are a significant factor in the dramatic rise in the prevalence of overweight and obesity. Regular exercise is considered to be key in weight management. Maintaining activity throughout life is important in avoiding weight gain. Participation in regular exercise expends calories, but it has also been shown to assist in appetite control. A combination of physical activity and dietary adjustments can maximise fat loss, preserve lean body mass and optimise health benefits.

Coronary heart disease

Coronary heart disease (CHD) is a major cause of death and ill-health. Rates in the UK are amongst the highest in the developed world. There is no single cause of coronary heart disease. It is considered a multi-factorial condition. However, the underlying condition of atherosclerosis is a degenerative condition of the arteries characterised by the deposit of fatty substances on the lining of the artery walls. Over time these fatty deposits build up and impair the flow of blood. If a narrowed artery supplying blood to the heart becomes blocked this results in a heart attack (myocardial infarction).

A number of risk factors increase the likelihood of developing CHD. Blood cholesterol level is an important risk factor, but so are other factors such as obesity, smoking, physical inactivity and high blood pressure. The major risk factors cited for the development of coronary heart disease are listed below:

* raised blood cholesterol

* raised blood pressure

* cigarette smoking

* inactivity

* obesity
* diabetes
* age
* gender
* family history
* previous heart attack.

> **Did you know?**
>
> Your risk of CHD increases with age and males are at greater risk. However, post menopause the risk equals out for males and females.

Physical inactivity and low fitness levels are considered to be independent risk factors for heart disease in both men and women. Unfit, inactive individuals have almost double the risk of dying from coronary heart disease. Physical activity also has a positive effect on other cardiovascular risk factors, such as high blood pressure and high cholesterol.

> **Did you know?**
>
> Inactive people have nearly double the risk of dying from heart disease than people that are active.

Exercise and hypertension

A regular programme of physical activity and exercise has been shown to be effective in reducing the risk of hypertension. The current guidelines for exercise prescription for the hypertensive are low to moderate intensity, with endurance activities forming the core of the programme such as walking, cycling or swimming, carried out at least three times a week. Prior to starting a new exercise programme, individuals with known hypertension should be cleared for participation by a medical practitioner.

Stroke

Stroke is a form of cardiovascular disease that affects the brain. A stroke occurs when blood supply to the brain is limited for any prolonged period of time, which results in the death of brain cells. The part of the brain affected and the number of brain cells damaged will determine the severity of a stroke. Minor strokes may result in loss of memory, disturbed vision or problems with speech, whilst severe strokes can result in major paralysis and death. The benefits afforded by physical activity in respect of decreased risk of stroke appear to be associated with activity and exercise of moderate to high intensity.

> **Did you know?**
>
> Highly active individuals appear to have a 25 per cent lower risk of stroke than inactive individuals.

Diabetes

Diabetes is a common **endocrine** disorder that currently affects over a million people in the UK. It is a condition that results from either a complete lack of insulin, produced by the pancreas, or a reduction in insulin production which the body is unable to use effectively to control blood sugar levels. Normally the uptake of glucose by the cells is controlled by insulin. When there is a lack of insulin, glucose cannot enter the cells to be used for energy. This leads to raised blood glucose levels, which gives rise to the common symptoms often observed before diabetes is diagnosed, such as increased thirst, the passing of large volumes of urine, weight loss, tiredness and blurred vision.

Types of diabetes

There are different types of diabetes, Type 1 and Type 2. With Type 1 diabetes, until recently referred to as insulin-dependent diabetes, the pancreas stops producing insulin completely. This type of diabetes usually occurs before the age of 40–45 years and is treated by insulin injections and diet. Type 2 diabetes develops when the pancreas produces some, but not enough, insulin to meet the body's requirements. This type usually occurs over the age of 40 years, although with increasing levels of overweight and obesity is now seen in individuals below this age. It is treated by diet alone or by diet and tablets, and in some cases insulin injections may also be required to stabilise blood glucose control. This type of diabetes is commonly associated with obesity, which causes insulin resistance. Insulin resistance may also occur during pregnancy, leading to the condition known as gestational diabetes.

Diabetes contributes to an increased risk of other diseases such as heart disease, kidney disease and stroke, and also increased risk of infections. Contrary to popular opinion, excess sugar in the diet is in itself not thought to lead to diabetes – unless it is associated with obesity as a result of excess calorie intake. Increased levels of physical activity and the achievement and maintenance of a healthy body weight have a critical role to play in both the prevention and treatment of diabetes, particularly Type 2 diabetes.

Physical inactivity can be a major risk factor in the development of Type 2 diabetes, with the active population having a reduced risk of up to 50 per cent compared to the inactive population. Type 2 diabetes is common in inactive and obese people. The preventative effect of physical activity is particularly strong for those at most risk, such as those with a strong family history or previous gestational diabetes. In those that are already diabetic, significant improvements in blood glucose control can occur with programmes of either aerobic or resistance training carried out three times per week, which appear to reduce their risk of mortality.

For those with Type 1 diabetes, a regular programme of physical activity and exercise can help maintain good blood glucose control by making insulin work more efficiently, and may reduce the risk of other chronic diseases, such as heart disease and cancer.

> **Key concept**
>
> Diabetic sportspeople who exercise regularly may need to consume greater quantities of healthy complex carbohydrate. In addition to careful control of total calorie and carbohydrate intakes the timing and regularity of meals and snacks is important to ensure that low blood sugar levels (hypoglycaemia) is avoided.

Cancer

Physical activity appears to be associated with a decrease in overall risk of cancer, but particularly cancer of the colon, and breast cancer after the menopause in women. To gain optimum benefits in terms of cancer protection, lifetime physical activity participation is required, but generally it is thought that the higher the level of physical activity participation the lower the overall risk. The mechanisms by which physical activity and exercise exert their effect in terms of cancer prevention are not fully understood, but it is proposed that physical activity may modify metabolic hormones and growth factors as well as regulating energy balance and fat distribution. Another theory is that physical activity speeds up the transit of food through the gut, reducing the time the intestinal tract is exposed to cancer-causing agents, but as yet there is insufficient scientific data to support these claims.

Osteoporosis

Osteoporosis, often considered a silent disease because it does not display any symptoms, is a degenerative bone disease characterised by thinning of the bones. With osteoporosis the bones become brittle and more prone to fractures. The most common sites for fracture are the hip, spine and wrist.

> **Key concept**
>
> 'Physical activity can increase bone mineral density in adolescents, maintain it in young adults, and slow its decline in old age'.
> (Chief Medical Officer's Report 2004)

Regular exercise can help to prevent osteoporosis. Like the heart and muscles, our bones can suffer if they are not exercised regularly. For optimum protection, regular weight-bearing exercise must exert a loading effect and stress the bone; such activities include jumping, skipping or jogging. Other healthy lifestyle habits to support the development and maintenance of healthy bones include:

* eating a well balanced and varied diet rich in calcium
* not smoking
* drinking alcohol and caffeine in moderation.

Mental illness and health

Mental health problems are increasingly prevalent, with anxiety and depression forming the most common causes of mental ill health in the UK. Physical activity can have a role to play in both the prevention and treatment of mental health disorders. Physical activity enhances mood, reduces anxiety and raises self-esteem and confidence. This is a growing area of scientific research, but surveys suggest that physically active individuals feel happier with life; even single bouts of activity can improve mood and energy.

Exercise and stress

Stress can be considered a physiological and mental response to things in our environment that make us feel uncomfortable. Chronic stress is thought to lower our resistance to disease and increase our risk of emotional disorders. Although high-intensity prolonged exercise can be seen to impose physical and mental stress on the body, there is evidence to suggest that low- to moderate-intensity exercise can reduce some types of stress. Those activities proposed to have a beneficial effect include aerobic activities, such as walking, swimming and cycling, but other activities focused on relaxation such as tai-chi, pilates and yoga are also beneficial.

Try it out

Active individuals report fewer symptoms of anxiety or emotional distress.

Undertake your own research, using the Internet and scientific journals, into the role of exercise in the management of stress. One of the factors you might want to look at is the effect of stress and exercise on immune function.

Try it out

Visit the NHS Direct website (www.nhsdirect. nhs.uk) to check out the advice offered on using exercise to manage the conditions identified in this section of the unit.

Summary

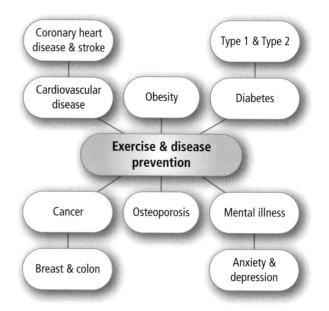

Jayne's current measurements:

Age – 40 years
Height – 1.67 m
Weight – 89.0 kg

Jayne was never overweight as a child and has had a lowest adult weight of 69.0 kg. She recently became more concerned about her weight when she was fitted for a new business suit and realised her waist size had gone up to 36 inches.

She is a managing director of a company. She is frequently required to attend lunch time meetings with clients. She smokes 20 cigarettes a day and wants to give up, but feels this will be difficult due to her work-related stress.

She lives with her partner and her eight-year-old son. She had no cause to consult the doctor until recently when she started to complain of increased back pain. The doctor noted that her blood pressure was slightly raised. She has a family history of heart disease. Her father died from a heart attack at an early age.

She does not participate in any formal exercise at present. She does, however, have a swimming pool and gym equipped with a treadmill, free weights and equipment to target the stomach at home. After visiting the doctor, who has cleared her to begin exercise participation, she is considering aiming for three one-hour exercise sessions per week.

1. What benefits would a regular programme of physical activity or exercise bring for Jayne?

2. How long would you expect it to take before Jayne would notice any benefits from participation in a regular programme of physical activity or exercise?

3. How suitable do you think her current exercise goals are?

4. How would you monitor her progress?

5. Are there any forms of exercise that would not be appropriate for Jayne at this time?

13.7 Exercise programmes for different clients

Basic principles of exercise prescription

The preparation and construction of an effective exercise programme should be based on the way the body adapts to different training regimes. Exercise programmes can develop one or many aspects of fitness, for example strength, aerobic endurance and flexibility. The following factors should be carefully considered in the construction of any physical activity or exercise programme:

* individuality

* specificity

* reversibility

* **overload.**

Individuality

Genetics plays a large part in determining how quickly and to what degree an individual will adapt to a specific exercise regime. Two individuals are unlikely to show the same rate and magnitude of adaptation in response to the same training programme. As a result, the principle of individual differences must be taken into account when designing exercise programmes and monitoring progress. The programme must not be too easy or too hard and must encourage the individual to stay with the programme.

Specificity

Adaptations to training are highly specific to the type of activity undertaken and the intensity to which it is performed. Specificity relates both to the muscle groups involved and to the energy sources utilised. Training for one sort of activity does not lead to fitness for all activities. Take a squash player who sprints around the court returning every shot, and keeps going long after his or her opponent looks exhausted and concedes defeat. Enter the same squash player in a long distance road race and he or she may manage to get round the course, but are unlikely to win the event. The individual may even get out of breath and have to stop along the way.

Similarly, there is little transfer of training from strength training to cardiovascular efficiency. A marathon runner, for example, would not spend much time lifting heavy weights, or doing short sprint intervals. The power lifter would not overemphasise distance running, or low-intensity resistance training, while prolonged long-distance running is unlikely to improve endurance swimming time.

Reversibility

Training effects are reversible. If the benefits of adaptation to an exercise programme are to be maintained and improved, then regular activity has to be adhered to. It is possible to *lose it by not using it'*. All components of fitness can be affected by non-activity. Once a level of fitness has been achieved, it can be maintained with less effort than was initially required for its development.

Overload

To achieve a higher level of fitness it is necessary to stress the body systems and place them in a state of overload, a point above and beyond that which is usually achieved. If this greater level is not achieved, adaptation will not occur. To avoid the problems associated with injury, illness and motivation it is important that the training load is increased progressively. Rest and recuperation are also important.

Consider the novice gym user, who at the start of their training programme can only perform six repetitions of a press up. After two or three weeks of training two to three times per week, they should be able to increase the number of repetitions beyond six. They can then think about including sets of repetitions.

Being physically fit is about having enough energy, strength and skill to cope with the everyday demands of your environment. Individual fitness levels vary greatly, from low levels required to cope with daily activities, to

optimal levels required by some performers at the top of their sport. Improving fitness will improve the physiological functioning of the body.

When preparing a training programme, the correct amount of exercise is needed to promote gains in physical fitness components. Training prescriptions should be tailored to the individual and the demands of the sport or activity. Consideration should be given to:

* fitness goals, which should be realistic

* mode and form of training

* how often it is to be undertaken

* how long and at what intensity

* maintenance to be effective.

These aspects relate to the FITTA principles of exercise prescription.

FITTA principles

The FITTA principles suggest that all training or exercise programmes should include:

* **frequency** of exercise refers to the number of times, usually exp ressed in times per week, that the exercise is to be undertaken

* **intensity** of exercise refers to how hard, or the amount of stress or overload that is to be applied

* **time** (duration) of exercise refers to how long the activity is to be carried out

* **type** of exercise refers to the mode of exercise performed.

* **adherence** to the programme should produce the desired adaptations in response to the prescribed training programme.

Different types of exercise provide different health and well-being benefits. Once fitness goals have been determined, the exercise undertaken must allow for the type of benefits that are desired:

* weight control

* stress management

* prevention of disease

* muscle definition

* maintenance of flexibility.

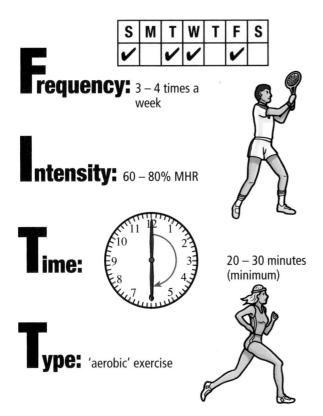

Frequency: 3 – 4 times a week

Intensity: 60 – 80% MHR

Time: 20 – 30 minutes (minimum)

Type: 'aerobic' exercise

FIGURE 13.16 *Principles of exercise programming*

Important factors to be considered are:

* convenience
* cost
* motivation
* enjoyment.

Did you know?

Around 70 per cent of women and 60 per cent of men in the UK are not active enough to gain the health benefits from physical activity. That is, they do not participate in activity of the appropriate intensity for the appropriate duration often enough to gain any benefits to their overall health and well-being.

Training techniques for aerobic fitness

Endurance training is a generic term that refers to any mode of low intensity, long duration activity, such as walking, running, rowing, swimming, cycling or skating, that aims to improve aerobic fitness. There are a number of techniques employed by athletes and sportspeople to develop this fitness component. These include:

* long, slow distance training
* interval training
* varied pace (**fartlek**) training
* circuit training
* cross training.

Long, slow distance training

This is a popular continuous form of training undertaken at a steady pace. The exercise intensity is sub-maximal and usually set at around 70 per cent of maximum heart rate.

Interval training

This is a common form of endurance training for athletes who have already established a good base of endurance and wish to attain higher levels of fitness. Set periods of work, usually at a relatively high intensity, are followed by periods of recovery. The length of the interval can vary from 30 seconds to 5 minutes and the recovery phase may be complete rest, a walk, or jogging. The recovery period, especially active forms of recovery, allows for the oxygen debt incurred during the work interval to be repaid. This mode of training develops both aerobic and anaerobic systems. As with fartlek training, a major advantage of this method is the variety of workouts it allows, assisting in maintaining the motivation to sustain training. The principles of interval training can easily be incorporated into a gym training programme to maintain health and well-being

Varied pace or fartlek training

'Fartlek' is a Swedish word meaning 'speed play'. This type of training varies the pace at specific intervals throughout the training and is usually applied to running. Continuous running at a steady pace is interspersed with changes in speed for varying durations. This form of training is similar to interval training, but less fixed in its work-to-rest ratios. It utilises a variety of terrains and gradients, such as woodland trails, golf courses, sand dunes, uphill and downhill. Again, one of the key advantages of this mode of endurance training is that variety and motivation can be maintained. Fartlek training can also be used effectively with a walking programme, for example by varying pace between lamp-posts.

Circuit training

Circuit training is a mode of exercise training in which a series of exercises are organised and performed in a particular sequence. Each exercise usually targets a different muscle or muscle group. Circuit training sessions can be planned to emphasise the development of cardio-respiratory or muscular endurance and as a result are useful for improving overall fitness. Exercises aimed at the development of muscular endurance, such as curl-ups, squats and press-ups, can be interspersed with aerobic activities, such as running, stepping and skipping. The resistance, number of repetitions and recovery period between each exercise will be determined by the fitness level of the participants. This mode of training can be adapted for individuals or groups. Again, it has the advantage of offering an infinite variety of training session possibilities in relation to its organisation and structure. It can be undertaken indoors, outdoors, with free weights or fixed weights in the gym and can be specifically tailored to meet the demands of individuals or groups.

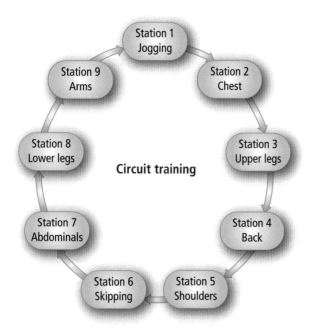

FIGURE 13.17 *A simple circuit format*

Cross training

Cross training is becoming increasingly popular for developing aerobic fitness. It combines a variety of different exercise modes, such as rowing and swimming, or swimming and jogging. Again, this can help to relieve boredom within the exercise programme and may reduce the risk of injuries due to overuse of the same muscles or body parts.

Key concepts

Muscular strength: is achieved by using high resistance with low repetitions.

Muscular endurance: is achieved by using low resistance and high repetitions.

Training techniques for muscle fitness

The fitness of muscles relates to their strength, size, power, and endurance capacity. To develop muscular strength and endurance the concept of 'progressive resistance overload' must be applied to the training process. Muscle improvements are gained as they respond and adapt to overload, the stress applied to encourage improvement. Progressive resistance overload means that, as the muscles strengthen and endurance increases, the load against which a muscle is working must be increased periodically for continued gains to be realised. The training programme may be planned to emphasise muscular strength, muscle bulk, muscular endurance or explosive power. Muscular strength is achieved by using high resistance with low repetitions. Muscle strength and muscle bulk are interrelated in that as strength increases, so does bulk. Resistance training undertaken to result in muscle bulking should include sessions focused on maximal lifting.

Muscular endurance is achieved by using low resistance and high repetitions. There are a number of techniques that can be employed to develop muscular strength and endurance including:

* circuit weight training

* specific strength training using a number of different systematic approaches.

Circuit weight training

Circuit weight training is based on low resistance with high repetitions and aims to develop muscular endurance and cardiovascular fitness by making the circuit continuous. Each exercise is performed for a set number of repetitions (15–25) or a set time period usually 30–60 seconds.

Specific strength training

Progressive resistance is applied to develop strength or endurance in specific muscles or groups of muscles. A variety of methods can be applied to achieve progressive resistance overload from a simple circuit to sets and pyramid systems.

Simple circuit

This is a series of exercises, usually 6–12, performed in rotation as a circuit, with 15–25 repetitions using a light resistance; the emphasis is on whole body conditioning. This is an ideal format for the novice weight trainer, providing the opportunity to become familiar with basic lifts, or for the athlete returning to training after the recovery phase.

Set systems

> ### Key concept
>
> *1RM = 1 repetition maximum:* the absolute maximum load you can lift in one contraction. It can be used to predict your 6 or 10RM (i.e. the heaviest weight you can manage to lift 6 or 10 times).

Single set system

A single set of each exercise is performed for 8–12 repetitions at 75 per cent 1RM. The American College of Sports Medicine (ACSM) recommend this approach for muscular fitness and suggest 8–10 exercises utilising the large muscle groups.

Basic sets system

This method can be used to provide an easy introduction into the concept of multiple sets of an exercise. It follows the circuit approach, but requires the performance of a designated number of sets, usually 2–4 for each exercise, before moving on.

Delorme Watkins (10RM)

This system is built around gradually increasing the workload while using the same number of repetitions (reps) per set. This method requires the establishment of the 10RM, best done through trial and error after a warm-up. A three-set format is then developed around the 10RM.

> For example:
> Set 1 – 10 reps at 50% of 10RM
> Set 2 – 10 reps at 75% of 10RM
> Set 3 – 10 reps at 100% of 10RM

Rest periods should be no longer than 90 seconds between sets and failure should occur in the last set if the 10RM has been correctly established.

Berger system (6RM)

This method is considered effective at promoting gains in muscular strength. In this method three sets of six repetitions each at 6RM are performed with up to 5 minutes rest between sets.

Pyramid system

This is an advanced method of promoting strength gains based around the establishment of the 1RM. The number of sets in a pyramid can vary, but the general principle of a gradual increase in resistance applies to build up to the final execution of 1RM.

> For example:
> Set 1 – 12 reps at 50% of 1RM
> Set 2 – 6 reps at 65% of 1RM
> Set 3 – 3 reps at 80% of 1RM
> Set 4 – 1 rep at 100% of 1RM

Super sets system

This is an advanced system with various approaches. One approach is based on performing two sets of exercises for the same body part using opposing muscle groups with no rest periods between these exercises.

Training for flexibility

Flexibility is often underrated as a fitness component. As previously discussed, it can be defined as the range of movement around a joint. It is in part determined by the shape and position of the bones that make up the joint, and the muscles and connective tissue that surround it. If the muscle and connective tissue are tight this will impede joint movement. Performing flexibility exercises will gradually lengthen the connective tissue and encourage greater relaxation of muscle fibres. Every muscle contains special sensory receptors. If these receptors are stimulated they inform the central nervous system about what is happening within the muscle. There are two main receptors stimulated during flexibility work, the muscle spindle and the golgi tendon organ. Both are sensitive to changes in muscle length, the golgi tendon is also sensitive to changes in muscle tension. Rapid stretching of muscle spindles results in a reflex contraction to prevent the muscle from overstretching. This 'stretch reflex' is counterproductive to effective stretching.

Exercising for stress management

Exercise should be viewed as a positive stress for the body. The choice of pleasant exercise surroundings can help to cancel out the negative stresses that accumulate in daily life. Taking part in an activity that is social can also help, such as participating in exercise to music.

Designing a physical activity or exercise programme

Exercise plans should promote the development of all components of health-related fitness. By setting yourself **SMART** goals you are much more likely to be successful.

SMART goal setting:

Specific	to wants or needs
Measurable	fitness test
Agreed	and recorded
Realistic	achievable
Time framed	to keep you on track

Creating exercise programmes for different objectives and clients

The older adult

Older adults, both men and women, can benefit from regular physical activity and exercise. Physical activity does not have to be strenuous for older adults to achieve health benefits, with significant health benefits gained from moderate amounts of physical activity, preferably taken daily. A moderate amount of activity can be achieved through longer sessions of moderately intense activity, or shorter sessions of vigorous activity, while additional gains can be made by increasing intensity, duration or frequency. It is important to note that previously sedentary older adults should begin with short intervals of moderate intensity activity, such as walking, and build

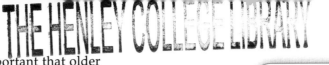
up gradually. It is also important that older adults consult their medical practitioner before beginning a new physical activity programme. In addition to aerobic activity, such as walking, swimming or dancing, older adults can benefit from muscle-strengthening activities. When designing exercise programmes for the older adult, the following considerations should be taken in to account:

* they are likely to be more unfit compared to younger adults

* they will progress at a slower rate

* maximum capabilities will be lower

* they are likely to have cardiovascular risk factors

* there is the possibility of fragile bones.

Benefits of a long term exercise programme for the older adult

* increased fitness and stamina

* increased muscle tone, strength and shape

* decreased body fat

* protection from osteoporosis

* decreased cardiovascular risk

* improved immune system

* increased psychological well-being

* increased social interaction.

Exercise to combat ageing

The UK has an ageing population. It is predicted that between 1995 and 2025 the number of people over 80 years of age will have increased by half. If older people do not remain fit and healthy this will increase the burden on our health care system.

Try it out

Using the Internet and scientific journals investigate the current physical activity patterns of older adults. What implications can you draw from your research?

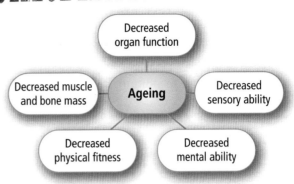

FIGURE 13.18 *The effects of ageing*

Think it over

1. Which aspects of fitness are affected most by the ageing process?

2. Is there an upper age limit to improving fitness?

3. List four considerations for exercise for the older adult.

4. List five benefits of exercise for the older adult.

5. List some appropriate exercise activities for the older adult.

Current fitness guidelines for the prevention of disease

To gain health benefits the Department of Health recommends at least 30 minutes of moderate exercise on five, if not all, days of the week. These are similar guidelines to the rest of the world, including the USA and Australia. This 30-minute-a-day recommendation should probably be viewed as the minimum to obtain health benefits, but it does not have to be in a single session. Several short bursts of activity can count towards the total. This approach may make it easier for some individuals to meet their daily physical activity target. Greater benefits will be gained from increasing the amount to 40–60 minutes each day, especially for those at risk of weight gain. The same recommendations apply to older people dependent on ability, but children are encouraged to achieve at least one hour every day of moderate-intensity activity.

What is 'moderate activity' and what type of activity should an individual undertake? Moderate means that you must get a little warmer and slightly out of breath. The more vigorous the activity the greater the cardiovascular health gains will be. In terms of type, it can be anything that raises your energy expenditure above resting level, enough to expend about 200 calories. It should bring about the symptoms already described, for example brisk walking, swimming, cycling, jogging, dancing, or heavy housework or gardening.

Exercise and weight control

There is little robust scientific literature about how much activity is undertaken by those who successfully manage their weight. However, the relatively low incidence of overweight and obesity in those who maintain active lifestyles suggests that regular physical activity and exercise have clear benefits. At least 30 minutes on five or more days of the week of moderate-intensity physical activity will represent a substantial increase in energy expenditure for most individuals. Assuming no corresponding increase in energy intake, a significant negative energy balance to facilitate weight loss will occur. The ACSM guidelines (2000) suggest that overweight and obese individuals should be encouraged to exercise on most, if not all days of the week, or for a minimum of 150 minutes per week, preferably 200 minutes. When designing exercise programmes for the overweight and obese the following considerations should be taken in to account:

* *mode:* low impact, such as walking or swimming

* *duration:* 40–60 minutes per day, although this may need to be in shorter bouts

* *intensity:* 40–50% VO_2 max.

Exercise for rehabilitation

Since the early 1990s many areas in the UK have operated 'exercise on prescription', also known as GP referral schemes. This is where a medical practitioner may refer an individual for exercise programming as a way to speed rehabilitation after illness and hopefully encourage the exercise habit. GP referral schemes work as partnerships between medical practitioners, including GP's practice nurses and other health care professionals, with local authority or private sector fitness facilities. The type of patient that might be referred for exercise on prescription include those with high blood pressure, obesity, depression and low back pain. Within such a scheme the patient would undergo a thorough health, fitness and lifestyle screening. If they were deemed to be low risk their physical activity and exercise programme would reflect this in terms of minimal supervision. Those deemed to be high risk would require greater supervision while carrying out their physical activity and exercise programme.

Try it out

Investigate the availability of exercise on prescription schemes in your local area. Your investigation should include the types of patient catered for, how long the programmes are run for and the qualifications of the staff that run them.

Summary

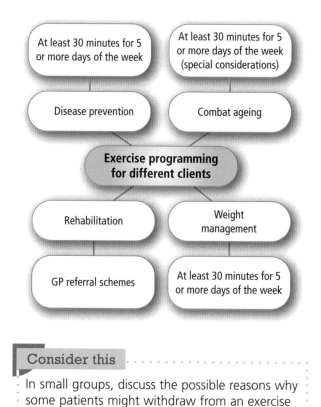

Consider this

In small groups, discuss the possible reasons why some patients might withdraw from an exercise on prescription scheme.

John is a 30-year-old businessman. He is married with two young children aged six and four years. Recently he has become increasingly concerned about his expanding waistline. He's always tired and has also noticed that he is having difficulty keeping up with his children on their weekend outing to the local park.

John works long hours, giving him little time to enjoy his membership of the local health club, and he is considering giving up his membership as he feels he is not getting value for money. Before the pressures of his work increased he used to enjoy playing football for the local Sunday league team.

Consider the following questions and activities:

1. How would you summarise John's lifestyle?

2. What potential barriers do you think there are to John adopting a healthier lifestyle?

3. What changes would you recommend to John's lifestyle?

4. Devise an exercise programme for John taking into account current recommendations for physical activity.

5. How can you ensure he will stick to your programme?

UNIT 13 ASSESSMENT

How you will be assessed

This unit is externally assessed. You will be assessed on your knowledge, understanding and skills relating to exercise and its role in maintaining health and well-being through a written examination. Your examination questions will be drawn from each of the seven sections of the unit. You will be required to analyse research data, including numerical data, relating to exercise; and to evaluate evidence, make judgements and draw conclusions. This unit will be assessed through a two-hour written test. Some specimen questions relevant to this unit are set out below. They will give you an indication of what form the test will take and the possible marks for each question (shown in brackets).

Test questions

1. Describe the concept of wellness. (5)

2. Identify and discuss five major benefits of regular physical activity and exercise. (10)

3. Why is it important to undertake a thorough health, fitness and lifestyle screening prior to formulating a physical activity and exercise prescription? (8)

4. Identify five different techniques for the measurement of body composition and discuss their relative merits for application to the sedentary population. (10)

5. Define the term VO_2 max. (2)

6. Describe two field techniques for the measurement of aerobic fitness suitable for use with previously sedentary subjects. (8)

7. Identify and discuss the guidelines that should be followed in order to minimise the risk of injury from increased physical activity and exercise. (6)

8. What key factors play a role in the maintenance of a regular programme of physical activity and exercise? (5)

9. What are the key elements of a physical activity or exercise prescription? (5)

10. What is overload and why is it important? (4)

11. Identify three training techniques that aim to improve aerobic fitness. (3)

12. Name three reasons why muscular training for improved strength and endurance should be included in an exercise programme. (3)

13. What are the major risk factors for the development of CHD? How can a programme of regular physical activity and exercise benefit these? (10)

14. Define stress and consider why the management of stress is important to maintaining health and well-being. What role can exercise play in the management of stress? (10)

15. Describe the current physical activity guidelines for the prevention of chronic disease. (5)

16. Why is it important for older people to maintain or increase physical activity levels? (6)

17. Identify five barriers to increased physical activity and exercise participation that might be encountered by the currently sedentary? Provide examples of how these might be overcome. (10)

18. What tools and techniques would you use to monitor progress of a participant's physical activity or exercise programme? (5)

19. Why is it important to include a warm-up and warm-down in the basic structure of any physical activity or exercise programme? (8)

20. What are the key features of a GP referral scheme? How might such schemes facilitate increase physical activity and exercise participation in the UK population? (10)

References and further reading

DoH (2001) *National Service Framework for Coronary Heart Disease, Diabetes, Mental Health and Older People* London: HMSO

Useful websites

www.csep.ca
   The Canadian Society for Exercise Physiology
www.dh.gov.uk
   Department of Health website

Additional material

Health Status Questionnaire

Name _____   Date _____

The following questions are designed to ascertain your readiness to participate in the practical exercise and physical activities outlined within this unit. If you answer **YES** to any of the questions below, you should have a thorough medical examination prior to participating in the practical tasks described within the unit.

- Have you ever had a heart condition or experienced chest pains or a sensation in your chest associated with exercise?

- Do you have a family history of heart disease below the age of 55?   Yes ☐   No ☐

- Have you ever suffered from high or low blood pressure?   Yes ☐   No ☐

- Are you taking any prescribed medication?   Yes ☐   No ☐

- Do you suffer from any respiratory problems such as asthma or shortness of breath with minimal exertion?   Yes ☐   No ☐

- Have you ever had any condition or injury affecting your joints or back that could be aggravated by exercise?   Yes ☐   No ☐

- Do you suffer from diabetes or epilepsy?   Yes ☐   No ☐

- Has your GP ever advised you not to participate in exercise?   Yes ☐   No ☐

Now please read the exercise advice below

When undertaking the exercise and physical activities described in this unit start at a slow pace and listen to your body. If you experience any signs of discomfort or stress terminate the activity immediately and seek medical advice as soon as possible.

Service users with disabilities

This unit covers the following sections:

15.1 What is disability?

15.2 Causes of impairments

15.3 Disability conditions

15.4 Practitioners and provision

15.5 Barriers

15.6 Aids and adaptations

15.7 Legislation

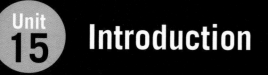
In this unit you will study a range of disability conditions, and a range of service provision to people with these conditions.

You will be introduced to different models of disability, together with legal definitions and the legal framework that now protects the rights of disabled people.

In the last twenty or thirty years, attitudes towards disabled people have been slowly changing, due to legislation and also the efforts of a number of people to promote a more positive image of disability. Furthermore, advances in science and technology are contributing to the greater independence and better health of many people with long-term disabling conditions. Nevertheless, there are still a number of barriers to inclusion for disabled people, many of which are due to the attitudes of non-disabled people; and financial constraints sometimes make advanced technology (and sometimes treatments) beyond the reach of some disabled people.

Professionals with knowledge of what is available, together with an awareness of what is possible, can make a tremendous difference to the lives of disabled people by working towards their greater empowerment in a number of ways.

Unit assessment

This unit is externally assessed by a written two-hour test. A more detailed guide to the assessment is given at the end of this unit.

15.1 What is disability?

Definitions of disability

Disabilities are usually considered in terms of three broad categories: physical disabilities, sensory disabilities and learning disabilities (also sometimes referred to as learning difficulties).

Key concepts

Physical disabilities: affect the body's main motor functions, i.e. the use of the large muscles of the arms and legs, head, neck and torso, and problems with some of the internal organs (for example, the bladder and bowel).

Sensory disabilities: relate primarily to problems with hearing and vision. Problems with hearing range from mild impairment to profound deafness. Similarly, visual problems range from visual impairments to complete blindness. There are also conditions that affect the sense of touch (anesthesia) and smell (anosmia).

Learning disabilities: affect a person's ability to interpret what is seen and heard, or to link information from different parts of the brain. This can lead to problems with spoken and written language, difficulty in co-ordinating limbs and body, limited attention span and hyperactivity, and sometimes the inability to make and sustain relationships with other people, even parents.

Of course, one individual may have more than one disability (for example someone who is deaf-blind), or disabilities from more than one of the broad categories (for example, a person with a learning disability who is also deaf).

It is also important to note that some conditions result in psychiatric or mental problems which can also be disabling, either physically or socially. Although this unit does not require you to be familiar with the causes and types of mental-health problems, it is important for you to be aware that for some people with disabilities mental health issues may also be important. At a very basic level, living with a disabling physical or sensory condition over a long period of time can result in depression, which causes additional problems.

Because disabled people are entitled by law to receive specific support from the state, a legal definition of what it means to be disabled has been deemed necessary (see page 140).

Models of disability

Throughout history, societies have made decisions about how to regard people with disabilities, and this has often led to disabled people being treated very badly indeed. The Elizabethan Poor Law, for example (set up by an Act of Parliament in 1601), saw disabled people as a 'problem' that paid officials had to deal with. To some extent, this approach has survived into the twenty-first century, although there are now many people (both disabled and non-disabled) who are working hard to counteract this view of disability as a 'problem'.

The medical model of disability

This view is, in some respects, a hangover from the old view of disability as a 'problem'. From this perspective, people are disabled as a result of the physical and cognitive impairments they have. These impairments prevent them from functioning like the rest of society who are, by definition, seen as 'normal'.

The medical solution to this is to intervene to cure people, or at any rate to rehabilitate them into society. This view sees disability as an individual problem, and it focuses on personal limitations. It is very much an 'impairment' view of disability. One consequence of this view is that if a disability cannot be 'cured', or if a person cannot be successfully rehabilitated, then he or she is seen as unable to play a full role as a member of society. This attitude thus devalues that person.

The social model of disability

Disabled people have been challenging the medical model of disability since the end of the nineteenth century. The British Deaf Association

(BDA) and the National League of the Blind (NLB) were set up at this time, and the NLB actually registered as a trade union in 1899. Such organisations aimed to promote the rights of disabled people to have equal status with non-disabled people. In more recent years many such organisations have been founded (for example the British Council of Disabled People in 1986, and Disabled Peoples' International in 1989).

The argument put forward by such organisations is that it is not the fact of having a physical, sensory or learning impairment as such that disables a person. Rather, it is the attitude of the rest of society towards that person that limits what he or she is able to do. This is a social model of disability.

If Nicholas (see Scenario above) had been born in the late 1990s, his life might have been quite different. His parents could have applied for equipment and adaptations to their home to allow him to live with them (for example bath hoists, bathing aids, ramps and widened doors to accommodate a wheelchair). Other support might be available in the form of social work intervention, or home nursing. Adapted computer equipment now exists to help with intellectual and educational needs. Day care can be supplied to support personal development, and it is no longer considered necessary for people with severe disabilities to be hidden away in institutions.

However, there is still some way to go before all barriers to the inclusion of disabled people into society are removed (see page 174).

Disability: the legal definition

The 1995 Disability Discrimination Act (DDA) defined a person as being disabled, if they have 'a physical or mental impairment which has a substantial and long-term adverse effect on their ability to carry out normal day-to-day activities' (Department for Work and Pensions (DWP) 2005). However, the DDA allowed for modification of this definition in the case of people with mental health problems and progressive conditions. This meant that some people with either mental health problems or certain chronic conditions were excluded from the protection afforded by this legislation.

However, the 2005 Disability Discrimination Act (DDA 2005) extended the definition of disability to make it more applicable to many people with mental health problems, by removing the specification that a mental illness must be 'clinically well recognised'. It also specifically extended the legal definition to people with HIV, cancer and multiple sclerosis *from the point of diagnosis* (rather than when the condition has an adverse effect on daily life). This is a very important change, which means that many more people are now protected by the DDA and the DDA 2005. The section on legislation (page 182) explains the provisions of the DDA and DDA 2005 in some further detail.

Key concept

Chronic: a term used to describe a condition that persists over a long period of time.

Summary

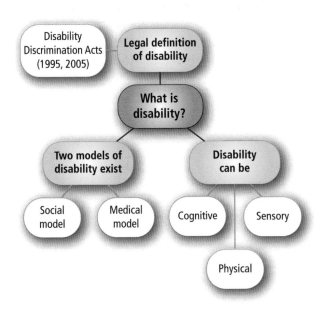

15.2 Causes of impairments

Disabilities are not conditions in themselves; rather they result from a number of causes which can be internal or external to the human body.

Table 15.1 sets out some of the key factors which can result in impairment to the human function, whether this is physical, sensory or cognitive.

The central nervous system

The brain and spinal cord together make up the central nervous system (CNS). Damage to any part of the CNS can result in bodily impairment or disability, the severity and nature of which depends on the extent of the damage and its prime location.

Figure 15.1 shows the key areas of the brain, and Table 15.2 gives a very simplified explanation of the bodily functions that these key areas control. The central sulcus is the large fissure along the centre of the brain. If specific areas of the brain are damaged, then the body's ability to perform functions normally controlled by these areas is impaired. However, it must be stressed that this is a very simplified view. Certain functions are located in more than one specific area, and the brain is also capable of compensating for damage to specific areas by taking over their functions elsewhere.

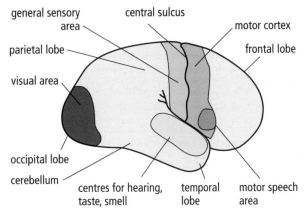

FIGURE 15.1 *The functional areas of the brain*

The one area of the brain that is unambiguously associated with a specific type of impairment is the motor cortex, which is situated at the back of the frontal lobe. Damage to the left-hand side of this area results in problems with movement to the right side of the body; damage to the right-hand side of the motor cortex impairs movement on the left side of the body.

Table 15.2 sets out the key functions of each part of the brain, indicating broadly the likely damage to bodily functions resulting from injury or impairment of each lobe of the brain. However, the reservations expressed above should be kept in mind. The brain is a very complex organism, and damage to any part may result in a range of symptoms and impairments.

CAUSE	EXPLANATION	EXAMPLE
Pre-birth		
Genetic	A gene may be faulty or missing	Cystic fibrosis (physical disability)
Chromosomal	There may be extra copies of chromosomes	Down's syndrome (learning disability)
Nutritional	Poor nutrition or taking of harmful substances by mother causes harm to the foetus	People damaged by **thalidomide** (physical disability)
During birth		
Trauma	May result from hypoxia (lack of oxygen) or physical injury	Learning disability as a result of brain damage
Post-birth		
Accidental injuries	Damage to the central nervous system (CNS), i.e. to the brain or spinal cord	Paralysis of lower part of body (tetraplegia); total paralysis (quadriplegia)
	Shock Exposure to loud noise	May cause psychological problems May cause deafness
Infectious diseases	Damage to key organs, such as the brain	Meningitis (physical disabilities)
Nutritional/lifestyle factors	Damage to key organs and/or bodily systems resulting from smoking, lack of exercise, obesity, dangerous substances (e.g. drugs)	Strokes, circulatory disorders (physical disabilities); existing conditions may be exacerbated (e.g. diabetes)
Environmental factors	Damage to key organs and/or bodily systems as a result of exposure to toxic substances, e.g. radiation, asbestos	Gulf War syndrome (physical and psychological problems) Asbestosis (physical disabilities)
Age-related causes	Progressive deterioration of key systems (e.g. circulatory, musculo-skeletal) Development of lesions in brain etc	Osteoarthritis (physical) Osteoporosis (physical) Dementias (psychological) Stroke (physical) Failing senses (hearing and visual problems)

TABLE 15.1 *Main causes of disabling conditions*

AREA	SOME FUNCTIONS POSSIBLY AT RISK FROM DAMAGE	NOTES
Frontal lobe	Motor functions (motor cortex) Emotions Changes to personality	Opposite sides of body are controlled
	Language/speech production	Left side of lobe
	Short-term memory, concentration, retaining information	May affect ability to solve problems

continued on next page

AREA	SOME FUNCTIONS POSSIBLY AT RISK FROM DAMAGE	NOTES
Parietal lobe	Sensation and perception Body orientation	
Occipital lobe	Visual perception	
Temporal lobe	Hearing, taste, smell Understanding speech	Damage may also affect memory
Cerebellum	Voluntary motor movement, balance, muscle tone	
Brain stem	Attention, arousal, consciousness Deep emotions (e.g. fear)	Conduit for all information to the rest of the body

TABLE 15.2 *Functional areas of the brain*

This is a very complex area of study. If you are interested, there are a number of websites where the functions of areas of the brain can be explored. At the time of writing, these include the websites of the BBC (www.bbc.co.uk/science), and of the Centre for Neuro Science, an American based service for people with brain damage (www.neuroskills.com).

Damage to the rest of the CNS can also cause impairment. If the spinal cord is broken or if the myelin sheath is damaged, as a result of a condition such as multiple sclerosis, then signals from the brain will fail to reach areas of the body beyond the point of damage. Impairment of bodily function will then result.

Did you know?

The term stroke refers to damage caused by problems in the blood supply to the brain. Ischaemic stroke results from blockage to blood vessels, whilst haemorrhagic stroke involves bleeding around or into the brain.

In both kinds of stroke, brain cells are damaged or die. The effects of stroke range from mild to severe, depending on which parts of the brain have been damaged and how badly.

Find out more at the website of the Stroke Association (www.stroke.org.uk).

Summary

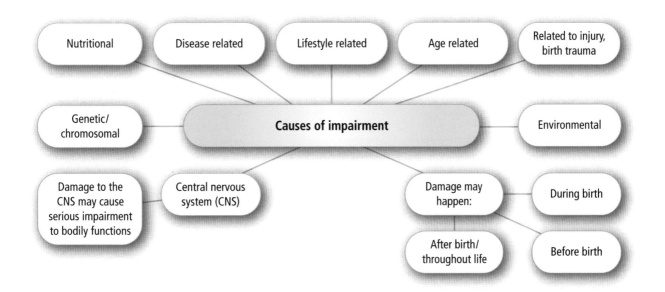

15.3 Disability conditions

In this section you will learn about the following disability conditions and their main treatments, together with the ways in which people with these conditions can be supported:

* Alzheimer's disease

* cerebral palsy

* cystic fibrosis

* Down's syndrome

* Duchenne muscular dystrophy

* Multiple sclerosis

* osteoarthritis

* spina bifida

In considering treatments and support for a condition, it is important to remember that shared decision-making is usually the best way forward for an individual. The website Best Treatments (which is compiled by the *British Medical Journal* and linked to the NHS Direct website) has an excellent series of articles describing how patients can get the best out of working with their doctors. Patients should expect to discuss all the options available to them, and to be able to ask for further information if necessary. The risks and benefits of all treatment options should be assessed, and patients should be helped to use findings from research to make a final decision, if they so wish.

Of course, some patients prefer to let the doctor make decisions on their behalf, but others prefer to remain in control of what happens to them, and to choose treatments that are in accord with their own views and values. Sometimes, people will opt for a

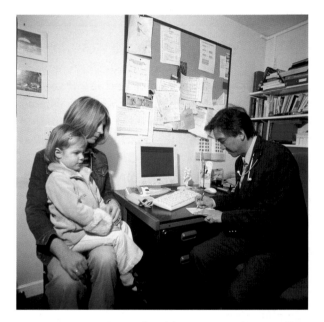

FIGURE 15.2 *Patients should expect to discuss all options available to them with their doctor*

treatment that is not fully endorsed by the medical profession (e.g. homeopathy); at other times, people may be determined to take a particular drug, despite the risks of unpleasant side-effects.

In the final analysis, disabled people (like everyone else) have the right to take as full a part in decision-making about themselves as they wish.

Alzheimer's disease

Description

There are over 100 types of dementia, but Alzheimer's disease (AD) is the most common, affecting about 500,000 people in the UK. This progressive condition involves chemical changes in the brain, including a deficiency of **acetylcholine.** These changes cause 'plaques' and 'tangles' in the brain's structure, resulting in death of brain cells. In time, this affects memory, understanding, communication and reasoning, although progress is often very gradual. Eventually, a person's ability to look after him or herself can be seriously impaired.

Physical and psychological effects

Alzheimer's is a progressive disease; the symptoms usually appear gradually and become more severe with time. Although three stages may be distinguished, in practice individuals may differ considerably. Some people may not have all of the symptoms while others may display aspects of different stages at the same time (e.g. a person may have memory loss with respect to names, but still be able to perform personal tasks quite adequately). In other cases, certain symptoms may appear and then disappear at a later stage.

Some of the characteristics of the three stages of Alzheimer's are set out in Table 15.3. Further information, including an extensive series of fact sheets, is available from the Alzheimer's Society website (www.alzheimers.org.uk). The psychological manifestations of Alzheimer's are set out in Table 15.4.

Progression

The three key stages of Alzheimer's, set out in Table 15.4, are broad categories; individuals may experience some or all of these typical symptoms.

CAUSES	SIGNS/SYMPTOMS	PROGRESSION	TREATMENT/SUPPORT
No single cause identified. Combination of: * age * environmental factors * diet * general health * (smoking, high blood pressure or high cholesterol) Sometimes genetic (small number of cases). People with Down's syndrome may sometimes develop AD. Head injuries may increase the risk.	*Early stage:* Confusion, memory loss, mood swings, loss of confidence	*Middle stage:* Existing symptoms more severe; also, inappropriate behaviour, dangerous behaviours, hallucinations *Late stage:* Possible total dependence (e.g. nursing care needed); complete memory loss; physical frailty; incontinence; loss of speech	No current cure. Drugs to slow progression: * Aricept * Exelol * Reminyl * Ebixol People with AD need: ongoing stimulation, meaningful activities, physical and emotional support. Some complementary therapies can help.

TABLE 15.3 *Alzheimer's disease: key facts*

KEY STAGES	MANIFESTATIONS
Early stage	Anxiety Agitation Depression Need for reassurance
Middle stage	Anger/aggression Frustration Emotional dependence
Late stage	Restlessness Distress, agitation May respond positively to affection, sensory stimuli (including music), animals

TABLE 15.4 *Some psychological symptoms of Alzheimer's disease*

Main treatments and support

Although there is currently no cure for Alzheimer's, a number of drugs are used to slow the progress of the condition. These can sometimes bring improvements in some symptoms, and help to stabilise a person's condition.

The drugs Aricept, Exelol and Reminyl are used to maintain levels of acetylcholine in the brain, a chemical often deficient in the brains of people with AD. The drugs are used for mild to moderate cases. The product Ebixa is sometimes used for people in the middle to late stages of AD. This drug impedes excess entry of calcium ions into brain cells. Too much calcium prevents brain cells from receiving neurological signals.

All these pharmaceutical products may have unpleasant side effects, and sometimes complementary therapies (CAMs) are used for people with AD. The Alzheimer's Society reports that some encouraging results have been noted from the use of nutritional supplements such as ginkgo biloba and vitamins (particularly Vitamin E), from some herbal medicinal products, and from aromatherapy and massage. Music therapy, too, may be beneficial, as may be acupuncture. Good general nutrition, together with supplements and antioxidants is also important in maintaining health.

These therapies are examined in greater detail in an Alzheimer's Society fact sheet, in which the need for further research is stressed. In choosing to use a CAM for someone with AD (as for any condition), you should always do some research beforehand, and check out the credentials and qualifications of any practitioner you intend to consult.

Key concept

CAMs: an acronym that refers to all complementary and alternative systems of medicine and therapy. These therapies are an alternative and/or complement conventional medicine.

Like anyone else, people with AD have the main psychological needs described so clearly by Kitwood (1997) and set out in Figure 15.3. The difference is that someone with AD may not have the inner resources to set about making sure that these needs are met. It is up to people caring for them to make sure that all of these psychological requirements are in place.

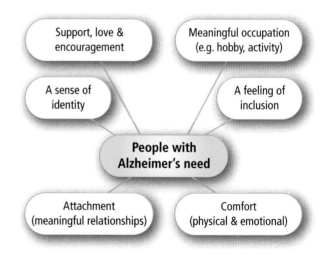

FIGURE 15.3 *People with AD require ongoing support to enhance their existing skills and abilities (Source: Kitwood 1997)*

The social worker explains that sometimes a task like dressing is easier when it is broken down into simple steps. She suggests that Archie should lay out Lilian's clothes for her in the morning, in the order that she should put them on. He should also lay out the breakfast items ready for Lilian to make tea and toast. She explains that it's good for people with dementia to be encouraged to continue to look after themselves for as long as possible, and Archie needs to give his wife praise and encouragement for what she does achieve, even if she doesn't manage to complete a task. The social worker also advises Archie to encourage Lilian to do other small household jobs with him, and to try to maintain a calm and reassuring speaking voice.

She also advises Archie that he needs to take time out for himself, as looking after someone with AD can be very tiring and frustrating.

Several times a week their son, Charlie, takes Lilian out: sometimes to the park, sometimes to a concert, as she loves music. This gives Archie a much-needed break.

Testing for Alzheimer's disease

There is no standard test. Elimination of other causes of symptoms is the first step:

* vitamin deficiency
* brain tumours
* thyroid malfunction
* infection
* side-effects of drugs
* depression.

Other possible input from:

* psychologist
* psychiatrist
* neurologist.

Tests include:

* blood tests
* memory tests
* brain scans.

Cerebral palsy

Description

The term cerebral palsy (CP) is used to describe an abnormality in which the parts of the brain that control movement have either been damaged, or have not developed normally. The word *cerebral* indicates that the problem is within the brain; *palsy* means paralysis. These abnormalities are present before the brain has finished developing.

CP is not one single condition. There are actually three main types, which are set out in Table 15.5. Scope, the national association for people with CP, describes it as 'diverse and complex', and stresses that no two people

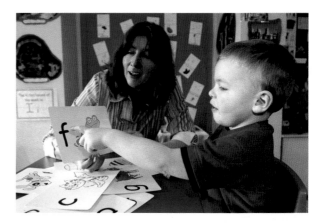

FIGURE 15.4 *Pre-school children learn through structured activities*

have exactly the same experience of the condition. People with CP display various symptoms and experience widely differing degrees of disability. Consequently, some people may have few physical difficulties, whereas others may have mobility problems, difficulties with personal care (e.g. eating), sensory problems (e.g. visual or hearing difficulties) and some associated learning difficulties. Some children may not show signs of the condition until they are over 12 months old, and sometimes even older.

CAUSES	SIGNS/SYMPTOMS	PROGRESSION	MAIN TREATMENTS/SUPPORT
Part of the brain fails to develop, either before birth or in early childhood. Multiple possible causes: * blocked blood vessel * premature birth * difficulties in labour * illness just after birth * infections (in pregnancy or early years, e.g. meningitis, encephalitis) * genetic disorder	*Spastic CP:* stiff, weak muscles; poor muscle control. *Athetoid CP:* loss of posture control; some unwanted movements; speech problems; eating problems. *Ataxic CP:* balance problems; shaky hand movements; speech difficulties. Some people have a combination of symptoms from the different types of CP. People with all types of CP may also experience: * visual, aural or cognitive difficulties * epilepsy	Brain impairment itself does not change, i.e. CP is not progressive. Bodily symptoms may get either less or more severe over time.	No cure, but early treatment can alleviate effects. Medical interventions include: * intrathecal baclofen therapy (ITB) * Botox injection * selective dorsal rhizotomy Therapies/support include: * physiotherapy * speech and language therapy * educational psychology * Portage educational programme * dietary therapy * occupational therapy

TABLE 15.5 *Cerebral palsy: key facts*

Physical and psychological effects

It is important to stress that CP affects each person quite differently. The main types of CP are listed in Table 15.5, together with a broad indication of the associated symptoms. A person may be affected in one limb (monoplegia), in both legs (diplegia), on one side of the body (hemiplegia) or in all four limbs (quadriplegia/tetraplegia), usually including the trunk and neck. The term triplegia indicates that three limbs are affected. There may sometimes be associated difficulties such as problems with constipation or sleeping; problems with speech, chewing or swallowing; difficulties in understanding the spoken word; epilepsy; problems with visual or spatial perception (e.g. distinguishing shapes), and some cognitive or learning difficulties. However, it should be stressed that many people with CP have average or above average intelligence and cognitive abilities. It is important not to generalise, and to provide the support and treatment that is appropriate to an individual's needs.

As with all chronic conditions, the prolonged daily necessities of living with physical difficulties can sometimes result in depression. This can be the same for carers of people with long-term conditions. Many people in these circumstances require additional support from time to time.

> **Key concepts**
>
> *Monoplegia:* paralysis of one leg
>
> *Diplegia:* paralysis of both legs
>
> *Hemiplegia:* paralysis of one side of the body
>
> *Quadri/tetraplegia:* paralysis of all four limbs

Main treatments/support

Medical intervention varies, but may include surgery to cut sensory nerve fibres in the spinal cord (selective dorsal rhizotomy), or treatment with relaxant drugs such as Baclofen (delivered by a pump implanted under the skin) or Botulinum toxin A (Botox).

People with CP are usually offered a wide range of supportive therapies and interventions, including physiotherapy, special educational support (such as the Portage programme), occupational therapy, and speech and language therapy.

Cerebral palsy: reducing the risk

* improved maternity services
* improved neonatal care (reduces risk of damage from lack of oxygen or jaundice).

Paradoxically, because of better early care, more babies with low birth weights are now surviving, resulting in a slight increase in the proportion of children with CP. Visit the website of the national support organisation (www.scope.org.uk). Publications and fact sheets can be downloaded from this site, which is a good starting-point for further research into cerebral palsy.

> **Key concept**
>
> *Neonatal:* relating to newly born infants.

Cystic fibrosis

Description

Cystic fibrosis (CF) is a genetic disorder in which a faulty gene results in the production of a defective version of a protein that carries salt and water. This protein normally carries salt and water across cell membranes, but because it is defective in people with CF, water is lacking and mucous secretions become very thick and sticky. This, in turn, causes problems in the body, in particular the lungs, pancreas and intestines.

Physical and psychological effects

The thick mucus produced in the body results in problems with the lungs, pancreas and intestines. A person with CF will typically have breathing problems and be susceptible to chest infections. Taking part in demanding sports may be a problem. The pancreas fails to

CAUSES	SIGNS/SYMPTOMS	PROGRESSION	TREATMENT/SUPPORT
Genetic: recessive gene results in defective protein	Thick, sticky mucal secretions affect: * lungs * pancreas * intestines Syptoms include: * poor food absorption * poor weight gain * chest infections/ coughs/breathing difficulties * abnormally large stools * salty sweat	As a person grows, the following may occur: * clubbing * barrel-shaped chest * nasal polyps Also risk of: * collapsed lung * bowel obstruction * cirrhosis of the liver * diabetes * secondary heart failure * pancreatitis * sterility (males) * difficulty conceiving (females)	*Physical* * physiotherapy * exercise * aerobic (for lungs), stretching (for posture and chest) *Diet* pancreatic enzymes, A,D,E vitamins, extra protein, etc. *Medication* Lungs: * bronchodilator * antibiotics * steroids * DNase *Digestive system:* * enzyme pills * high energy drinks/ supplements *Bones Vit D:* * biphosphonates * and calcium *Liver:* * ursodeoxycholic acid * transplantation *Gene therapy* * ongoing research

TABLE 15.6 *Cystic fibrosis: key facts*

produce enough enzymes, which in turn causes digestion problems and poor absorption of nutrients from food. Maintenance of a healthy body weight is thus often an issue for people with CF.

In childhood and adolescence, young people may experience additional anxieties at school, because of the ways in which they differ from their colleagues. Being small, constantly coughing, and having to take medication regularly during the course of the day may be a cause of embarrassment. Having to take time out for daily physiotherapy can also mark out a child

as 'different'. Adolescence brings additional pressures, particularly if sexual maturity is delayed. However, with additional practical and emotional support (especially from teachers, friends and family), growth into maturity and a confident adulthood can be assisted.

Progression

CF, as such, does not change, but its manifestations may become more severe if not properly managed. Individuals with CF are prone to a number of physical problems. Recurring respiratory infections, the 'clubbing' of finger and toe nails (due to decreased oxygen levels in the blood), and the barrelling of the chest cavity may develop over time. Some people even experience lung collapse.

Telescoping of the bowel (intussusception) may occur, resulting in further reduction in food absorption. Pancreatitis, secondary heart failure, diabetes and liver cirrhosis are all potential complications. Finally, men with CF are usually sterile, whilst women have difficulties in conceiving.

Main treatments/support

Chest physiotherapy is an essential part of the treatment regime, from diagnosis onwards. This aims to stop mucus from blocking air tubes in the lungs. The number and length of sessions varies from one per day, to four times per day; initially done by adult carers (after instruction by a physiotherapist), older children and adults can administer this treatment for themselves. Daily exercise is also an important part of living with CF, particularly activities that cause breathlessness, and also stretching.

Attention to diet is especially important. A person with CF will need additional pancreatic enzymes and vitamin supplements, and adults need to eat twice as much protein as those who don't have the condition. Medication is helpful in the management of CF, and a list of the major types of drugs used is given in Table 15.6. Lung transplantation is a very radical treatment which is used only in very severe cases. Finally, gene therapy is currently being researched, but this is at a very early stage.

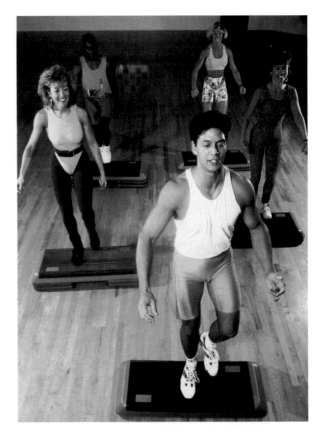

FIGURE 15.5 *Exercise is particularly important for people with CF as it helps to prevent deterioration of the lungs and improves physical bulk and strength*

Down's syndrome

Description

Down's syndrome (also called Down syndrome) results from a chromosomal abnormality. People with this condition have an extra copy of chromosome 21 in their cells, and there are three variants: Trisomy 21, Translocation and Mosaic. All three involve chromosome 21. It is not possible to predict whether or not a potential parent will produce an egg or a sperm with the extra copy of chromosome 21. The reason for this abnormality is, as yet, unknown, and the extra chromosome may come from either parent. Down's syndrome (DS) is found throughout the world, and is not specific to any race or class. Older mothers have a greater chance of having a child with DS, but in practice most babies with the condition are born to mothers under

TEST STAGE	TEST TYPE
Prenatal	Chorionic villus sampling (CVS) (analysis of cells taken from the placenta)
Postnatal	Heel prick (at birth – about a third of babies in UK are routinely tested in this way) Sweat test (for high salt levels) DNA analysis Lung X-rays

TABLE 15.7 *Testing for cystic fibrosis*

35 years, due to the higher fertility of younger women.

Children born with DS have a distinct physical appearance (see Table 15.8). They develop more slowly than other children with respect to both physical and cognitive skills. However, it must be stressed that people with DS and their families do not see themselves as 'victims' or 'sufferers'. With the right help and support, many people with this condition can achieve their full potential, can work and often make a significant contribution to society.

Physical and psychological effects

People with DS have a distinct appearance, with a flat facial profile, small mouth and sometimes protruding tongue, and distinctive eyes that slant upwards and outwards. They generally have poor muscle tone, and may have a greater susceptibility to certain medical conditions (see Table 15.8, and Progression, page 153).

Key developmental stages (e.g. walking, talking, the ability to feed oneself, etc.) will generally be later than for other children.

CAUSES	SIGNS/SYMPTOMS	PROGRESSION	MAIN TREATMENTS/SUPPORT
Genetic abnormalities associated with chromosome 21	* hypotonia (reduced muscle tone) * flat facial profile * distinctive eyes * small mouth, tongue often protrudes * sandal gap * short fingers, broad hands, single palm crease * below average birth weight and length	Children will develop more slowly than other children Life expectancy now up to 60–65 years or more (with medical and other support) **Potential medical problems:** * heart defects * gut problems * thyroid gland problems * cataracts/sight problems * hearing problems * poor immune system (coughs/colds/infections) * leukaemia * Alzheimer's* **Associated learning difficulties:** * slower acquisition of communication, personal, social skills * reading, writing delayed	* medical treatments as appropriate * physiotherapy * speech therapy * occupational therapy * special educational support

* The Down's Syndrome Association note that 'the incidence of dementia in people with DS is similar to that of the general population, only it occurs 20–30 years earlier.' However, other sources stress that there is a significant connection between DS and AD.

TABLE 15.8 *Down's syndrome:key facts*

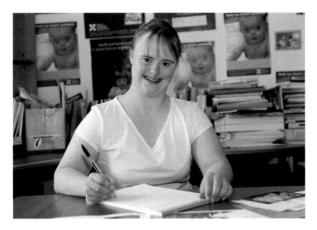

FIGURE 15.6 *Many people with Down's syndrome make a significant contribution in the workplace*

Cognitive, personal and social skills may be slower to develop, and children with DS will usually need special educational support. Support to develop life skills often continues into adulthood.

However, it has already been noted that people with DS do not see themselves as 'victims'. Rather, they see themselves as unique individuals whose development is simply different from that of people who do not have this condition. With support from groups such as Mencap, and also from developments such as the government initiative *Valuing People* (see www.valuingpeople.gov.uk), people with DS and their families now expect to enjoy a range of life and work choices. Many are in work, and are more than capable of making a contribution to society.

Progression

Down's syndrome may be regarded as 'stable but with changing needs', using the terminology of the *National Service Framework for People with Long-term Conditions*. The condition itself does not change. However, as an individual grows and develops, specific medical or other needs may occur. Although this particular National Service Framework relates specifically to people with neurological conditions, its authors make it clear that the framework and its provisions are also relevant to people with other types of long-term condition (DoH 2005).

People with DS may be more susceptible to a range of conditions, all of which are listed in Table 15.8. In later life, some may develop leukaemia, or even Alzheimer's.

Main treatments and support

There are a number of medical conditions that are more common in people with DS. Therefore, it is important for people with the condition to be screened regularly for developments such as hearing and vision problems and hypothyroidism. In addition, regular medication reviews and comprehensive medical assessments are highly desirable, together with all the usual health screening offered to the general population (such as cervical smear tests or breast screening). Preventive measures such as immunisation should also be taken.

Attention to a balanced diet and the provision of regular daily exercise is also of great importance.

Key concept

Immunisation: stimulation of the body to create antibodies to a disease, by introducing a weak or inactivated version of the disease organism.

The incidence of psychiatric problems in people with DS is the same as for the rest of the population. Some mental health practitioners are now specialising in work with people who have learning disabilities as well as psychiatric problems.

Throughout life, other developmental needs may be met in a number of ways. At times, input from practitioners such as speech or occupational therapists may be provided. Special attention is given to the educational development of children and adults with DS, both in mainstream school, special units or schools, and then later in day units, special centres or in mainstream colleges. There is now a much greater emphasis in assisting people with DS to develop to their full potential, in empowering them to make life choices, to live independently and to take paid employment if so desired. The wishes of people with DS and their families and/or carers are very important, and all decisions will involve everyone, not least the person with DS. The resources section of this unit lists a number of excellent websites which provide a good starting point to explore the issues set out in this section.

TEST STAGE	TEST TYPE
Prenatal screening	Tests offered include: Blood test (triple test) Nuchal translucency test (ultrasound) Chorionic villus sampling (CVS) (analysis of cells taken from placenta) amniocentesis (analysis of fluid from around the baby in the womb)
Postnatal diagnosis	Blood test (karyotype analysis of chromosomes)

TABLE 15.9 *Testing for Down's syndrome*

Duchenne muscular dystrophy

Description
There are a number of muscular dystrophies, all of which are caused by a faulty gene which results in a very low or absent amount of the muscle protein, dystrophin. This brings about a progressive condition in which the muscles waste, and the nervous system deteriorates.

In Duchenne muscular dystrophy (DMD), the faulty gene is passed on by the mother. It is the most common form of the condition in children and affects only males, appearing between the ages of two and six years. DMD is named after the nineteenth century French doctor, Duchenne de Boulogne, who pioneered research into the condition. (Note: In some forms of MD, the faulty gene is not inherited, but abnormality develops post-natally.)

Physical and psychological effects
The physical effects of DMD become more severe over time (see below, Progression). The main problems experienced by boys with this condition are muscle wastage and a deterioration of the nervous system. This results in increasing problems with both **gross** and **fine motor skills**.

Living with a chronic condition such as DMD is inevitably tiring and can sometimes cause depression, both for the person who has the condition and for his carer. At times, additional emotional support may be needed, together with the provision of respite care.

Progression
As DMD is a progressive disease, the effects become apparent gradually over time. A boy with DMD will gradually find it more difficult to climb stairs, or to pick himself up off the floor after a fall. Although support will be given in the form of orthoses, walking aids and wheelchairs, gradually the boy will become less mobile, and will then begin to lose upper limb function. Heart and breathing problems may become an issue, as spinal curvature may result in greater strain on internal organs, and on the body in general. Poor posture may aggravate these problems.

Main treatments and support
Medical interventions are made as problems develop, although sometimes these are preventative (as in the case of vaccination to minimise the chances of influenza) or the provision of orthoses (to minimise the development of muscle contractures).

If spinal curvature (scoliosis) becomes a problem, a decision may be made to correct

> **Key concept**
>
> *Vaccination:* the procedure by which a dead or weakened version of a disease is injected into a person, to challenge the immune system to produce antibodies to fight that particular disease.

CAUSES	SIGNS/SYMPTOMS	PROGRESSION	MAIN TREATMENTS/SUPPORT
Genetic: Mother passes on faulty gene	* muscle weakness * deformity of arms, legs and spine * muscle spasms and stiffening, weak hands, foot drop * clumsiness, frequent falls, spinal curvature, waddling gait, difficulties in walking, climbing stairs, etc.	* may need to use a wheelchair by age of 12 * breathing/heart problems in later stages * possible chest infections * weight loss and fatigue * shortened life-expectancy (late teens/early twenties)	*Medical/surgical interventions:* * surgery (spinal curvature) * gastrostomy (eating problems) * nasal ventilation (breathing problems) * orthoses (help muscle contractures) * antibiotics (chest and other infections) * steroids (slow down muscle wastage) * vaccination (against flu, pneumonia) * drug-therapy and/or pacemaker (heart problems) *Other interventions:* * physiotherapy/breathing exercises * other exercise * healthy diet * aids/adaptations * social work support * speech therapy * occupational therapy * special support at school * complementary therapy

TABLE 15.10 *Duchenne muscular dystrophy: key facts*

this surgically. If eating by mouth is difficult, a gastrostomy may be performed (insertion of a tube into the stomach). Steroids may be prescribed to slow down muscle wastage; whilst drug therapy or the insertion of a pacemaker may be used to alleviate heart problems (common in the later stages of the condition). If a boy has breathing problems, nasal ventilation may be used, often at night.

Key concept

Scoliosis: curvature of the spine.

Physiotherapy is a very important component of the care package to someone with DMD, and can help with a number of functions, including breathing and muscle flexibility. The provision of a healthy diet is vital as is a generally healthy lifestyle that includes gentle and appropriate exercise (both too much and too little exercise can be detrimental). Aids and adaptations will be necessary to meet individual needs, whilst boys of school age will require extra support at school. This might be in terms of accessibility to classrooms, toilets and other facilities, the provision of adapted IT hardware and software (as appropriate) to aid learning, and a general recognition of an individual's special learning needs. Occupational and speech therapy may be appropriate at certain stages, whilst social work support to a boy and his family will ensure a continuing appropriate package of care.

Finally, some people find that complementary therapies are helpful. Acupuncture can help with pain relief, and massage can improve circulation, alleviate tension in contracted muscles and also bring some relief from pain. Issues associated with complementary therapies are explored in AS Unit 9.

TEST TYPE	REASON
Muscle biopsy	To identify dystrophic fibres
Blood tests	To detect high levels of the enzyme creatine kinase
Electrical studies	To identify carriers
Genetic testing	Can be done either prenatally, or before conception.

TABLE 15.11 *Testing for Duchenne muscular dystrophy*

A series of very detailed fact sheets on all aspects of DMD is available from the Muscular Dystrophy Campaign website (www.muscular-dystrophy.org). This website makes an excellent starting point for further study of this condition.

Multiple sclerosis

Description
Multiple sclerosis (MS) is a neurological disorder in which the central nervous system (CNS) is damaged. A substance called myelin, which normally protects nerve fibres, is damaged or lost, and the body is unable to repair this damage. The term 'sclerosis' means 'scars', and these scars or lesions may be found both on the spinal cord and in the brain. As a result, messages from the brain to the rest of the body are impeded, leading to a number of symptoms (see Table 15.12). At present there is no cure for this condition.

> **Key concept**
>
> *Central nervous system (CNS):* the brain and spinal cord together comprise the central nervous system.

There are a number of possible causes for MS, although no specific cause has been definitively identified at present. It is possible that some people have a genetic predisposition to the condition (although it is certainly not inherited). Other research suggests that a bacterium or virus may trigger an autoimmune reaction, causing the immune system to attack the body itself. It is interesting that MS is more common in northerly countries such as Britain, the USA, Canada and Scandinavia than in countries closer to the equator. There are four types of MS:

* benign
* relapsing-remitting
* primary progressive
* secondary progressive.

Physical and psychological effects
The main potential signs and symptoms of MS are listed in Table 15.12. In reality, each individual with the condition will experience a unique combination of physical symptoms. Some people are affected very mildly, whilst others may have severe symptoms and difficulties, with drastically reduced mobility and dexterity, and severe pain.

As with any chronic condition, the long-term stresses involved in working around physical difficulties on a day-to-day basis can sometimes cause depression.

Progression
MS usually first appears between the ages of 20 and 40, although it can occur at any age. However, it is rarely seen after the age of 60, and before puberty. Women are affected more than men (the ratio is 3:2, women to men). Table 15.13 summarises progression patterns for the four types of MS.

Main treatments/support
There are a number of drug therapies available for the management of the symptoms of MS, some of which are listed in Table 15.12. However, it should

CAUSES	SIGNS/SYMPTOMS	PROGRESSION	MAIN TREATMENTS/SUPPORT
Not determined. Suspected factors: * Genetic (e.g. a specific gene combination) * Environmental (e.g. viral infection)	* fatigue * balance problems, vertigo, dizziness * visual problems * neuropathy * pain * loss of muscle strength * loss of dexterity * stiffness, spasms, weakness * incontinence * frequent urinary tract infections * anxiety, depression, mood swings * cognitive problems (e.g. concentration) * speech problems	Varies individually. Onset may be gradual. Remissions may be long initially.	Drug therapies to reduce relapses: * interferon beta, glatimer acetate Drug therapies to ease symptoms: * iummunoglobin, steroids, amantadine, tizanidine, baclofen, gabapentin Other treatments/support: * multidisciplinary care from MS nurse, physiotherapist, occupational therapist, continence advisers, dieticians, psychologist * nutritional therapy * other CAMs New developments: * stem cell treatment (current research)

TABLE 15.12 *Multiple sclerosis: key facts*

TYPE OF MS	PROGRESSION PATTERN
Benign	Mild episodes; full recovery.
Primary progressive	Gradual progression of symptoms over time.
Relapsing-remitting	Episodes of MS symptoms followed by recovery (remission). Unpredictable, and symptoms can be mild or severe.
Secondary progressive	May develop from relapsing-remitting MS. Severity of attacks may worsen, or deterioration may be steady.

TABLE 15.13 *Progression in MS*

be noted that some of these are still considered to require further research. The therapy chosen will vary according to the type of MS, and the patient's personal circumstances. Some people with MS take no medication at all. Appropriate treatment should be chosen in conjunction between the patient and the neurologist. Physiotherapy is sometimes used to help manage problems of mobility, posture, fatigue and balance. Other specialists who may help an MS patient to manage his or her condition include the specialist MS nurse, occupational therapists, continence advisers, dieticians and psychologists.

Many people with MS use complementary therapies (CAMs) to alleviate their symptoms. The National Institute for Health and Clincial Excellence has published guidelines on the management of MS (NICE 2003). This includes the recommendation that certain CAMs may be helpful to people with the condition, although the guidance also note that there is currently 'insufficient evidence to give more firm recommendation'. The MS Society also notes a number of complementary therapies that have been found to be useful by people with the condition. However, it is important to note that it is vital to check out any complementary therapy thoroughly before committing to treatment, as there are a

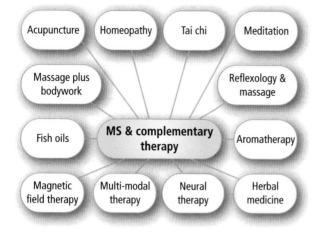

FIGURE 15.7 *Some useful therapies in MS*

number of unscrupulous people masquerading as *bone fide* practitioners, and some treatments which are not properly researched. There are a number of excellent guides to choosing and using complementary therapies, three of which are listed in the resources section of this unit (Barnett 2002, Pinder (ed.) 2005, Zollman and Vickers 2000).

Did you know?

Nutritional therapy involves eliminating foods to which the body is intolerant, and then taking supplements to aid healing or to help manage symptoms.

Find out more by accessing the website of the British Association for Nutritional Therapy (www. bant.org.uk).

Osteoarthritis

Description

'Arthritis' is a general term referring to inflammation in the joints. There are a number of different kinds of arthritis, of which osteoarthritis is the most common.

In this condition (which affects only the moving joints), cartilage deterioration causes the bones within the joints to rub together. This in turn results in pain and swelling. Bone cells may regrow unevenly and cracks may develop in some parts of the joint, whilst knobbly bone growths may appear elsewhere. The synovial membrane which lines the capsule (the tissue that surrounds the joint) will

TEST TYPE	SIGNIFICANCE
Discussion of symptoms	
Testing bodily reactions	Movement, reflexes, balance, co-ordination, speech etc.
MRI scan (magnetic resonance imaging)	To detect lesions to brain and spinal cord
Visual Evoked Potential Test	Electrodes placed on scalp; measure speed of conductivity of message from brain
Blood tests	To reveal antibodies
Lumbar puncture	Analysis of spinal cord fluid, for antibodies
Inner ear tests	To check balance

TABLE 15.14 *Diagnosing multiple sclerosis*

become inflamed. Finally, all these developments may cause the misalignment of the joint. The parts of the body most commonly affected by arthritis are the knees and hips, hands and spine. Osteoarthritis is frequently diagnosed in people aged 40–60, and becomes progressively more common thereafter.

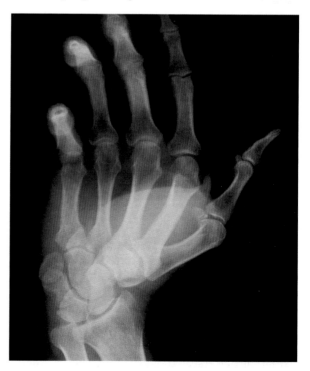

FIGURE 15.8 *X-ray of an osteoarthritic joint*

CAUSES	SIGNS/SYMPTOMS	PROGRESSION	MAIN TREATMENTS/SUPPORT
Not known. Genetics and lifestyle currently being researched. Risk factors: * age * gender * obesity * physical stress at work * previous damage (e.g. sport, accident)	Affects joints only: * pain * stiffness * swollen and/or knobbly joints * joint instability * muscle weakness Can lead to: * mobility problems (gross motor skills) * problems using hands (fine motor skills)	May gradually worsen with age, wear and tear. If associated with heart disease, or other chronic condition, symptoms may worsen However, some people do lose symptoms over time.	* paracetamol * creams and gels * NSAIDs (e.g. Ibuprofen) * Cox II selective inhibitors * knee and hip replacement (arthroplasty) * injection to knee joint (steroids, hyaluronic acid) * osteotomy (removal of bone) * diet * supplements (glucosamine, fish oil) * physical aids (shoe wedges, sticks, etc.)

TABLE 15.15 *Osteoarthritis: key facts*

Physical and psychological effects

Depending on the severity of their condition, people with osteoarthritis may experience problems with both fine and gross motor abilities.

> ### Key concepts
>
> *Fine motor ability:* the ability to co-ordinate the movement of the fingers in detailed activities such as writing, painting, cooking, etc.
>
> *Gross motor ability:* the ability to co-ordinate the larger muscles in activities such as walking, climbing stairs etc.

They may not be able to walk very far unaided, or to climb stairs. They may have problems with personal tasks such as bathing, washing hair or dressing; even eating can be a problem if the joints in the hands are painful or swollen.

Unlike other forms of arthritis, osteoarthritis affects only the joints. However the constant strain of living with pain, stiffness and physical disability can sometimes cause depression. Similarly, if someone is unable to go out to visit friends or take part in social activities, a feeling of social isolation may result.

Progression

The symptoms of osteoarthritis may get worse over time, although with good management (such as weight reduction, appropriate diet and exercise) their severity may be controlled. If someone has another chronic condition (such as heart disease) which further reduces mobility, then the likelihood that osteoarthritis symptoms will become more severe increases.

According to information published by the British Medical Journal on the Best Treatments website, for some people symptoms actually get better over time (see www.besttreatment.co.uk).

Main treatments/support

As with many chronic conditions, a strategy (or combination of treatments) is probably the most effective way of managing symptoms. Pain can be controlled by a number of medications, some of which are available without prescription (e.g. paracetamol). Doctors will usually recommend that a person with mild symptoms uses paracetamol or a non-steroidal anti-inflammatory drug (NSAID) such as Ibuprofen. Stronger drugs, known as Cox II Selective Inhibitors, may be used, although these sometimes have unpleasant side-effects. Topical treatments, such as creams or gels, are also used to control pain or swelling.

> ### Key concept
>
> *Topical treatment:* a treatment that is applied to the body at the site of the problem, e.g. a cream or gel.

For severe pain, cortocosteriods or hyaluronic acid may be injected into the joint. In extreme cases, surgery may be recommended. Knees or hips may be replaced (arthroplasty), or bone in the knee may be removed (osteotomy).

Exercise is generally recommended for the maintenance of joint flexibility, and the prevention of muscle atrophy. Swimming and cycling are considered helpful. Specific exercises, designed in conjunction with a physiotherapist, can be used to target and strengthen certain muscles. Sometimes, specific exercises are recommended in conjunction with other physical therapies such as warm baths or spas, and special packs to warm the joints. Sometimes, cold sprays or ice packs are used to reduce soreness. Physical aids to reduce pain and aid movement are set out in Figure 15.9.

A balanced diet to prevent weight gain can alleviate the pressure on weight-bearing joints. Some nutritional experts recommend that people with osteoarthritis should avoid food from the deadly nightshade group of plants (potatoes, tomatoes, aubergines and peppers) as these can exacerbate symptoms. Supplements, such as glucosamine and fish oils, have also proved effective in some cases, although research into the effectiveness of such products is ongoing.

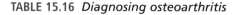

TEST TYPE	SIGNIFICANCE
Check on symptoms	Joint pain/stiffness Mobility/movement problems Other physical problems
Check on joints	Movement/size/shape X-ray data
Blood tests	To eliminate similar conditions
Joint fluid analysis	White blood cell count/crystals
Case history	Previous damage/work history/infections/ other family members

TABLE 15.16 *Diagnosing osteoarthritis*

> ## SCENARIO
> ## Joe needs help
>
> Joe is 70 and has osteoarthritis. He lives on his own, as his wife passed away two years ago.
>
> He has difficulties in using his hands, and is now experiencing walking difficulties. He also finds it hard to get in and out of the bath. Furthermore, the pain in his right hip is becoming more severe.
>
> 1. What further medical treatment might the doctor now suggest for Joe?
>
> 2. What else might be done to make Joe's situation easier?

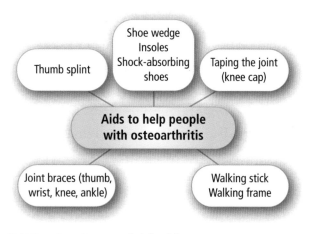

FIGURE 15.9 *Osteoarthritis aids*

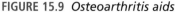

Spina bifida

Description

A person with spina bifida is born with a fault on the spine. The term actually means 'split spine', and in this condition one or more of the vertebrae (the small bones which form the backbone) do not close fully around the spinal cord, leaving the nerves within the spine unprotected. This fault is most common around waist level.

> **Key concept**
>
> *Hydrocephalus:* an accumulation of cerebrospinal fluid around the brain.

There are, in fact, three types of spina bifida (SB). Firstly, there is SB occulta (hidden form), which is both very mild and very common. In this form, the spinal cord is undamaged, and there are few consequences for the patient. The other two types of SB (SB cystica) are meningocele and myelomeningocele, both of which involve the presence of a cyst on the spine. In meningocele, the fluid in the cyst actually protects the spinal cord, and there is little disability as a result. Myelomeningocele is much more serious, as the cyst contains nerves and part of the spinal cord, which is thus damaged. It is this form of the condition which results in the greatest disability.

Some people born with SB also have hydrocephalus, an accumulation of cerebrospinal fluid (CSF) around the brain. Hydrocephalus can also occur in older children and adults. Hydrocephalus brings with it a number of difficulties, some of which can be disabling. ASBAH, the national association for people with SB in the UK, considers that as a neurological condition, SB is best defined as 'stable but with changing needs'. This is one of four definitions of types of neurological condition for people with chronic illness set out in the *National Service Framework for Long-term Conditions* (DoH 2005).

Physical and psychological effects

People with SB usually experience problems with balance and walking, and some need to use a wheelchair. Sometimes, people have problems with bladder and bowel control. Hydrocephalus may exacerbate problems with co-ordination of movements, particularly fine motor movements (i.e. using fingers and hands). Pressure on the brain may affect concentration, reasoning and learning ability, whilst pressure on the optic nerve may affect vision. There may sometimes be problems with breathing, speaking or swallowing.

CAUSES	SIGNS/SYMPTOMS	PROGRESSION	MAIN TREATMENTS/SUPPORT
Exact cause currently unknown: genetic and environmental factors likely to be involved	* paralysis, loss of sensation below point of damage to spine * bowel, bladder problems An associated condition may be hydrocephalus, which can affect: * co-ordination * concentration, reasoning, learning * vision * breathing, speaking, swallowing	'Stable, but with changing needs' (ASBAH) Ageing can bring associated problems, in particular: * weight gain * pressure sores * blood pressure problems * reduced mobility	* early surgery to repair defect to spine * shunt to control CSF * physiotherapy * urinary catheter * physiotherapy * special teaching for children * emotional support

TABLE 15.17 *Spina bifida: key facts*

Living with a physical disability can sometimes be very tiring, and many people who are in this situation may experience depression. This can be the same for carers of people with a long-term condition. Many people in these circumstances require additional emotional support from time to time.

Progression

It was noted above that SB can be described as a condition which is 'stable but with changing needs'. Clearly, an individual's needs change at each stage of life. For example, children with SB may require additional teaching support, especially if their condition is associated with hydrocephalus. Young adults may require additional physical and emotional support if they decide to live independently, or to go to college or university.

Medically, adults with SB may develop hydrocephalus, which may bring associated symptoms and disabilities (see above). As the body ages, people may experience weight gain (due to relative physical inactivity), pressure sores, blood pressure problems and reduced mobility.

Main treatments

For a serious spinal defect, surgery is usually performed shortly after birth to repair as much damage as possible. If hydrocephalus is present, the CSF will be drained surgically. For children and adults, physiotherapy is used to maximise mobility. A 'shunt' can be used to reduce levels of CSF. People with difficulties in passing urine may use a catheter regularly.

Visit ASBAH for detailed information on the nature of spina bifida, how it is treated and managed, and for some inspiring case studies about people who are living with the condition (www.asbah.org).

Disability conditions: detection and prevention

Advances in science now make it possible for the likelihood of the transmission of genetic abnormalities (from parents or grandparents to children) to be predicted. In other instances, the existence of genetic abnormalities can be detected whilst a child is still in the womb. Whilst these advances make it possible for people to avoid having a disabled child, they can also bring ethical dilemmas.

Genetic counselling is available for couples who are likely to be at risk of having children with genetic or chromosomal disorders. If there is a family history of, for example, Duchenne muscular dystrophy, couples may opt for genetic counselling (to assess the potential risk to themselves of having a child with the condition) before deciding to have a child (or more children). A radical way of preventing the conception of children with genetic problems is for a woman to be sterilised; whilst some couples may opt to abort a foetus if a disorder is detected by an antenatal test.

A more complex and expensive option is egg-screening, whereby a woman's eggs are removed and tested, those with genetic abnormalities are rejected, and the remaining eggs are artificially fertilised and re-implanted into the woman. All of these options have associated practical and ethical difficulties, as set out in Table 15.19.

As this table shows, knowledge often brings with it the need to make difficult decisions, and many people find themselves in the position of having to consider where they stand in relation to some very big issues. It would be a good idea for you to take some time to think through your own position on some of the issues highlighted in the summary of this section.

TESTING FOR SPINA BIFIDA	REDUCING THE INCIDENCE OF SPINA BIFIDA
* antenatal blood test (for faulty LPP1 gene) * ultrasound scans	* folic acid supplements before and during pregnancy * diet rich in natural folic acid during pregnancy * screening for people who already have a child with SB, or who have SB themselves

TABLE 15.18 *Spina bifida: reducing the risk*

	PRACTICAL CONSIDERATIONS	ETHICAL CONSIDERATIONS
Genetic counselling	* some conditions are not detectable until after a child is born * screening is expensive	* people may still choose to be parents, despite the risks * people with impairments have as much right to live as other people
Sterilisation	* difficult to reverse	
Abortion	* it may be hard to be sure that a disability condition is really present	* a foetus has a right to life * potential emotional harm to parents * some religious objections
Egg-screening	* expensive * time-consuming	* some religious objections * could be regarded as 'genetic engineering': people with impairments have as much right to life as others

TABLE 15.19 *Prevention and detection of disability conditions: some practical and ethical considerations*

Summary

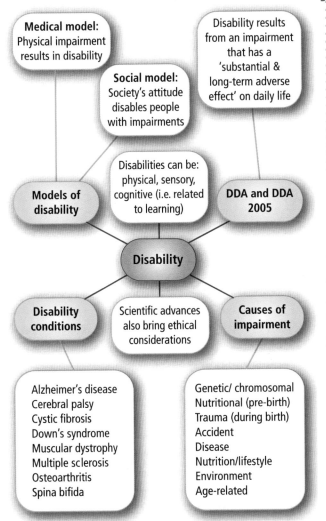

Medical model: Physical impairment results in disability

Social model: Society's attitude disables people with impairments

Disability results from an impairment that has a 'substantial & long-term adverse effect' on daily life

Disabilities can be: physical, sensory, cognitive (i.e. related to learning)

Models of disability

DDA and DDA 2005

Disability

Disability conditions

Scientific advances also bring ethical considerations

Causes of impairment

Alzheimer's disease
Cerebral palsy
Cystic fibrosis
Down's syndrome
Muscular dystrophy
Multiple sclerosis
Osteoarthritis
Spina bifida

Genetic/ chromosomal
Nutritional (pre-birth)
Trauma (during birth)
Accident
Disease
Nutrition/lifestyle
Environment
Age-related

Consider this

A hard decision

Stacey and Tim want to have children, but there is someone in Tim's family with cystic fibrosis. They are worried that if they conceive, their child might have this condition.

1. What options are open to them?

2. What personal and ethical questions may need to be resolved by couples in Stacey and Tim's situation?

15.4 Practitioners and provision

The current emphasis on the provision of care to people who need services is that this should be *multi-disciplinary* in nature. This means that professionals from all disciplines should work together to provide 'joined-up' services tailored to meet individual needs. There is also now a *mixed economy of care*, whereby services can be provided to one person from a number of different sources and suppliers (see Criteria for assessing needs and eligibility, page 169).

Mixed economy of care: the notion that care can be provided by a range of different service providers including statutory providers (e.g. NHS), voluntary and charitable organisations (e.g. Mencap) and private, profit-making businesses (e.g. BUPA).

Multi-disciplinary working: the practice whereby professionals from different disciplines work together to provide care to individuals and/or groups.

Health, social care and other practitioners

You should always check your local situation with regard to services provided for disabled people; remember, too, that the ways in which services are provided are reviewed and reorganised periodically. It is a good idea to check the current situation at the time you are conducting your studies. Figure 15.10 shows the people who might give support at the time of writing.

Children's Trusts are coming into being (2006) and all areas should have such Trusts by 2008. Local authorities must take the lead, in collaboration with local Health Authorities and Primary Care Trusts. The idea is to provide strong partnership arrangements between bodies providing services to children. Each area will design its own unique local arrangements, so Children's Trusts will not all be exactly the same.

Table 15.20 gives a general indication of where key health professionals work and who supplies their services. However, in practice you may find some different arrangements from those listed here. Services delivered 'in the community' are those delivered outside hospital or residential settings. These may include GP surgeries and health centres, people's homes, day units, private clinics etc.

What's available where you live?

Do some research to find out what's available for people with disabilities in your area. Remember to check out:

Council Services (e.g. 'Social Services', Adult Community Care, Children's Services Authority/ Children's Trusts)

Other Council services (e.g. housing, education)

Health services (including hospital-based, and those provided in the community by the local Primary Care Trusts (PCTs))

Services provided by charities/ voluntary organisations (e.g. MENCAP, Scope, etc.)

Other service providers (e.g. Connexions, Jobcentre Plus, Benefits Agency)

Private service providers.

Remember that services for children are currently (2006) being reorganised into Children's Services Authorities. This will be a gradual process, and some authorities may continue to use the older terms for services (e.g. Social Services) for some time.

1. Are there any examples of services being provided from a multi-disciplinary team?

2. What evidence for a 'mixed economy of care' can you find in your locality?

3. Did you find any professionals working in unusual settings (e.g. a physiotherapist working with people with learning difficulties)?

Support from carers

Sometimes, a disabled person may rely heavily on another person for his or her care. This person is usually known as the carer, and may be responsible for a range of caring responsibilities, including providing physical, emotional and social care and support. The carer is often a close relative, sometimes a friend or neighbour.

Even when carers are devoted to their relatives or friends, the stress put onto them can be very great. People with dementia, for example, may forget where they are, or even the names of people close to them. They may ask the same questions repeatedly, or get lost when they go out.

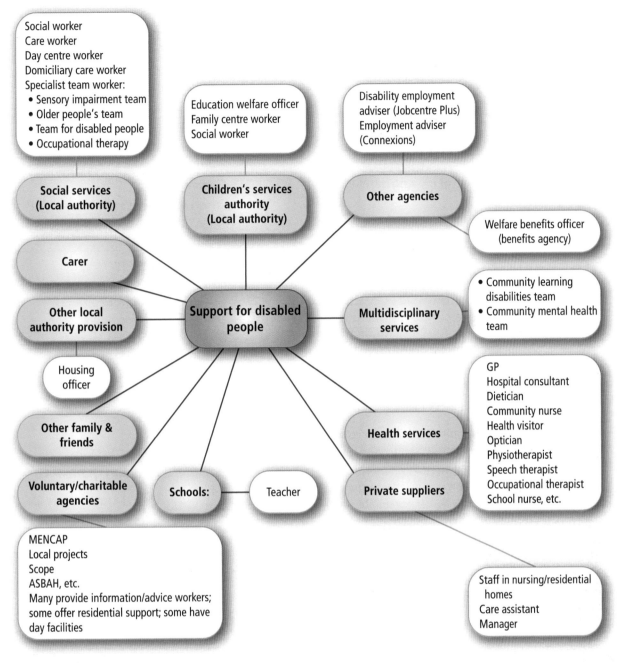

FIGURE 15.10 *Sources of support for disabled people*

In the last ten years, carers from all over the UK have been working together to gain recognition and support for the work that they do. In 1999, the Government published a *National Strategy for Carers*, acknowledging their value and recognising their needs (DoH 1999). Many authorities now have a Carers' Charter, setting out the rights that

TITLE	ROLE	LOCATION/TYPE OF ORGANISATION
GP	Assessment, advice on and treatment of illness and medical conditions.	*Community* NHS
Specialist consultant	Assessment, advice on and treatment of illness and medical conditions.	*Hospital, private practice* NHS or private.
Nursing staff	General nursing care.	*Hospital or community* NHS/private/charitable and voluntary.
Community nursing staff: district nurse, health visitor	General nursing care/advice.	*Community* Often in patient's own home, GP surgeries, health centres. NHS
Dietician	Advice on nutrition to maximise health and wellbeing.	*Hospital, community.* NHS, some private.
Physiotherapist	Physiotherapists work to maximise movement potential through a range of approaches and methods. Direct treatment includes manual therapy, exercise and electrophysical treatments.	*Hospital, community, private practice, patient's home* NHS/private/charitable and voluntary organisations.
Occupational therapist	Assessment/treatment of physical, psychological or social problems using specific, purposeful activity to prevent disability and/or promote independent function in daily life.	*Hospital or community* NHS or private.
Speech therapist	Assessment/treatment for people with speech, language and communication problems (e.g. people who have had a stroke).	*Hospital, community, patient's own home* NHS or private
Continence adviser	Information and practical help for people with incontinence problems.	*Hospital or community* NHS
Complementary therapists	Therapy via art, drama, acupuncture, homeopathy, osteopathy, etc.	*Hospital or community* NHS or private
Care manager	A social worker who has the designated role of assessing need and producing a care plan. The care manager will also ensure that services are provided according to the care plan, and will monitor and evaluate service provision and the effectiveness of the plan.	*Hospital or community* Local authority Note: Some social work teams may be hospital-based.
Social worker	Assessment of and planning to meet need.	*Hospital or community* Local authority, also private agencies, some charities also employ social workers.
Specialist social worker	As for social worker, but with a specialist responsibility (e.g. older people, disabled people).	As for social worker. *continued on next page*

TITLE	ROLE	LOCATION/TYPE OF ORGANISATION
Care worker	Provides daily physical care, often in a residential or a day care setting. Also gives support for intellectual, emotional and/or social needs.	*Residential and/or day care settings* Local authority, voluntary or charitable organisations, some agency workers (private).
Home help (domiciliary care worker)	Practical support to someone in his or her own home. May include help with personal tasks such as washing, shaving, bathing, etc.	*Service user's own home* Often supplied by private companies or agencies.
Day centre worker/support worker	Support to users of day facilities. Such staff may have a range of job titles. Support can be practical; can also include support with intellectual, emotional and social needs.	*Day care centres or units often in community, but can be attached to hospitals* NHS/ local authority/ charitable/ voluntary organisations.
Housing officer	Advice and some practical support to tenants of local authority or housing association premises.	*Community* Local authority, housing association, charitable/voluntary organisations.
Teacher	Although their main role is to educate, teachers are often concerned with the well-being of their pupils in other ways. Specialist teachers (e.g. for deaf students) will give expert support to a student's cognitive development.	*In schools* Local education authority, charitable/voluntary organisations, private and/or special schools.
Education welfare officer	Performs social work–type role to children in schools.	*Schools and elsewhere in the community* Local education authority

Note: This table gives a general indication of where key health professionals work and who supplies their services. However, in practice there may be some unusual or different arrangements from those listed here. Services delivered in the community are those delivered outside hospital or residential settings. These may include GP surgeries and health centres, peoples' homes etc.

TABLE 15.20 *Support for disabled people: job roles*

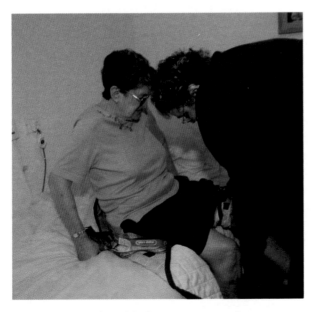

FIGURE 15.11 *A disabled person may rely on another person for his or her care*

carers have. These rights include being consulted and involved at every stage of service planning and delivery, and also having their own needs addressed.

TYPE OF PROVISION	ADVANTAGE	LIMITATIONS
Home care	Helps to maintain independence in own home.	May be costly to service user (means tested).
Day care	Provides social, emotional and intellectual support to service user. Provides respite for carer.	May not be available as often as user wishes, or in a convenient locality. May be costly to service user.
Respite care	Provides respite support for carer.	Service user may not be happy in respite facility, even for a short time.
Residential/nursing home care	Provides secure environment; guaranteed physical comfort, plus some intellectual, emotional and social support.	Independence may be compromised. May be costly to service user.
Special schools	Provides education geared to particular needs of students (e.g. deaf teachers working with deaf students).	May isolate students from the community. May be costly to run.
Special educational units in mainstream schools	Students have benefits of both types of education; students don't become isolated from their peers.	Students may be stigmatised by mainstream students (if not managed properly).
Welfare benefits	Provides financial assistance.	System is complex, some benefits are means tested. Receipt of benefit restricts a person's freedom to work.
Independent Living Funds (ILF)	Government funds providing payments to severely disabled people for specific purposes.	Limited to personal and/or domestic care. Many other services cannot be paid for from these funds.
Direct payments	Cash payments from Department of Health to allow eligible individuals to purchase the care they need. Can tailor-make own packages of care.	System is still not running smoothly (2005). Lack of information, bureaucracy, paperwork, reluctance of professionals to hand over such control to disabled people (CSCI 2004).
Disabled Services and Financial Services Teams (DSFST) (formerly PACT Teams). Schemes include: ✳ Access to Work ✳ Work Preparation ✳ WORKSTEP ✳ Job Introduction Scheme ✳ New Deal for Disabled People (NDDP)	Available via Jobcentre Plus: Advice and information on gaining employment, or remaining in employment after onset of a disability. Access to training/education. Personal support from Disability employment advisers (DEA)	Some schemes have specific eligibility criteria. Some disabled people are concerned they will lose benefit, especially if employment does not work out.

TABLE 15.21 *Provision for disabled people: advantages and limitations*

Criteria for assessing needs and eligibility

The process of assessing need in social and health care is currently very well defined in government policy and guidance. This guidance is associated with several key Acts of Parliament which give a framework to the help and services that people are entitled to receive.

Section 29 of the National Assistance Act (1948) states that 'local authorities have responsibilities and duties to promote the welfare of people with sensory, physical or mental difficulties'. Local authorities must do this by making accurate assessments of people's needs. The 1986 Disabled Persons Act stated that if a disabled person, or his or her representative, were to ask for an assessment, the local authority has a duty to carry it out. This legislation was strengthened by the NHS and Community Care Act 1990, which says that if a person is disabled, he or she has an automatic right to an assessment and should be informed of this.

Both the law and associated guidance make it clear that the three areas to be assessed are need, risk and services. The resulting decisions are to be set out in the form of a **care plan.** Such care plans must record:

* the objectives to be met for the service user
* how this is going to be achieved (the implementation plan)
* what to do if things do not go according to plan (contingency arrangements)
* how unmet needs will be identified and taken into account.

Separate legislation and guidance covers children with special educational needs (see page 170). This system is dependent upon good quality assessments of need and risk. Local authorities have rules that set out how money and resources should be allocated to people with additional needs. Such rules are called **eligibility criteria.**

Basically, the more disabled a person is, the greater is his or her entitlement to receive all the services needed. In 2003, the government introduced *Fair Access to Care Services* (FACS),

Key concepts

Care plan: a formal document that sets out everything that needs to be done to meet someone's needs. This document sets out the objectives or goals of the plan, together with the services that will be provided to meet these objectives.

Eligibility criteria: the rules that explain a person's entitlement to receive services. The greater a person's needs and threats to independence, the greater is their entitlement to receive services.

a system that sets out four categories of eligibility for services: critical, substantial, moderate and low (DoH 2003).

SCENARIO

Help in taking a bath

Mrs Green is 68 and lives with her husband. She has severe arthritis, which means that although she can manage to give herself a wash, she cannot get into the bath.

She is able to perform all other personal care tasks, but unless she receives some help she will have to give up taking baths. However, her hygiene and health are not at risk.

Although Mrs Green is fairly low risk in terms of the FACS eligibility criteria, it is clear she could be helped by the provision of specialist equipment. In her case, an assessment would be carried out (probably by an occupational therapist or a physiotherapist from an Older Person's Team), and it is likely that a bath hoist would be ordered and installed. The assessment would also probably include Mrs Green's ability to perform household tasks, to walk and to travel (e.g. on public transport). After six weeks, the care manager allocated to support Mrs Green would check whether or not the hoist had been installed, and if she was able to use it safely and with confidence.

If Mrs Green was found to have any further needs, these would then be built into a revised care plan. The local authority would keep an eye on her at least every 12 months to see if either she or Mr Green had any further requirements.

Children with special educational needs (SEN)

Part 4 of the Education Act (1996) made provision for the educational needs of children with disabilities, including identification, assessment and recording of these needs, and then meeting and reviewing them. If a child has a Statement of Special Educational Needs, this gives him or her a legal right to have these needs met.

In 2001, the Special Educational Needs and Disability Act amended both the 1996 Education Act and the 1995 Disability discrimination Act, recognising the importance of education to disabled children (and adults). This new legislation enhances the rights of parents to ask for a place at a mainstream school if their children have statements of special educational needs.

Up to the age of 19, a child has special educational needs if she or he has learning difficulties and needs special help. A Practical Guide for Disabled People and Carers (DoH 2003) states a child has learning difficulties if:

* he or she has 'significantly greater difficulty in learning than most children of the same age' or

* 'has a disability that stops or hinders him or her from using educational facilities of a kind provided for children of the same age in schools within the local authority's area'.

The process of making this assessment of special educational needs is often referred to as **statementing,** and documents such as care plans often make reference to **statemented children.**

The care management process

It is the local council's responsibility to establish its own detailed eligibility criteria, in order to determine whether a person's level of need is critical, substantial, moderate or low. This stage of assessment has to be made first, in order to work

> ### Key concepts
>
> *Statementing:* the process of making an assessment of Special Educational Needs for a child, under the provisions of legislation.
>
> *Statemented child:* a child who has had a Statement of Special Educational Needs made about him or her.

out how complex the next level of assessment has to be. The *Fair Access to Care Services* (DoH 2003) identifies four types of assessment:

* initial assessments

* assessments to take stock of wider needs

* specialist assessments

* comprehensive assessments.

In the case of Mrs Green (see above), the council may have decided just to do a specialist assessment, focusing on her physical disabilities and the needs arising from these.

However, individual needs can be very complex, extending beyond physical issues and difficulties. A good assessment will also take into account a person's intellectual, emotional and social needs (see below, Life quality factors and principles, page 172).

In addition to the FACS guidance, there is also government guidance on care planning for older people, for children, for people with learning difficulties and for people with long-term conditions.

The *National Service Framework for Long-term Conditions* (DoH 2005) says that provision of a person-centred service is an essential quality requirement. Although this document focuses mainly on people with neurological conditions, its recommendations are universally applicable to anyone with a long-term condition. The concept of a person-centred care is also found in the *National Service Framework for Older People* (DoH 2001), and in the *Valuing People* (see www.valuingpeople.gov.uk) recommendations for planning services for people with learning disabilities. The care management process is a cyclical one, as Figure 15.13 shows.

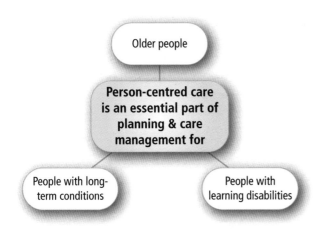

FIGURE 15.12 *Person-centred care*

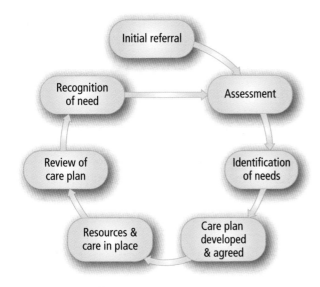

FIGURE 15.13 *The care management process*

You are not required to have an in-depth knowledge of the care management process in order to satisfy the requirements of this unit. However, it is important to recognise that any treatment or intervention designed to satisfy the needs of a disabled person must be carefully planned (in consultation with everyone concerned, including the disabled person, his or her carer(s) and all relevant professionals or staff). A detailed care plan must then be made, which should be monitored regularly to ensure that everything is being done according to the plan and that things are working out satisfactorily. Finally, the plan should be evaluated, and either new provisions made, or existing interventions should be continued or discontinued, according

to the changing needs of the disabled person concerned.

SCENARIO

Checking things out

Vikram is the care manager for Stella, who has learning difficulties. After consultation, a care plan has been devised, whereby (among other things) Stella works for three hours every Friday in the local charity shop.

On the first day of this arrangement, Vikram phones the Transport Section of the council to make quite sure that the coach will pick Stella up and take her to the charity shop. At the end of the first day, he calls the shop manager to check on the day's events. The shop manager knows that she must ring Vikram every week for the first few weeks so that they can discuss Stella's progress and any problems she may have.

Vikram will also make sure that Stella is asked how she feels about working in the shop, and he arranges to see her after the first day and then at monthly intervals (unless a problem arises, in which case he will see her straight away).

A full review and evaluation of Stella's situation at the shop will take place after six weeks.

When evaluating a care plan or intervention it is vital that a balanced view is taken. In the above scenario, for example, after thinking it over and discussing it with others, including Stella,

Vikram may decide that some things might have been done better, as well as identifying things that might have gone very well. This process of thinking about something is also known as **reflection.** It is impossible to evaluate something without spending some time reflecting on it.

> **Key concept**
>
> *Reflection:* the act of thinking about something objectively.

When Vikram spoke to Stella and the shop manager, he discovered that Stella was very worried about handling money, although the other shop assistants knew that she needed help with this, and she was never left alone to deal with payments. It was decided (with her agreement) that Stella would be given some additional money-skills training at the day unit. Until she felt more at ease about handling money, she would work mainly in the stockroom as she enjoyed cleaning and sorting the clothes and other goods, and felt very confident about doing this kind of work. These changes to the way the care plan was implemented were possible because Vikram monitored the situation carefully, and engaged everyone in meaningful evaluation of how things were developing.

Life quality factors and principles

Making a care plan and providing services to a disabled person involves much more than seeking to meet his or her immediate physical, sensory or cognitive needs. Consider the scenario opposite.

Esther does not simply have physical needs, although these are currently considerable, as she is unable to walk unaided. However, because she has lost self-esteem and is no longer able to go out with her friends, she is currently lacking the social and emotional support that she would enjoy from group membership. She lacks stimulation, in that she is unable to go to the theatre, or even to read. Esther therefore has needs which are physical, intellectual, emotional and social. These four

broad categories can be usefully remembered with the acronym P-I-E-S. Any assessment of need for a disabled person should take all of these four areas into account (see Figure 15.14).

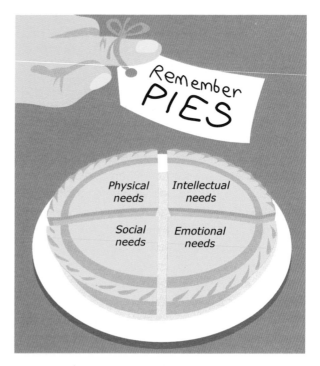

FIGURE 15.14 *P-I-E-S categories*

The concept of person-centred care was introduced in Unit 11 (page 25). As the name suggests, this concept emphasises that the person should be at the very centre of all planning activity and that all kinds of need should be addressed (not simply physical needs). The *Valuing People* (see www.valuingpeople.gov.uk) initiative, for people with learning disabilities, takes the concept even further in that it stresses that service users should be helped to make a contribution to and have a place in the community, and also to get what they want out of life. *Valuing People* refers to this as Person Centred Planning (PCP). It embodies many excellent principles that are equally important for people with all kinds of disability.

In Unit 1, Effective Caring, the concept of life quality factors was discussed. These principles need to be adhered to when planning an intervention on behalf of a disabled person, as this contributes to the goal of achieving a person-centred approach to care. The care value base that was devised in 1982 provides guidelines for professionals to ensure that appropriate services are delivered, and that individual needs and preferences are taken into account. The care value base affects the following three main areas:

❋ fostering equality and diversity

❋ fostering people's rights and responsibilities

❋ maintaining confidentiality of information.

Figures 15.15 and 15.16 set out the main psychological and physical life quality factors. These represent needs that any person-centred care plan should seek to address.

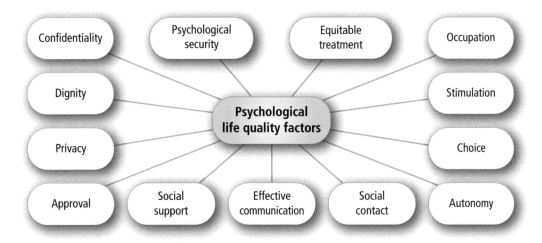

FIGURE 15.15 *Psychological factors that affect the quality of life*

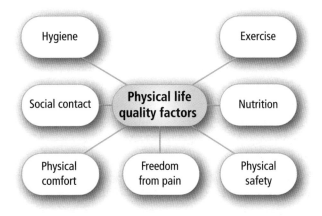

FIGURE 15.16 *Physical factors that affect the quality of life*

Summary

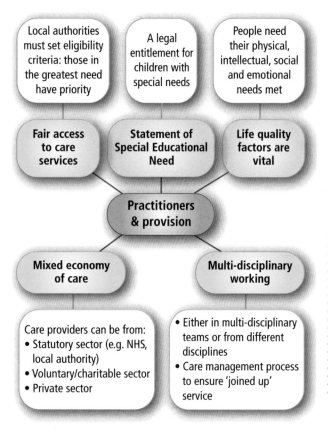

- Local authorities must set eligibility criteria: those in the greatest need have priority
- A legal entitlement for children with special needs
- People need their physical, intellectual, social and emotional needs met

- Fair access to care services
- Statement of Special Educational Need
- Life quality factors are vital

Practitioners & provision

- Mixed economy of care
- Multi-disciplinary working

- Care providers can be from:
  - Statutory sector (e.g. NHS, local authority)
  - Voluntary/charitable sector
  - Private sector

- Either in multi-disciplinary teams or from different disciplines
- Care management process to ensure 'joined up' service

Consider this

Preparing for life at home

Peter is 37 and has lost his sight in an accident. Having spent some time in hospital, he has recovered enough for plans to be made for him to go home. However, he is no longer able to do his old job because of his loss of sight.

1. What kinds of need is Peter likely to have?

2. Which professionals are likely to be involved in Peter's Care Plan?

3. What kinds of service and support might Peter need, and who might supply these services?

15.5 Barriers

Barriers to education

The following scenario is based on a real experience.

This story describes how Martin was allowed to go to the school of his choice only after key

SCENARIO

Going to the school of my choice

Martin, who has mild learning disabilities, was in a mainstream primary school, but it was time for him to leave. His mother, Margaret, wanted him to go to a mainstream secondary school.

She knew that Martin's school reports were full of 'labels' about what he could not do, and also about behavioural issues. She decided that she wanted the new school to see who Martin really was, so she sent this school a copy of Martin's personal development plan (see page 170) and a video of him.

The head teacher of the secondary school told Margaret that if he had just seen the primary school's report, without the plan and video, he would not have believed that Martin could go to a mainstream school (Sanderson *et al* 2002).

decision-makers (including the head teacher) had been shown the video that Martin had made about himself. In this video, Martin was able to present himself fully and in his own way, as someone with capabilities and who could make a contribution to the school. If he had not been helped to prove otherwise, a decision would have been made based on the forms and reports on Martin that said he should not have a place in a mainstream school. The educational system itself very nearly acted as a barrier to Martin's progress. This story provides another illustration of the social model of disability. It was not the case that Martin could not make the most of the experience of going to a specific school: rather, the assumption was made automatically that this was not the right place for him, simply because he had a learning difficulty.

Students with disabilities may opt to go to a specialist school. Some parents of deaf children, for example, feel very strongly that they will do better in an environment where the use of signing is the preferred method of communication (see page 182). The point is that everyone is entitled to the education of choice, and that no assumptions should be made about what someone might want.

Getting to the preferred school or college is not the only barrier faced by students with disabilities. Some educational establishments still have a long way to go before all students have easy access to every aspect of educational life. However, since 1995 developments in legislation have improved the rights of both children and adults with special needs (see Legislation, page 182, and Children with Special Educational Needs, page 170).

Barriers to employment

Sometimes, people with disabilities are prevented from gaining paid work because of the attitudes of potential employers. Employers may feel that disabled people cannot do the job, and may also be unaware that they can obtain financial assistance to adapt the workplace to meet the needs of disabled employees. In practice, it is perfectly possible for people with disabilities to make a great contribution to any business or organisation, given the right support and working arrangements.

SCENARIO

Tapping into talent

Wally had been a qualified plumber for over 30 years when an accident at work left him totally blind.

His employer did not want to lose his experience and expertise, however, and made it possible for him to carry on working with the help of an assistant.

Wally can diagnose some problems by listening, and visual clues are explained to him by his mate. Working as a pair, they give good service to the employer, who is glad not to have lost a valuable worker. Wally's assistant is also learning more about the trade by working alongside him.

Unemployed people with disabilities are entitled to benefits, but the benefits system can be very difficult to fathom. Many local authorities have benefits advisers to help people to understand their entitlements and fill in the forms. However, being in receipt of benefits also restricts the amount of paid work that a person can take on. Consequently, many disabled people are afraid to take on any sort of work for fear that their benefits will be adversely affected. There is also a fear that any employment may not work out, and that it will be a difficult and lengthy process to get back onto benefits once these have been given up. The whole issue of employment versus benefits is thus a very difficult area for many disabled people, who sometimes find themselves caught between a rock and a hard place.

Try it out

What's going on?
Access the website of the Employers' Forum on Disability (www.employers-forum.co.uk). What initiatives are currently ongoing to promote the employability of people with disabilities?

Barriers to physical access

If you are reading this as a non-disabled person, please try the following three exercises, which are designed to allow you to experience something of what it feels like to be blind (Exercise 1), deaf (Exercise 2) and physically disabled (Exercises 3 and 4).

Try it out

How does it feel?
1 Link arms with a friend and close your eyes. Walk around the room without opening your eyes, letting your friend warn you when you are approaching obstacles. How would you feel about doing this without someone to lean on?

2 Switch on the TV and turn the sound right down. How far can you understand what is going on?

3 Sit in a public place (like a railway station or your local high street) and imagine that you are in a wheelchair, or that you have some difficulty in walking. Look around you carefully. Can you see any obvious obstacles to moving around freely?

4 If possible, borrow a wheelchair, and allow yourself to be pushed around in it for half an hour or so. What do you notice about the attitude of people you meet? How do you feel about this experience?

If you already have a disability of some kind, then it is likely you have an understanding of the kinds of physical barriers that people with physical and sensory difficulties experience on a daily basis. In 1995, the Disability Discrimination Act (DDA) established that disabled people have rights of physical access to almost every kind of public service, for example hospitals and banks. This means that businesses and public services are now legally obliged to make their premises and services accessible, by installing facilities such as ramps or power-operated doors, and loops for people with hearing problems.

However, the Act also says that businesses and service providers are expected to make 'reasonable adjustments' with respect to the needs of disabled people. In practice, there are still many situations in which barriers to access have not yet been removed (see Legislation page 182, for more on this and the Disability Discrimination Act, 2005). Sometimes, the removal of such barriers is simply a matter of better organisation, as the scenario demonstrates.

In this example, the hospital where Kim is currently being treated is very old, and is due to be replaced by a brand new building in the next twelve months. There will be ten MRI scanners in the new hospital, as opposed to the existing

SCENARIO
A step too far?

Kim has MS, and has an appointment to have her third MRI scan to check on her progress. She has been to the same scanner unit on two previous occasions in the last 18 months.

When she arrives at the hospital, she finds that rather than being scanned in the main facility, which is on the ground floor, she is asked to go outside into the car park to the mobile scanner, which is on the back of a trailer. The steps up to the scanner are very steep and wobbly, and she is unable to get up them. The scanner in the main facility is fully booked for that day, so she is given an appointment for another date and told to come back.

What steps could the health authority have taken to prevent this from happening?

two machines. Kim understands that the mobile scanner currently provides a much-needed service. She cannot appreciate, however, that no one has thought to put a note on her records that she cannot manage to climb steps. It might not be reasonable to expect the health authority to put a ramp up to the mobile scanner, given the tight space that it operates in, and given the

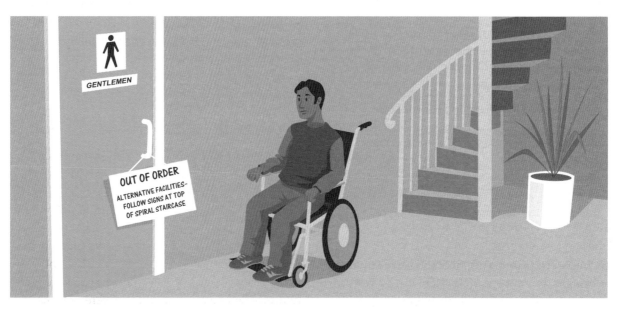

FIGURE 15.17 *Strange but true: sign seen on door of disabled toilet in a seaside hotel*

short lead-in time to the provision of a brand-new facility. However, it is certainly reasonable to insist that staff include notes about mobility and other physical and/or sensory problems on each person's record, so that mismatches of this kind are avoided.

The following scenario provides another example of how forward planning and the allocation of a small amount of funding can improve access in a public setting.

SCENARIO

Is there a Mrs Jenkins here?

Mrs Jenkins is profoundly deaf. She has picked up an infection and because she is worried, she goes to her local hospital A&E Department to be checked out.

No one is available to go with her to help interpret, so she has to go by herself. There are rows of chairs facing one wall in the waiting area, but the door through which staff come and go to call each patient to see a doctor is positioned to the left-hand side of the rows of chairs, and towards the back of the room. Consequently, if a patient is sitting down in one of the front rows of chairs, this door is not visible.

The only way individuals know that it is their turn to see the doctor is when a staff member puts a head round the door and calls out a name.

Mrs Jenkins does not know that this is the system; she also cannot hear her name called. Consequently, she misses her turn. Time goes by, and as her daughter is soon due back from school, she leaves without being seen.

In this situation, the system in the waiting area could have been improved by installing an electronic sign, warning people that their meeting with the doctor was imminent. Blind people using the waiting area would also be helped by the installation of an associated audio-system to make sure that names could be heard. In fact, everyone would benefit from this kind of improvement.

Improving access and reducing environmental barriers require a positive and creative approach, as well as the allocation of funding. Managers and staff who do not have disabilities need to learn to look at their working environment differently in order to bring about meaningful and sensible changes. Consulting service users with disabilities would be a good first step.

Similar observations apply to access to public transport. Many bus companies have now introduced dedicated wheelchair spaces and priority seating for disabled passengers. Some train companies now have carriages which have more disabled toilets than ordinary ones, and in which all doors are electronically operated. However, some parts of the public transport system still require attention: London's underground network, for example, is still very hard to negotiate by people with disabilities. Clearly, a lot of work has been done to make a very antiquated system accessible: stations with easy access between platform and street are now clearly marked on tube maps, for example, but not all stations have this due to existing architectural or design features. Travel on the underground at peak times remains difficult for people with mobility problems, or those who are blind. However, the DDA requirements now mean that large transport companies must make every effort to make reasonable adjustments to their premises and vehicles, so that easier access is available to disabled passengers.

Barriers resulting from prejudice and discrimination

Many people with disabilities will say that the attitudes of other people often act as barriers that prevent them being included in society. Ways in which the negative attitudes of potential employers can prevent disabled people from obtaining work were discussed above (page 175). Sometimes, disabled people are excluded from taking part in social or educational groups because non-disabled people treat them differently. The following scenario shows how this can happen.

A number of things were going on here. Firstly, the group had made a number of assumptions about Chris, based solely on the fact that he was deaf. Thinking of him as deaf, rather than as a person who happens to be deaf, is known as **labelling.** The students had seen only his disability, and had made no attempt to find out about his abilities. This had led them to **stereotype** him as someone who, because of his deafness, could not do certain things. The scenario opposite shows how someone with a physical disability can be labelled.

In this situation the store manager is guilty of labelling Jo. He has seen only the wheelchair and not the person in it. Of course, he was right to help her with her access problem: the situation could have been dangerous for both Jo and the people around her if no one had attempted to manage the crowd. However, the manager's choice of language reveals that at a subconscious level he sees her as a wheelchair 'case' who is also a problem.

Think it over

What's in a word?
Write down all the words you have heard to refer to people with disabilities.

How many of these words are positive, and how many have negative connotations?

In practice, the attitudes of non-disabled people towards disability issues range from complete indifference through a continuum to the other end of the scale, which is pity and an overwhelming insistence on giving 'care' and sympathy. In fact, disabled people do not need sympathy; they need empathy, which is a very different quality.

Key concepts

Labelling: classifying someone in a fixed way that refers only to one aspect of that person, e.g. physical appearance, ethnicity, disability, etc.

Stereotyping: a fixed way of thinking that involves generalisations and expectations about an issue or a group of people.

Empathy not sympathy: people with disabilities often resent being treated with overwhelming concern (sympathy). Rather, they appreciate it when others make an effort to understand their needs, do what is required and then allow them simply to get on with things. This understanding is known as empathy.

Empowerment: giving power to others

Achieving a position of empathy requires the ability to listen, and also an attitude shift. Try the following exercise, and answer the questions honestly.

Try it out

What's your attitude?
Which of the following words best describe your attitude towards people with disabilities:

pity   fear   uncertainty

compassion   sympathy   disgust

understanding   empathy

1. Are there any other attitudes or feelings you have that are not listed here?

2. Do you have different attitudes towards people with different kinds of disabilities?

3. Do you feel that you need to rethink the way that you have viewed people with disabilities?

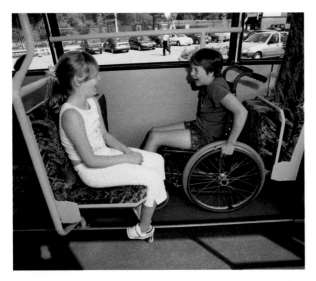

FIGURE 15.18 *Disabled people appreciate empathy rather than sympathy*

Summary

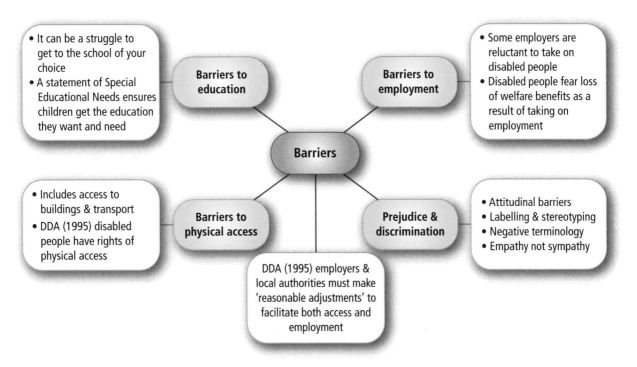

- It can be a struggle to get to the school of your choice
- A statement of Special Educational Needs ensures children get the education they want and need

Barriers to education

Barriers to employment

- Some employers are reluctant to take on disabled people
- Disabled people fear loss of welfare benefits as a result of taking on employment

Barriers

- Includes access to buildings & transport
- DDA (1995) disabled people have rights of physical access

Barriers to physical access

Prejudice & discrimination

- Attitudinal barriers
- Labelling & stereotyping
- Negative terminology
- Empathy not sympathy

DDA (1995) employers & local authorities must make 'reasonable adjustments' to facilitate both access and employment

Assistive technology has made some very advanced aids to daily living available, including electronically controlled living environments, 'smart houses' and 'telecare' systems to monitor an individual's condition or to give early warning of a medical or other emergency.

15.6 Aids and adaptations

Technological advances in recent years have resulted in the development of a vast number of aids to assist people with physical and/or sensory difficulties, whilst buildings can be adapted to accommodate their needs, both in terms of access and usage. This practical help is now known as **assistive technology,** and there is at least one postgraduate course in the UK specialising in this discipline (King's College, London), which is becoming increasingly sophisticated as technology develops.

The design and manufacture of prosthetic devices (to replace and imitate the function of lost limbs), and surgical interventions such as cochlear implants (for deaf people) have increased the options open to people with physical or sensory difficulties.

However, although many disabled people choose to make use of such devices, it should not be automatically assumed that disabled people will always wish to be as 'normal' as possible. The contemporary artist disabled Alison Lapper, for example, who was born with very short legs, has stated that she prefers to walk on her own limbs, rather than using prosthetic legs which she finds uncomfortable. She is proud of her own body, and her artwork is intended to be a celebration of her appearance. Similarly some parents of deaf children opt not to have cochlear implants to 'improve' their hearing. Doing this might result in the loss of a Deaf identity, something which is extremely important to many members of the Deaf community.

Instead of lamenting their lack of 'normality', many disabled people have moved on to taking a pride in their identity, even to the point of celebrating their difference. This important point should be kept in mind when working with people with disabilities, who may make some decisions that are surprising to non-disabled people.

The term 'adaptation' is normally reserved for significant structural alterations to buildings, or to vehicles. However, you might want to quibble about the categorisation of some of the items in Table 15.22, particularly since assistive technology is resulting in some devices which might be said to be both an aid and an adaptation (e.g. household devices controlled by integrated computer systems). The distinction between aids and adaptations is not vital; the outcome of their use is the important factor.

> ### Key concepts
>
> *Aid:* any device used to assist a disabled person with daily life, work, personal tasks etc. This might be a Zimmer frame, a hearing aid, Braille or an audio book.
>
> *Adaptation:* a term normally used for the process of making significant structural alternations to buildings, or mechanical alternations to cars, to make them more user-friendly to disabled people. Examples might be the building of a ramp to allow access to a building, or the provision of hand-controls to a vehicle.

TO ASSIST WITH	AIDS	ADAPTATIONS
Mobility	* walking frames, sticks, crutches, surgical footwear * wheelchairs * callipers or splints * prosthetic limbs	* adapted cars * ramps, stairlifts, widened doors, automatic doors * lowered controls in lifts
Daily living	* shower seats * extended taps * special cutlery, utensil cuffs * pick-up aids	* lowered work-surfaces, walk-in baths, bath-lifts/hoists, handrails, grabrails * electronically controlled environments; 'smart houses'
Work	* IT equipment, e.g. speech sensitive software, large key pads, adapted chairs	* ergonomic workstations, adaptations as per mobility (above)
Communication	* hearing aids, low vision aids * surgical intervention, e.g. cochlear implants * use of communication systems, e.g. British Sign Language or Braille	* telephone/television adaptors * visual and auditory messages in public places (e.g. lifts, public transport), hearing loops * telecare systems
Leisure and creativity	* wheelchairs adapted for sport * specially adapted creativity tools, e.g. mouth-held paintbrushes	

TABLE 15.22 *Aids and adaptations*

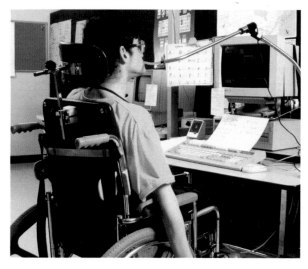

FIGURE 15.19 *The provision of appropriate assistive technology can empower disabled people to take control of their own lives*

SCENARIO
Disabled or different?

Lynne, who was born deaf, has been offered a cochlear implant to enable her to hear for the first time. Her mother Rachel, who was also born deaf, is objecting to the operation. She argues that Lynne can communicate perfectly well with her friends by using British Sign Language (BSL). She is also a proficient lip-reader and can make herself understood to non-deaf people. Lynne, who is now 11 years old, attends a special unit in a mainstream school (where there is a deaf teacher), and she is currently thriving there.

Rachel feels that if Lynne were able to hear, she would lose her identity as a member of the Deaf community. Furthermore, she might not be fully accepted by hearing people, as she still might have some kind of hearing impairment even after the operation.

1. What do you think of Rachel's point of view?

2. What would you advise her to do if you were involved with the family in a professional capacity?

3. Why do you think that some disabled people embrace having a disability as part of their identity?

Summary

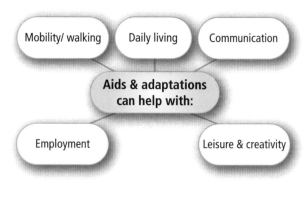

Mobility/ walking

Daily living

Communication

Aids & adaptations can help with:

Employment

Leisure & creativity

Consider this

A home of my own

Rob is 35 and has spina bifida. To get around outside, he has a wheelchair which is either pushed by a family member, or self-propelled. Indoors, he gets around by sitting on the floor and then propelling himself with his arms. He can get up and downstairs by himself in this way, but finds it tiring.

He is an excellent cook, and enjoys making huge meals for himself and his family. He also spends a lot of time on his computer, playing virtual reality games and also making contacts all over the world via the internet.

There are now plans for Rob to get his own flat.

1. What kind of premises might suit Rob's needs best?

2. How would the premises need to be adapted to accommodate him?

3. How will having his own home contribute to meeting Rob's needs?

15.7 Legislation

Since 1990, the way in which care services are provided has changed considerably. Before that date, the majority of services were provided directly by local authority departments. Subsequently, legislation has resulted in a change in emphasis with respect to care provision, so that there is now a mixed economy of care (see page 163). Social Services Departments now act mainly as assessors and purchasers of care and commissioners of services, and the actual input of support is coming more and more from other providers. This applies equally to everyone in receipt of services, not just to people with disabilities.

In recent years, other legislation has strengthened the rights and entitlements of people with disabilities and their carers. The new legislation stresses that people should be cared for in the community as far as possible. This might mean remaining in their own homes, or moving from large institutions (such as long-stay hospitals or residential units) into smaller, more homely provision (such as sheltered accommodation or supported living). The legislation and associated guidance also expects that people with disabilities should be empowered, as far as possible, to live fulfilling lives, going to work if they wish, and pursuing their education and personal interests in the same way as anyone else.

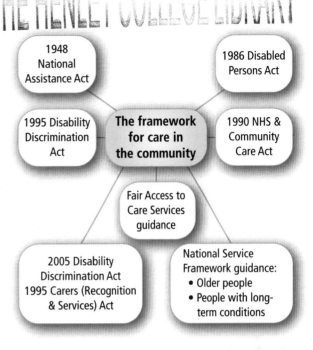

FIGURE 15.20 *Care in the community framework*

Full details of how care in the community works, including the ways in which need is assessed and prioritised, the care planning and management cycle and practitioners who contribute to the mixed economy of care can be found in Section 15.4, page 163.

Key concepts

Care purchaser: the organisation that controls the funding to buy care – usually the local authority or the PCT.

Care provider: any organisation that delivers a service e.g. A home meals delivery company, an NHS Trust, a voluntary organisation, a social services department.

What if?

What are the advantages and disadvantages to a disabled service user of remaining in his or her own home to receive care? What are the corresponding advantages and disadvantages to care managers?

The following section summarises developments relating to care in the community, and then explores the provisions of the Disability Discrimination Acts (1995 and 2005) in some detail.

Community care

Figure 15.20 sets out some key aspects of the legal framework (and associated guidance) for care in the community.

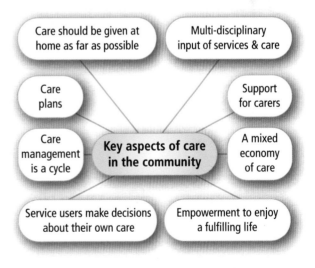

FIGURE 15.21 *Care in the community – key aspects*

The law and disability

The legal definition of disability under the 1995 and 2005 Disability Discrimination Acts was discussed above (page 140). The provisions of the

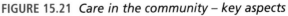

1995 Act have been implemented incrementally since that date, and the 2005 Act further strengthens the protection and rights afforded to disabled people. Associated legislation is the Special Educational Needs and Disability Act (2001) (SENDA), which applies specifically to educational providers. In Northern Ireland this is covered by the Special Educational Needs and Disability Order (NI) 2005 (SENDO). Together, these pieces of legislation apply to four areas of daily life: employment; education; access to goods, facilities and services; and the management, buying or renting of land and property.

Main areas of provision

It is important to remember that legislation and associated guidance and/or regulations change over time. The information in this section relates to the law at the time of writing. You should always check out the latest guidance or legislation (for your part of the UK) at the time when you are conducting your studies. Very simply, the law states that the following provisions apply in these four areas of daily activity:

* it is unlawful to treat a disabled person less favourably than someone else on the grounds of their disability

* employers, education providers, providers of goods and services must make 'reasonable adjustments' so that disabled people can work, study, buy goods and use services as freely as anyone else

* from December 2006, all public bodies have a Disability Equality duty to actively promote equality of opportunity for disabled people.

Making reasonable adjustments might include:

* giving extra help where needed

* making changes to the ways in which services are provided

* improving access to premises

* providing aids or special equipment.

Try it out

Who is out there?
Explore the Internet to find out what organisations exist in your part of the UK to promote the rights of disabled people.

The cumulative effect of this legislation is that the responsibility for being pro-active and including people with disabilities now lies with employers, education providers, and providers of goods and services. Whereas in the past, disabled people might end up taking the initiative on a particular issue (e.g. going to law on a particular issue of discrimination), the law now expects large public bodies to prove what steps they are taking to promote accessibility and inclusion with respect to disabled people. Disabled people should now expect employers to do everything reasonably possible to make sure that they can take on (or keep) employment. It is also in the interests of companies providing goods or services to make sure that the needs of disabled customers are provided for.

What is a reasonable adjustment?

Jim is deaf. He works in a large warehouse where fork-lift trucks are used continuously.

His deafness makes it impossible for him to anticipate possible danger, as he cannot hear the fork-lift vehicles approaching.

His employer has solved this problem by installing mirrors at key points in the warehouse aisles, particularly at corners and junctions. Jim can now see around dangerous corners and thus has warning of approaching vehicles.

The fact of having a deaf colleague has also made all staff in the warehouse more safety conscious – which has made the workplace safer for everyone.

Inclusion at school

Gemma is 13 years old and has cystic fibrosis. She needs to self-treat regularly during the day with physiotherapy, and also to do daily exercises. She takes food supplements with her meals.

What provisions can the school make to ensure that Gemma can attend, and take part as fully as possible in school life?

The head discusses Gemma's needs with her and her parents. Gemma's form teacher is also involved. The school has a designated medical room, and it is arranged that this room is available for Gemma at set times during the day. Here, she can do her own physiotherapy in privacy. The school nurse is on hand to assist at times when Gemma takes medication. Gemma's food supplements are stored securely in the kitchen, so that these are readily available for her when required. The head teacher asks Gemma how she feels about other people knowing about her condition. Gemma decides that it is best if her classmates know about her needs, and about how the condition affects her. Thus, everyone understands that there are times during the day when Gemma needs to go off to organise her self-treatment; they are also considerate when she gets out of breath during exercise.

It is important to recognise, however, that this scenario describes the options chosen by Gemma. Someone else with the same condition may choose different ways of meeting daily needs, and may have different views on what other people need to know. Each person is different and requires a personally-tailored set of provisions. You should never make assumptions about what an individual needs or wants. In terms of the law, the school is legally obliged to make reasonable adjustments, which respect Gemma's needs and wishes, so that she can take part in school life as fully as possible. From December 2006, the school is also required to actively promote policies of equality of opportunity for disabled people.

Getting out and about

Nicki has mobility problems, and uses a specially adapted car for long journeys.

She can transfer from her car to a wheelchair, but access to buildings is sometimes problematic.

Nicki enjoys meeting her friends, and they often go to their local pub for lunch. Fortunately, the brewery has taken its obligations under the DDA very seriously, and is also keen to make sure it gets the custom of disabled people and their friends and families. A ramp has been installed to the premises, together with a buzzer that can be used by disabled customers who may need assistance. The buzzer sounds in the bar, and a member of staff immediately goes to see what help is needed. Nicki can thus be confident she can access the pub (and her friends) without too much difficulty.

Summary

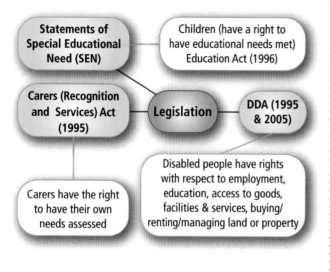

- Statements of Special Educational Need (SEN)
- Children (have a right to have educational needs met) Education Act (1996)
- Carers (Recognition and Services) Act (1995)
- Legislation
- DDA (1995 & 2005)
- Carers have the right to have their own needs assessed
- Disabled people have rights with respect to employment, education, access to goods, facilities & services, buying/renting/managing land or property

Consider this

Planning for the future

Ruth is preparing to leave hospital after a stroke which has left her with weakness down the left-hand side of her body. Her husband and family are keen to have her home, and she has been assessed as capable of living at home with the right support and input.

1. What are likely to be the key elements of Ruth's care plan?

2. What role is informal care likely to play in this plan?

3. What support can Ruth's husband expect?

4. What are the advantages to Ruth of receiving care in the community (as opposed to care in a residential home or hospital)?

UNIT 15 ASSESSMENT

How you will be assessed

Your knowledge, understanding and skills concerning clients with disabilities will be assessed by a two-hour written test, which will be externally marked.

There will be four compulsory questions, which will test:

* your knowledge of disability conditions

* how you apply your knowledge to specific situations (as described in scenarios)

* how well you select appropriate aids, adaptations and services for users

* how well you evaluate the appropriateness and quality of treatments and services.

You will also need to demonstrate a familiarity with the life quality factors and principles described in AS Unit 1 Effective Caring.

The following specimen paper gives an indication of what form the test will take, and the kinds of question that may be asked.

Test questions

Answer all questions. Each question carries 20 marks. Marks for each question part are shown in brackets.

1. Terence is 81 years old, and lives with his wife, Selina, who is his main carer. His memory has been deteriorating for some years, and he can no longer remember the names of friends and neighbours. He is often confused by tasks like shopping and paying for goods, and now has some difficulties with remembering how to do personal tasks like shaving and dressing. He gets lost easily, and no longer goes out alone.

(a) Name one medical condition that is likely to have caused Terence's symptoms. (1)

Terence has been prescribed Aricept to slow down the deterioration in his condition. Twice a week he attends a day unit run jointly by the NHS and Social Services. His wife has been given advice on practical ways to help Terence on a daily basis, and she has help on a daily basis to get Terence washed and dressed.

(b) Name three practitioners likely to have been involved in setting up and/or delivering Terence's Care Plan. (3)

(c) What support is available to carers like Selina? Name a piece of legislation and a national organisation that would help. (6)

(d) What psychological factors are important to people with long-term needs like Terence? Name three factors that will contribute to his sense of wellbeing. (10)

2. Angela has a long-term condition that requires her to use a wheelchair. She also has some problems in using her hands, which become weak after a certain amount of use. Thus, she can use a keyboard for a limited period of time. She is at her best between 10.00 am and 4.00 pm, after which her condition makes her very tired. However, she has excellent interpersonal skills, together with extensive experience as a housing adviser for her local council, answering telephone queries from the public, and also interviewing council customers face-to-face. She has just taken on a new job in a similar role for another council Housing Department.

(a) The Disability Discrimination Acts (1995 and 2005) require employers to make 'reasonable adjustments' to make it possible for disabled people to work. Name four ways in which Angela's new employer might be expected to make such provision. (10)

(b) Explain how Angela might face attitudinal barriers at work. (10)

3. Down's syndrome is a condition that results from a chromosomal abnormality.

(a) What specific chromosomal abnormality causes Down's syndrome, and how is this transmitted? (4)

(b) List four signs or symptoms of Down's syndrome. (4)

(c) Describe how Down's syndrome can be detected. What ethical considerations are raised by the pre-natal detection of this condition? (6)

(d) How has society's attitude changed towards people with learning difficulties in the last 20 to 30 years? (6)

4. Lilian is 77 and has been in hospital following a fall in which she broke her hip. She has been suffering from osteoarthritis for some years, and although her hip has now healed, her ability to walk has been drastically curtailed having sustained a fracture and spent some time in hospital.

Lilian badly wants to go home. She lives alone, but has two daughters who live nearby who are more than willing to make sure their mother has everything she needs.

(a) Suggest two practitioners who might be involved in assessing Lilian for discharge from hospital, and say how each one might help. (4)

(b) What additional services might be necessary to help Lilian resume her life at home? (4)

(c) What benefits will Lilian get from living in her own home? (6)

(d) What benefits will Lilian get if she goes into residential care? (6)

References

Barnett, H. (2002) *The Which? Guide to Complementary Therapies* London: Which? Ltd.

CSCI (2004) *CSCI study finds people are being denied choice and control in their lives by bureaucracy and 'failure of imagination'* Commission for Social Care Inspection Press Release, 24 August 2004 (accessed via www.csci.org.uk/media, 18/01/06)

DoH (1999) *Caring about Carers: a National Strategy for Carers* London: Department of Health (can be accessed via DoH website)

DoH (2001) *National Service Framework for Older People* London: HMSO

DoH (2003) *Fair Access to Care Services: Guidance on Eligibility Criteria for Adult Social Care* London: Department of Health (accessed via DoH website)

DoH (2003) *A Practical Guide for Disabled People and Carers: Where to find Information, Services and Equipment.* London: Department of Health

DoH (2005) *The National Service Framework for Long-term Conditions* London: Department of Health

DWP (2005) *The Definition of Disability*, DDA 2005, Factsheet 1. London: The Department for Work and Pensions (accessed via DWP website)

Kitwood, T. (1997) *Dementia Reconsidered: the person comes first* Maidenhead and New York: The Open University Press

NICE (2003) *Multiple Sclerosis: Management of Multiple Sclerosis in Primary and Secondary Care*, Clinical Guideline 8. London: National Institute for Clinical Excellence

Pinder, M. (ed.) (2005) *Complementary Healthcare: a guide for patients* London: The Prince of Wales's Foundation for Integrated Health

Sanderson, H., Jones, E. and Brown, K. (2002) *Essential Lifestyle Planning and Active Support* (accessed via website of Northwest Training and Development Team)

Zollman, C. and Vickers, A. (2000) *ABC of Complementary Medicine* London: BMJ Books

Useful websites

www.alzheimers.org.uk
   Website of the Alzheimer's Society. Information and advice.

www.arthritiscare.org.uk
   Website of Arthritis Care. Information and advice about arthritis. Links to branches in UK regions.

www.asbah.org
   Website of the Association for Spina Bifida and Hydrocephalus. Information and advice.

www.bbc.co.uk/health
   Health section of BBC website.

www.besttreatments.co.uk
   Website set up by British Medical Journal (BMJ) and NHS direct. Reviews 'best treatments' for a wide range of conditions.

www.carersuk.org
   Website of Carers UK, an organisation that supports and promotes the rights of carers.

www.cftrust.org.uk
   Cystic Fibrosis Trust. Information and advice.

www.csci.org.uk
   Commission for Social Care Inspection

www.down-syndrome.info
   Website of the Down syndrome information network. On-line library, access to information and advice.

www.downs-syndrome.org.uk
   Website of the Down's Syndrome Association. Information and advice.

www.directgov.uk
   Government website with useful section for disabled people.

www.drc.gov.uk
   Disability Rights Commission (for people in England, Scotland and Wales). This organisation actively promotes the rights of disabled people, both collectively and individually.

www.dwp.gov.uk
   Department for Work and Pensions website; useful information both for disabled people and employers

www.employers-forum.co.uk
   Website of the Employers' Forum, a body that actively promotes employment for disabled people, and helps employers to make this possible.

www.equalityni.org
   Equalities Commission for Northern Ireland, which fulfils a similar role to that of the

Disability Rights Commission in England, Scotland and Wales

http://inclusion.uwe.ac.uk/csie
Centre for Studies on Inclusive Education. Information about the statementing of children with special educational needs.

www.intellectualdisability.info
Website developed by St George's University of London in collaboration with the Down's Syndrome Association. Articles on many aspects of intellectual disability, including Down's syndrome.

www.jrf.org.uk
Website of the Joseph Rowntree Foundation.

www.lsc.gov.uk
Learning and Skills Council

www.mencap.org.uk
Website of MENCAP, the organisation that campaigns for, and gives advice and support to people with learning disabilities and their families.

www.mssociety.org.uk
Multiple Sclerosis Society. Information and advice. Links to regional branches.

www.msrc.co.uk
Multiple Sclerosis Resource Centre. Information and advice.

www.muscular-dystrophy.org
Website of the Muscular Dystrophy Campaign. Many factsheets and articles about MD.

www.nhsdirect.nhs.uk
Information on medical conditions and treatments provided by the National Health Service. Latest developments in health care are described. Links to other useful sites such as Best Treatments.

www.nwtdt.com
Northwest Training and Development Teacher for lifestyle planning and active support

www.opsi.gov.uk
Office of Public Sector Information. Also has useful links to the Scottish Parliament, the Northern Ireland Assembly and the National Assembly of Wales

www.portage.org.uk
National Portage Association. An educational system for pre-school children

www.scope.org.uk
Website of Scope, a national organisation dedicated to supporting the needs of people with cerebral palsy.

www.skill.org.uk
National Bureau for Students with Disabilities.

www.stroke.org.uk
The Stroke Association

www.valuingpeople.gov.uk
Government-sponsored website dedicated to the *Valuing People* initiative. This initiative aims to empower people with learning disabilities to take part in decision-making about their own lives.

Early years education

This unit covers the following sections:

16.1 The roles of learning, child-rearing, genetics and maturation

16.2 How early years learning takes place

16.3 Techniques for enabling learning

16.4 Theories of development, learning and education

16.5 Assessment in early years education

16.6 Issues in early years learning and education

The
Chiltern
College

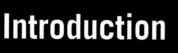

This unit looks at the content, practice and theory of early years education from 0–8 years. The unit will increase your understanding of the needs of young children and will help you to plan an early years learning situation for your assessment.

Good early years provision is dependent on the knowledge and expertise of the staff working in the area. Despite many early educators such as Rousseau (1712–1778), Froebel (1782–1852) and Montessori (1869–1952) recognising the importance of early years education, the UK has not been a leader in providing comprehensive early years education. This was mainly due to attitudes towards women. Until World War Two it was strongly felt that, until children went to school, the best place for young children to be was in their own homes. Most women did not work outside the home – their role was to care for the family.

However, since 1940, attitudes have changed. This was partly due to the war, when women were suddenly needed to carry out jobs to keep the country going during the war years while the men were away fighting. In more recent years, the structure of the population has been changing, with a smaller workforce and a larger dependent population. This has meant that modern governments have needed to develop ways to encourage more women back into work and this has led to a number of initiatives including supporting early years education outside of the home. This has resulted in an increase in employment opportunities in early years education.

It has also resulted in a raised awareness of how children learn, including activities and environments which help stimulate learning. This unit will help you to develop this understanding as well as giving you ideas for working with young children.

Unit assessment

This unit is assessed through a piece of coursework. You will have to choose an age group and two different topic areas from a list which is reproduced at the end of the unit. You have to research the topic area and plan a suitable learning experience for the age group you have chosen. You will then have to evaluate your learning plan. All the work is presented in the form of a report. A full explanation of the piece of work which needs to be carried out is given at the end of the unit.

16.1 The roles of learning, child-rearing, genetics and maturation

How children grow and develop is a fascinating subject and there are a wide range of theories and ideas about how humans acquire their various skills and abilities. Human development has been studied from conception, through early childhood and adolescence and into adulthood. This unit will deal with the development of children from birth to eight years.

Nature versus nurture debate

The first influences on development are biological. In the last century some biologists argued that many of an individual's skills, such as intelligence and personality, are genetically inherited in the same way that genetics determine the colour of a child's eyes or hair. This is known as the **nature** view.

Others disagreed with this view and argued that individuals are a product of all the different experiences they have – it is the effect of these experiences that will determine the person. These theorists believed that individuals have a free will and that as they grow they can change and be changed by their environment. This is known as the **nurture** view.

In essence, the nature side of the debate believes the skills humans have are innate but the nurture side believes they are socially learned skills.

Think it over

Do you think that intelligence, personality and how aggressive a child is, is the result of:

* nature

* nurture

* both?

Nowadays most people believe that both nature and nurture contribute to the development of an individual. It is also worth remembering that, even among people who agree that both nature and nurture have a role, it is not always clear which elements of development are governed by

which influence. Therefore, there is a continuing debate about whether particular skills, traits and even diseases are inherited or a result of lifestyle choices and/or environmental factors.

Humans are born with many abilities, but the way an individual develops and the person they become is influenced by the experiences they have and the people they mix with. Factors such as culture, economics, influence of friends and family values will all combine to influence the person a child becomes.

Maturation

Another biological influence on children is the rate at which they grow and mature. The process of physical growth is known as **maturation.** All normal foetuses develop at roughly the same rate. After birth, most babies will learn to use their hands, move their heads, crawl and walk at roughly the same time as this is genetically determined. Children can only adapt their behaviour when they are maturationally ready – therefore, while babies may be able to stand alone holding onto something at six months, they cannot walk unaided for another five to six months and trying to teach them to do so would not be successful as they are not maturationally ready.

Key concept

Maturation: genetically programmed physical growth and development.

Humans do not mature very fast. All people pass through the same stages of maturation in the same order, i.e. children crawl before walking and walk before running; but children do not all mature at the same rate. Therefore, some children will achieve milestones before others. The speed of maturation is determined by a child's genes.

There are differing opinions as to whether certain skills such as language and intelligence develop through fixed, clearly identifiable stages or whether development is continuous, with small developments each day. For skills to develop in stages, the following attributes will be evident:

* each stage will feature a particular kind of behaviour which does not occur in a previous stage

* the kind of behaviour and thinking in each stage will be different from the previous one

* all children would go through the stages in the same order at approximately the same age.

If this is applied to language development, clear stages can be seen.

1. The first stage of language acquisition is the babbling stage, which generally begins at four months. It disappears when more language skills are developed.

2. At around one year, children are able to use single words to communicate with others. When children acquire words they can explain what they want and ask questions. These skills are not evident earlier.

3. From around 18 months, children are able to use simple sentences.

Think it over

Do you think children's development of a sense of right and wrong is continuous development or fixed stages of development?

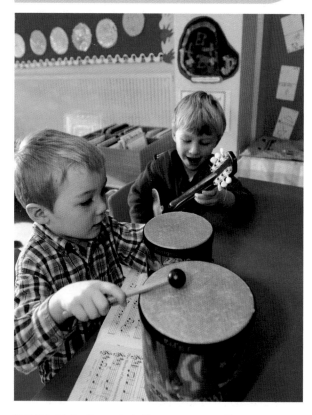

FIGURE 16.1 *Genetic influences can affect musical abilities*

There are other skills where it is believed that there is more genetic influence on ability – for example music. Musical children often have a strong music tradition in their families.

Social factors affecting development

A child's ability to learn is influenced by a number of different external factors which are often outside their control. From an early stage, these factors can have a significant effect on the child's life chances.

Home and family

The family unit is seen as a small mirror image of the wider society. It is through the family unit that the child is introduced to the norms and values of the society in which they live. Children will believe that the way things are done in their own family is the way all families operate. Therefore, the influence of the home on a child's development is huge and has lasting effects.

Language and communication

The home determines the language that is learned and the way language is used to communicate and to express feelings and ideas. Bernstein (a researcher into language development) referred to two language codes – the elaborate and restricted codes. Children who could use the elaborate code were able to communicate more effectively in wider society and therefore make progress, whereas children who could only operate the restricted code could not progress as easily because they could not make themselves clearly understood. The elaborate code is the one that is used in education, business and other aspects of life. Therefore, a child familiar with this type of language is likely to fit in more easily to 'accepted' society.

Equally, the family sets the norms of the type of language which is acceptable, e.g. if a child is brought up in a family which swears in every sentence, they will believe that this is the correct way to talk – until they meet other children. This will affect the child's perception. However, the influence of the family is very strong and children find it hard to make changes which go against the norms of their family life.

Effects of family size

The number of children in a family may affect the child's experience. Children with older brothers or sisters may achieve goals earlier as they copy their siblings. They may also feel more comfortable in groups than an only child, as they are used to being with other children. Language skills may be more advanced for their age as they learn from the language used by their brothers and sisters. On the other hand, older children may speak for younger ones and therefore these children may be less confident with their speech. In a large family, it may be expected that the older children 'look after' the younger children and provide activities for them.

Education

The family will also influence the attitude to education. Some families value the importance of good education and recognise it as a key to social success and economic stability in adult life. Such families would encourage learning as a positive experience and build this into the toys and games they provide for their children. They are also more likely to use early years provision as an opportunity for extending the child's learning and social skills, as this would be seen as an important preparation for school.

Children from this type of background will have a stronger start at school. They are likely to be supported through their education as their parents show an interest in what they are doing.

Some families feel education is a waste of time. Research has shown that there are some families where the parents have never worked and therefore they do not value education. Children from these backgrounds are less likely to attend pre-school education and consequently may find themselves ill-prepared for the demands of school. This lack of grounding is hard to catch up and children may find it difficult to learn at the same pace as other children in their age group. In areas with high levels of poverty, funding has been provided through schemes such as 'education action zones' or 'excellence clusters' to provide additional support for children and help them overcome these early barriers.

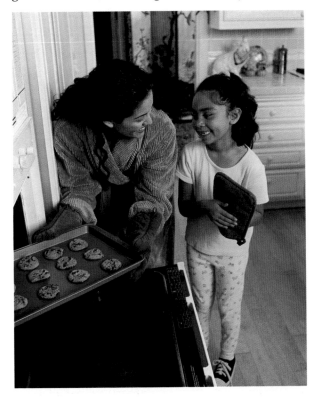

FIGURE 16.2 *The home environment is important in a child's development*

Environmental factors beyond home and family

The surroundings in which a child lives can affect their behaviour and the opportunities available to them. A child living in an urban area will have very different opportunities from a child living in a rural area.

Access to early years education

Urban areas are likely to have more access to early years care settings, and have plenty of different learning opportunities for children such as museums, playgrounds and other interesting places.

They are likely to have a better transport network, so parents can get children to their activities easily.

Rural areas often lack locally-based activities and parents may need a car to get to the nearest playgroup or nursery. Often, rural early years settings are based in church halls in the village. These settings generally have to be prepared and packed away each day and therefore the resources will be different to those in a full-time, purpose-built nursery setting.

The urban environment

On the other hand, some urban areas may have significant pockets of poverty. Inner cities can be very unhealthy; many are congested and polluted from car exhausts and industrial by-products. Many inner city areas have poor housing conditions which also influence health. For example, children living in high-rise flats do not have access to a garden, and therefore may lack the opportunity to play outside.

Statistics show that there are more one-parent families living in inner city areas who have limited access to family support networks. People often feel socially isolated even though they are living in an area of high population, as neighbourhoods in today's society do not include the extended family network that existed in the past. This may reduce the opportunities for interaction between children and adults.

The government has recognised that these issues are having a significant effect on children and their life chances. They are investing money in significantly deprived areas through the Sure Start scheme (introduced in 2002) with the aim of increasing access to good early years education.

Poverty isn't just restricted to urban areas. Rural areas can also have significant pockets of poverty and deprivation. In rural areas, some families find they cannot access facilities if they do not have the money to afford a car or other transport.

Economic factors

Family income has a significant effect on the opportunities a child may have. Money will influence the area where children live, the quality of the food their parents can afford to buy, the toys they have access to in the home and the learning opportunities they experience outside the home. A family with a high disposable income (the income they have left to spend after the essentials of housing, electricity, gas and food are paid for) will have more opportunities for outings, holidays and clubs. Most activities or groups cost money so to give children wider experiences such as swimming lessons, dancing, or even Cubs or Brownies, parents need money available.

Decisions have to be made about wants and needs. There are certain things which can be classed as a need and must be paid for, e.g. heating,

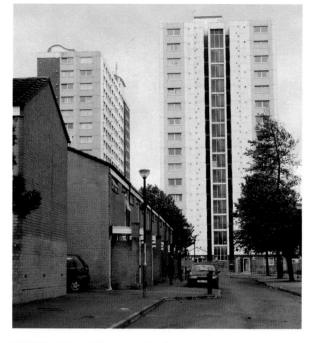

FIGURE 16.3 *Living in a high-rise flat limits the opportunity for outside play*

food and housing. There are other expenditures which could be classed as a want, such as social activities, designer clothing, and money for alcohol or cigarettes. However, individuals will classify different things as needs – some individuals who smoke may feel that having money to buy cigarettes is a need, whereas others would not see it as essential expenditure.

The wants and needs of any society is influenced by the norms of that society, so what families in the Western world see as essential would be very different from the needs of families in developing countries who are struggling to survive.

Summary

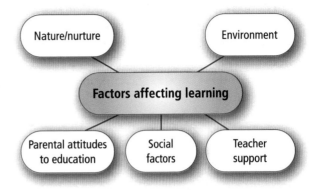

Try it out

Make a list of your own 'needs' and 'wants'. Compare them to others. How many of them are essential to survival and how many are linked to a lifestyle choice?

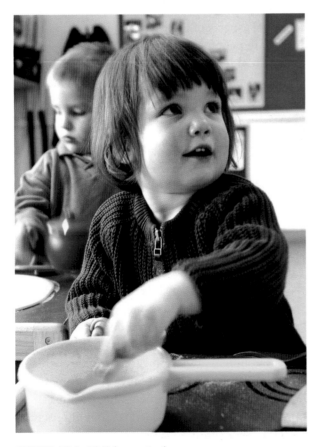

FIGURE 16.4 *Children at play*

16.2 How early years learning takes place

Much early years learning takes place through play. Children learn through play, which affects all aspects of a child's development. Play is widely accepted as being crucial to the development of the child. It is through play that children learn and understand many things about the world around them. Professionals working with children need to understand the value of play and how it helps children to learn.

Key concept

Play is considered to be one of the primary needs of the child. Play is often called a child's 'work'. It is a common behaviour of children in all countries and cultures. Children naturally want to play, although children also learn to play. Therefore, both nature and nurture contribute to the development of skills needed to play effectively.

Providing play which engages children's interest and is appropriate for their level of development takes time and effort. The key to successful play in the early years is the adult – in both the home and the professional situation. Adults can provide the environment and materials for successful play to take place. This doesn't mean that they direct the play in a rigid way, just that they have the skills to support and sustain play.

Play is a learning experience. Some theorists believe it allows children to practice the roles they will need to take on in adulthood. Susan Issacs (1885–1948, see Table 16.6) saw play as a child's life and the way by which children come to understand the world in which they live. Figure 16.5 outlines how play contributes to a child's development.

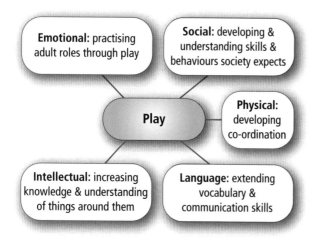

FIGURE 16.5 *How play contributes to a child's development*

Features of play

True play in younger children has a number of different features. It is:

* started by children themselves, for example role play of mothers and fathers, or playing in a puddle of water after rainfall in the garden

* designed by children themselves – they choose how to play and what to play – they use the resources available to them to satisfy their curiosity

* something children choose to do because they like to do it, not for an end product or reward

* natural, something that all children seem able to do without instruction or lessons

* spontaneous, which means children can involve themselves in it without guidance or instruction from an adult

* voluntary, in so far as children can choose whether or not to join in.

Children play because it provides a way to explore their environment, develop communication skills and express pleasurable feelings. It combines action and thought, and in so doing gives the child a sense of satisfaction.

Play provides the opportunity for a child to learn in different ways. Young children will drive their learning and use the situations and opportunities available to them to satisfy their curiosity and need for learning. Young children often use questions to do this – persistent use of 'why' or 'what' is one way in which young children learn.

Young children tend to learn through trial and error or by observation or modelling. Trial and error, or experiential learning, takes place where a child keeps experimenting with something until he or she achieves it. This can take more time and it is possible that the child may give up but it is a good learning experience. Social learning is often called observational learning. Children will not copy all behaviours that they see, but they may be influenced by the behaviour of adults who are important to them. They are more likely to model aspects of their behaviour on these important people. Younger children rely more on experiential learning and modelling, while older children are able to learn from verbal instruction and do not always need concrete examples to ensure learning.

The role of adults

Adults have a key role in supporting children's learning. Part of their role involves giving instruction, but designing learning situations and providing materials and activities that allow learning to happen are often far more important. Adults have to find a balance between standing too far back and letting children discover and learn on their own, and becoming too involved and taking control of the situation.

The adult has an important role in planning the environment and organising activities, which will stimulate children's interests and promote learning. Adults need to ensure that learning opportunities are stimulating and that interesting materials and equipment are provided to help the children learn effectively. Materials and equipment should be presented in a manner which encourages the child to explore them and discover their properties for themselves. This will encourage them to ask 'what' and 'why' questions. The adult can respond to these and further support learning through clarifying ideas and correcting misunderstandings. Children learn through this direction and effective planning.

Summary

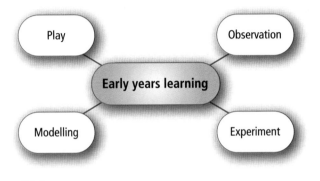

Consider this

Think about how children of different ages play. Compare and contrast the way in which a younger child learns through play, but an older child might carry out an activity from verbal instruction only.

Evaluate the role of the adult in each of these situations.

Consider this

Which type or types of learning are taking place in each of the examples given below?

* A child is pouring 250 ml of water from a thin beaker to a wider beaker and looking at the amount of water in each. The child is trying to decide which beaker contains more water.

* A child has grown mung beans on tissue paper and is considering the conditions needed to grow a daffodil bulb.

* A child has visited a castle and has read a story about the life of people living in a castle in medieval times.

* A child carries out a marbling activity after being shown how by an early years worker.

Comment on how each learning experience could be developed to incorporate other types of learning.

16.3 Techniques for enabling learning

Table 16.1 outlines a variety of ways in which children learn. Details of each of these types of learning occur throughout this unit but the table gives an overview.

Development and learning

Learning is complex. Children develop in a number of areas which include cognitive development; language development; physical development; emotional development and social development. Much of this development in the early years is through play.

Cognitive development

Cognitive development is the development of understanding and concepts. Through play, children develop an understanding of concepts. They are able to explore different materials such as wet and dry sand, experiment in different ways and solve problems. This exploration begins with the young baby playing with his or her fingers and toes, and continues as the child is able to grasp objects and explore them with the mouth in a more controlled manner. Children will start to understand cause and effect as they experiment with objects that they can move or make a sound with.

Play helps children to group or categorise objects according to different criteria. Through creative activities, they develop an understanding of shape, colour and form.

Language development

Language is the key way in which we communicate. With each new area of play, each fresh activity or toy, a new set of words will be needed to describe the play that is taking place. Play is a very powerful tool for developing language, particularly as much play in later childhood is based on social relationships and language will be needed to develop and sustain these. All forms of play allow a child to practise language, and role play in particular allows children to try out new words and sentence

METHOD OF LEARNING	EXPLANATION
Discovery or experiential	Children learn effectively through first-hand experience or finding out for themselves. It is believed that if children actively experience learning then they are more likely to remember and learn. Many early theorists such as Frobel, Steiner and Piaget believed children should be able to explore and find out for themselves (see pages 216-7). They based their learning theories on this idea.
Modelling	Modelling is the imitation of behaviour. It is clear that children often learn through copying the behaviours of people who are important to them. This is known as social learning theory and it is one way in which children learn about the norms and values of the society in which they live. (See Unit 12 for more details.)
Reinforcement	Reinforcement reflects the idea that children learn through their actions being reinforced, either positively or negatively. If children's actions and behaviours are positively encouraged and reinforced, they are likely to repeat those actions or behaviours. Positive reinforcement brings pleasure. If actions or behaviours are punished, for example through being told off, or another punishment, children are not encouraged to repeat the behaviour. This type of learning underpins operant conditioning (see page 206).
Verbal instruction	Children learn from verbal instruction. Adults have a key role in imparting information to children and the amount a child can absorb increases as a child gets older. However, it is widely believed that a child needs to be actively engaged in order to learn. Verbal instruction, in large amounts, can be very passive and therefore the value in terms of learning can be poor.
Researching and reading	Children's knowledge and creative thinking are developed through books and stories. Children can get a lot of enjoyment from books, as well as social, intellectual, linguistic and cultural benefits.
	Researching is another way children can acquire knowledge. There is much information available on the Internet and in written form. A child who is able to research and find out has access to a wealth of information and ideas.
Reflection and analysis	Thinking about ideas and concepts can help children accommodate them. Children need to assimilate or take on board ideas and concepts they have learned in order to move to the next stage of learning. As children get older, their memory capacity increases. Children can use their knowledge and the 'rules' they have acquired from previous experiences to apply to a broader range of problems. This helps them extend their knowledge and understanding.

TABLE 16.1 *The ways children learn*

structures. Adults have an important role to play in extending children's language through introducing new words into the play situation.

Children learn the language for problem solving by asking why, how and what as they explore. The adult can encourage this by answering a child's questions and encouraging further questioning. As children get older, they will use language to explain what they are doing and their intentions for their play.

They will use language skills to negotiate with other children. From six or seven years, children use language to explain the rules of their games and ensure that players keep to the rules.

Physical development

Physical development includes the development of gross and fine motor skills.

> ### Key concept
>
> *Gross motor skills:* skills which require larger muscle movements and control such as running, throwing, hopping and skipping.
>
> *Fine motor skills:* smaller, more precise skills such as drawing, cutting, painting or colouring.

Play can develop co-ordination and control of bodily movements as there are often opportunities to run, jump, skip and hop which develop muscle tone and balance. Catching and throwing help to develop gross and fine motor skills. Physical activities also develop confidence in a child.

Emotional development

As children develop, they begin to experience the wealth of different emotions every human being has. Play is often useful as a vent for a child's emotions, both positive and negative. For example, an angry child can let anger out on his or her toys rather than other children or adults, and through this will learn to control anger constructively. Equally, a child may show love and affection through role play. Quiet activities may prove an effective outlet for a child who needs time and space to be alone.

Social development

All children live as part of a society and learning its norms and values so that they are able to fit in and function is an important part of development. A child will learn to interact with others through play. Play situations such as nursery or playgroup will also help them develop the skills necessary for relating effectively to both adults and children – they will learn social skills such as sharing and taking turns. They will become aware of the feelings of others and begin to be able to take those feelings into account.

Stages of development

All children go through different stages of development, and develop at different paces. A key role of the early years setting is to provide opportunities for learning and development which are appropriate for the child's developmental stage but also help them move toward the next stage. The stage of development will determine the types of activities provided. Activities will be heavily influenced by both the way children play and their level of understanding.

The stages of play are linked to age. However, children develop at different speeds and some may take longer to go through a particular stage than others. In addition, greater adult support may be needed to move some children from one stage to another and this will be reflected in the activities planned.

The background and experience the child has may also influence the activities provided and the way a child responds to them. A child from a large family may find it easy to play co-operatively with other children in a nursery situation whereas a single child may find settling in more difficult. Table 16.2 shows the main stages of play.

The stages of play are not necessarily separated, a child who is able to play with other children may also like to play alone at times. Early years workers need to remember that not all children develop at the same rate. It is important that they know the children they are working with and plan accordingly.

Respecting the individual

It is important when planning activities to recognise that all individuals are different. The Children Act (1989) clearly states that the needs of all children must be met regardless of age, gender, race, religion or ability. One way in which this is tackled is through equal opportunities and anti-discriminatory policies.

TYPE	AGE	EXPLANATION
Solitary	0–2 years	Children play alone. There is little interaction with other children.
Spectator	2–2.5 years	Children will watch other children playing around them, but do not join in.
Parallel	2.5–3 years	Children play alongside each other, but do not play together.
Associative	3–4 years	Children begin to interact and co-operate with others in their play. There are signs of them beginning to develop friendship groups and preference for playing with certain children. Play is usually in mixed sex groups.

TABLE 16.2 *The main stages of play*

These exist in many childcare settings as staff try to ensure every child is included in all activities. This affects the play provision and the way staff encourage children to join in.

There are certain groups in society who can be discriminated against, including females, ethnic minorities, people with disabilities and people from disadvantaged backgrounds. Often these groups are portrayed negatively in the media. This can affect a child's self-esteem, and therefore it is important that toys, games, posters, books and other equipment in the childcare setting are carefully chosen to avoid stereotypes. It is also important to include differentiation techniques which ensure an activity has a range of challenges, so children of all abilities will find it rewarding.

Differentiation within an activity allows all children to achieve the activity to the best of their ability. An example would be asking a child to describe their favourite meal. All children, whatever their ability, could attempt this, but the more able child might describe flavours, textures and colours whereas another child might just name the foods on the plate.

Many childcare providers put equal opportunities into action through an anti-discriminatory policy. This encourages staff to look at their own ideals and values and adjust them to ensure all children have equal access to opportunities provided.

Encouraging children to play

Children can be encouraged to learn in a number of ways. It is often said that there is no 'right way' to educate children as they are very adaptable and can benefit from a wide range of approaches. Whichever approach is used, adults have an important role in the process as they can help enhance both the learning experience and the learning potential of activities in different ways.

This can include supporting play and providing materials which encourage rich play activities, thus enabling children to learn from the play opportunity and extend it to its full potential. It may also involve providing information about experiences children haven't yet had or things they need to know. The role of the adult in children's learning and play is one of finding the right balance between standing too far back and letting the children play alone and becoming too involved and taking control of the situation.

The adult has an important role in planning the environment and organising activities which will stimulate children's interests and promote learning. They need to make sure that both indoor and outdoor play areas are stimulating and that there are enough interesting materials and equipment for the children to play effectively. Materials and equipment should be presented in a manner which encourages

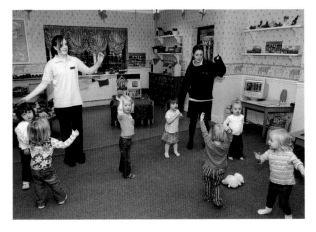

FIGURE 16.6 *Adults can support children's learning through play*

the child to explore them and discover their properties for themselves. This will encourage them to ask questions so the adult can support learning by clarifying ideas and correcting misunderstandings. Children learn through this direction and effective planning.

Children do not always have the understanding or imagination to take an activity forward. Therefore, an adult may need to extend a child's play by offering ideas which the child may take and develop further. In this situation, the adult is **facilitating** the play and through careful observation and listening is able to suggest ideas which make the activity more challenging. For example, in a junk modelling activity, an adult might help make an activity more challenging by asking what might happen if the child adds another piece of junk to the model. In doing this, the adult will extend the discussion with the child and allow them to think through and explain ideas.

An adult may also facilitate the play by helping children to remain in role or stay in their story in imaginative play. They may do this by providing props to help the pretend play, for example, two dolls so two children can play 'babies'. They may offer ideas, for example, where children are playing 'cars' by lining up chairs in a car layout, then the adult may ask 'Where is the car taking you?'. This may encourage them to develop the activity perhaps into a shopping trip or outing to the zoo.

Adults may also need to demonstrate certain skills to children as they develop and learn. For example, an adult may need to demonstrate a particular painting technique to children before they try the activity themselves. Once this skill is acquired the children can explore it on their own. Adults sometimes act as role models, working alongside the children to help them develop a new skill. An example of this might be in a cooking activity where the adult works with the children to make a food item, being a role model for them for aspects such as hygiene and safety.

Adults can use questioning cleverly to help support play. Questions can be used to develop different skills. Table 16.3 illustrates how questions can do this.

SKILL	QUESTION
Explaining	How are you going to use this?
Prediction	What do you think will happen if you put all those bricks in the bowl of water?
Recall	What did we see yesterday when we were digging the garden?
Recall a process	What did we need to do before we started cooking when we made biscuits?
Understanding	How will you put this train set together?

TABLE 16.3 *Questions help develop skills*

No matter what toys and activities are provided, some children find it difficult to play. An adult may need to support a child in their play and help them to join in any activity which is going on. Shy children often need an adult with them in the initial stages of play until their confidence grows. Children can be encouraged to play alongside other children first, rather than playing with them, to move gradually into a group play situation.

For example, an adult might encourage a child to play in the sandpit by asking them if they would like to make a sandcastle alongside another child. This may then develop into co-operative play.

SCENARIO

George

Mary, an early years worker has noticed that George, a quiet three year old, seems to be playing a lot on his own. He will sometimes play alongside other children or stand and watch other children play, but does not join in. What should Mary do?

Adults can provide information about experiences they have had or roles that they do. Often adults in well-known job roles such as the ambulance, police or fire crew will visit a nursery or school to talk about what they do. This helps children understand the world around them and the things that happen each day. They may then incorporate these ideas into their play.

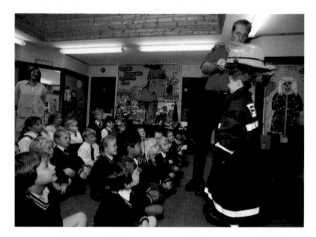

FIGURE 16.7 *Adults can support children's learning through explaining their job roles*

Positive feedback

One key role of the adult is to provide feedback to children on what they are doing. Children need both praise and recognition. This should be freely given and not necessarily linked to an achievement or result. Positive feedback can be given for working well or carrying out a task as requested. This type of positive feedback can encourage children to co-operate, as all children like to please. If praise is linked to a particular event or achievement, it should be as immediate as possible after the event.

Positive feedback is essential in encouraging young children to learn and keep persevering with the activity they are doing. Early years workers may comment as they are supervising children – for example saying 'your game looks fun' when a group of children are playing 'cops and robbers' together. Such comments should not interrupt the game, but allow the adult to comment on the fact that the children are playing well together. Giving positive praise should help children recognise their own efforts. Eventually they will inwardly recognise their own efforts and this will give them self-satisfaction.

Structured tasks

Structured tasks are directed activities which are sometimes used in early years settings, particularly if staff want children to experience or learn a specific skill. Often this activity is introduced by the adult with verbal instruction or demonstration or a mixture of both. The children will then follow this by practising the skills explained or demonstrated with the aim of perfecting the skill. An example of this might be a cooking activity. The practical, first-hand experience helps children to learn and remember the skills involved. Questioning and discussion with the adult will often be part of this process and can help the child to remember the skills being learned.

Summary

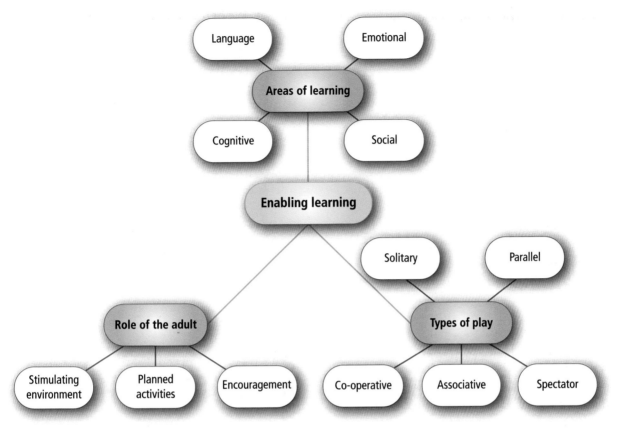

16.4 Theories of development, learning and education

To be able to understand how children learn, it is important to appreciate the difference between development and learning. The term development relates to the way in which a child functions. It relates to general development. It is spontaneous which means that it happens naturally. For example, a two-year-old child can run and jump but will not yet be able to skip.

Learning, on the other hand, occurs in specific situations and can be defined as a permanent change in behaviour brought about by previous experience. Some things are easier to learn than others and the kinds of things people learn contribute to making each person different.

Key concepts

Development: the natural way in which a child develops general functions.

Learning: a permanent change in behaviour brought about by experience.

There is a close link between development and behaviour. Generally, if children are encouraged in their general development, they will learn. There are examples where children have been held back in their learning because their general development was stifled, for example, in orphanages where children were kept in their cots for long periods. Both their general development and intellectual development were held back as they could not explore or learn.

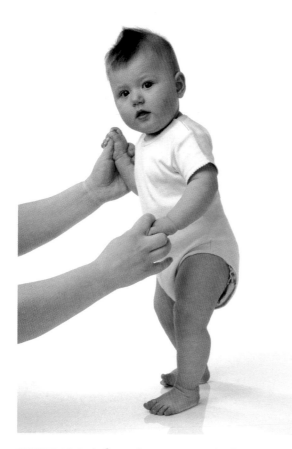

FIGURE 16.8 *Infants have a genetically inbuilt response to try and walk, but experience and learning are necessary for this ability to develop*

The simplest form of learning is probably associative learning where a stimulus causes a reaction or response. In other words, there is an association between the two actions. One example would be putting a coat on (response) when it starts to rain (stimulus). Another example might be eating (response) when a child feels hungry (stimulus).

Think it over

Think of other examples of associative learning.

There are many theories of learning. Some describe the process of learning as a gradual, continuous process, where every day we learn something new and this affects the way we think about the world. Others see learning as a series of stages which are passed through in a logical sequence, each one having to be achieved before the next can begin. To explore this further, we will look at different theories of learning.

Operant conditioning

The term **operant conditioning** is used to describe learning as a consequence of our actions. Pleasant outcomes are likely to reinforce the occurrence of the behaviours that created them. Behaviour operates on the world and so Skinner (1904–1990), an American biologist and psychologist, used the word 'operant' to describe behaviours which create learned outcomes.

Key concept

Operant conditioning: learning to repeat actions which have a reinforcing or strengthening outcome. In other words, people learn to repeat actions which have previously felt good or are associated with 'feeling better'.

Early research on this theory was carried out in the early nineteenth century by E. L. Thorndike. Thorndike put a cat in a box and food outside the box. In order to get the food the cat had to escape, but to do this it had to perform some act such as pulling a string. Eventually, by chance, the cat would achieve this. Thorndike then repeated his experiment the next day and timed how long it took the cat to get out of the box. After a few trials, the cats could escape immediately. Thorndike called this the 'Law of Effect'. He believed that any action that produced a good effect would become stamped into the mind of the animal. In 1898 Thorndike wrote an article in which he explained the 'Law of Effect'. The 'Law of Effect' means that actions are governed by their consequences. Animals and humans will learn to repeat actions which produce good effects and to avoid repeating those which have bad outcomes.

This theory was developed further by Skinner who developed the Skinner box, which was a box containing a lever and a food tray. He used it to study how rats and other animals learn. Like Thorndike's cats, the rats soon learned to press the lever to get a pellet of food. Skinner also found that a number of things other than food could be used as rewards.

Skinner described anything that made the animal repeat the response as a 'reinforcer'. He also discovered that removing discomfort might act as a reinforcer. If a response caused pain to stop, this was also learned quickly by animals. The main purpose of reinforcement is to shape and then maintain certain behaviours. Therefore, a reinforcer can be anything that causes behaviour to be repeated. The reinforcer may please people personally – it may be money for doing a task, or personal satisfaction for doing something for someone else. In early years, the reinforcer for a child might be positive feedback and praise. Children like to please and interest and praise can reinforce behaviour and actions in the same way as food or money.

Skinner believed there were primary and secondary reinforcers. Primary reinforcers are things that satisfy a physical need such as sleep or food. Secondary reinforcers are things humans have learned are worth having, such as money. His theory stressed the importance of reinforcing a new 'desirable' behaviour pattern to replace 'less desirable' behaviour. Skinner argued that punishment is an inefficient way to influence people because it blocks a response without supporting an alternative behaviour. It is important to remember that the use of punishment is contrary to care values and codes of practice in care work. Many people believe that the deliberate use of punishment is unethical and the use of physical punishment is likely to be illegal.

Social learning theory

Social learning theory suggests that children learn by observing and imitating the behaviour

of others. While it is accepted that children learn a great deal from reward and punishment, social learning theory believes modelling or copying behaviour that is observed in others has a greater effect. If children see behaviour which leads to something positive happening, they are likely to try to copy it.

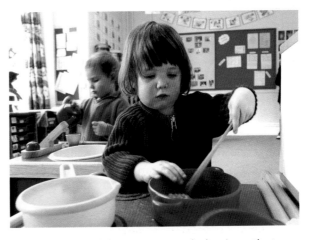

FIGURE 16.9 *Children may copy behaviour that they see*

Social learning is sometimes called observational learning. This does not mean children copy everything they see, but they will model aspects of their behaviour on people they believe to be important (see Unit 12 for further details). Every child is different and will copy different things. Therefore, as the environment in which they live affects learning, children will develop differently.

Albert Bandura, a social psychologist (born 1925), explored social learning theory in detail. He believed much of an individual's personality and behaviour is learned. Much of this will happen in childhood, as children are likely to model and imitate the behaviour of others.

Bandura did an experiment using an inflatable plastic doll called a Bobo doll (Bandura *et al* 1963). Children were shown a film of an adult attacking the doll, hitting it with mallets and shouting at it. However, there were three different endings:

* Ending 1: the adult was rewarded with sweets

* Ending 2: the adult was told off and smacked for his aggression

* Ending 3: no reward or punishment was seen.

Children were shown one of the endings and then allowed to play with the doll. The results showed that those who saw the adult being rewarded with sweets, or saw no consequences, were aggressive towards the doll, whereas those who saw the adult being punished were less likely to be aggressive.

Bandura concluded the aggressive behaviour that had been seen had two effects on the children. Firstly, it taught them new ways to be aggressive, and secondly it increased the amount of aggressive behaviour in the children. The work has been criticised as it was felt that children were not familiar with Bobo dolls and therefore may have believed that they 'played' with them in the correct way. Nevertheless it highlights the way in which behaviour can be learned through imitation.

Think it over

How might this example affect the types of television programmes and films young children are allowed to watch?

Social learning theory is often used to explain how children learn social norms. It can highlight how the norms of behaviour in different cultures are passed from adults to children (see Unit 12 for further details). It can also show how children learn **schemata** for attitudes and stereotypes through the observation of adults and modelling their behaviour. For example, a child who has an adult role model who expresses negative views about different ethnic groups is likely to learn this response and express similar negative opinions and views.

Key concept

Schema (plural: schemata): a pattern of behaviour or actions which children acquire to use in similar situations, for example, crossing the road. A child learns to look right and left before crossing a road and also not to cross between parked cars or near junctions. It doesn't matter where a child learns this; they will apply it to crossing any road, in any town or country.

Cognitive development

A major contributor to our understanding of **cognitive development** and how a child's intellect develops is Jean Piaget. He was a Swiss psychologist (1896–1980), who spent much of his life studying children in great depth. He based many of his theories on studies of his own children and felt that children are actively involved in developing their own knowledge so they can understand the world around them. To do this successfully, Piaget believed children used a number of thinking processes to allow them to adapt to their environment. The development

Key concepts

Cognitive development: development of mental functions such as the ability to think logically and abstractly, to reason, to understand concepts, to concentrate, to remember and recall information and to use problem-solving skills.

Intelligence: all aspects of cognitive development, including language.

of these thinking processes is called 'cognitive development'. All these mental functions are linked together and also linked closely with language development.

Schemata

Piaget believed that children develop a number of patterns of behaviour or actions, which they then apply to similar situations. This helps them categorise things into manageable and understandable groups.

Many patterns of this sort are developed. For example, a young child may always use a spoon to eat with. When first given a knife and fork, the child will need to learn that food can be picked up with other implements, and will amend the pattern of understanding to accommodate this new information. Piaget called this type of pattern 'schema' (plural 'schemata'). As the child grows older, the schema for eating will develop to include other eating implements such as chopsticks.

Think it over

Think about other examples of schema where humans develop ways of dealing with situations which may then be developed, depending on the circumstances.

As children develop, they add more complex schemata to their thinking. Piaget believed that the progression from very simple thinking in early childhood to the more complex thinking of adolescence is achieved through three basic processes.

Assimilation

Assimilation means taking in and understanding new information. To be assimilated, new information needs to connect to or attach to something a person already knows. Therefore, the amount of new information a child can assimilate will depend on the level of understanding the child already has. For example, a child may have a cat as a pet and think that all cats are the same. She may then see another species of cat, such as a Siamese, which she will label as 'a cat' and add to her schema on cats. She will then start to understand that cats can be different shapes and sizes.

Did you know?

It is believed that one of the reasons babies sleep so much is that their brains need to assimilate all the new information they are taking in from the world around them.

Accommodation

Accommodation occurs when a child takes in new information which causes a change to an existing schema. An example might be that a child who always has milk in a blue bottle thinks that all blue bottles contain milk. If the child is then given milk from a green bottle, he or she will accommodate the new information that milk does not always come from blue bottles.

Equilibration

Equilibration occurs when all pieces of information fit into the schemata a child has developed. Disequilibration occurs when the pieces do not link up. Piaget thought this might occur when a child moves from one stage to another, as more major reorganisation of schemata occurs. A child may have to abandon an idea because it no longer fits in, and take another idea on board.

Piaget's stages of development

Through his observations, Piaget saw that children make similar mistakes at similar ages. He therefore suggested that a child passes through four stages of development, which are roughly age-related. Piaget believed that these four stages are sequential, which means that a child has to pass through each one in order to reach the next. Piaget did not believe it was possible to teach a child in one stage about concepts from a more advanced stage. Therefore, Piaget believed that activities developed for different age groups should reflect their stage of development.

Piaget demonstrated that when a child is shown the same number of buttons presented differently, the appearance influences the child's answer as to whether there are more or fewer

Conservation: in Piaget's theory, a child who understands conservation will know that, no matter what shape something is made into, unless it is added to or something is taken away, the amount remains the same.

buttons. If the experimenter lines up two sets of five buttons equally, then lengthens one line in front of the child, a child who is unable to conserve will say that the longer line contains more buttons.

Piaget showed that this pattern occurs with other concepts besides number. In other experiments two identical glasses are filled with water, one is then poured into a taller, thinner glass; or two equal balls of dough or plasticine are shown to a child, before one is moulded into a different shape. A young child will believe that the quantities differ according to appearances.

Many modern researchers have built their ideas on Piaget's work. However, Piaget's ideas have been criticised for a variety of reasons, particularly because researchers have since shown that children reach the stages at earlier ages. Despite this, his work is still valued and is often

STAGE	WHAT HAPPENS	EXAMPLES
Sensorimotor stage (0–18 months)	Babies learn about their world through their senses and physical activity. Babies use schemata which have been developed using trial and error methods. Babies are learning to control their movements and so play involves repeating and varying movements as they acquire more control. Babies also enjoy being able to make things happen and observing cause and effect. A baby will think that something has gone if he or she cannot actually see it – babies do not understand **object permanence**. Babies and toddlers in this phase are extremely egocentric, which means that they can only see things from their own point of view.	Babies explore objects using their mouths. A baby will be interested in a baby gym because of the repetition that is possible. If, playing ball with a baby, you hide the ball under a cloth, the baby will think the ball has gone.
Pre-operational stage (18 months– 7 years)	Children use symbols to represent experiences. Children begin to pretend within their play and use objects to represent something else. Memory begins to develop and a child will mention absent people and things. Children come to understand the concepts of past and future. Children try to share knowledge and experiences. Children at this stage are still egocentric. Children are still influenced by the appearance of objects.	For example, using a broom as a horse.

continued on next page

STAGE	WHAT HAPPENS	EXAMPLES
Concrete operational stage (7–12 years)	From the age of seven, children begin to understand concepts such as conservation and can use mathematical skills such as addition, subtraction, and multiplication. Children of this age can understand that things may belong to more than one category and that categories have logical relationships. They begin to develop inductive logic, which means that they can link their own experience to general principles. They deal best with things they can see or manipulate, and are less successful in discussing abstract ideas or possibilities.	A child will be able to categorise dogs and cats, but also realise that dogs and cats both belong to the category of pets. A child may know that if you add one more car to a line of cars and count them, there will be one more than before. So the general principle is that addition always increases something
Formal operational stage (12 years–adulthood)	Children are able to deal with abstract concepts and relate experiences to others of which they have no first-hand knowledge. They can imagine themselves in different situations and roles. They can apply deductive logic to solve problems, which means they can think through similar experiences they have had and apply them to an unfamiliar situation. They become aware of abstract ideas, such as fair play. Abstract ideas are theoretical, and cannot be physically demonstrated.	This is the stage that most adults are in, but it is worth remembering that some people never reach this stage of development, for example if they have learning difficulties. It is also true to say that people can have well-developed formal operational thinking in one area of life but not in another in which they are less skilled.

TABLE 16.4 *Stages of development*

seen as a breakthrough in the way we understand how children think and learn. See Unit 12, pages 59–66, for more information on Piaget.

Other theorists on cognitive development

Vygotsky (1896–1935)

Vygotsky was a Russian theorist whose ideas had great influence in the 1990s and continue to influence educational theory today. Vygotsky thought that play helps children to understand and accommodate what they have learned, because they are free from any constraints when they play and can explore ideas fully. He believed

play allowed children to move from their present stage of thinking to a higher level.

He also thought that the role of the adult was important. He believed adults could stretch children so that they further developed ideas and thinking through their play. As well as being aware of a child's current stage of development, Vygotsky looked at what a child could do in the next stage. He called this the 'zone of potential or proximal development' and focused play experiences on this. An example in language development might be that a child does not seem to be able to verbalise certain ideas when asked individually, but can contribute in an effective way to a group discussion on the topic. In a play situation, a child may not be able to do a puzzle on their own but can with the support of an adult guiding them or when working with more able peers.

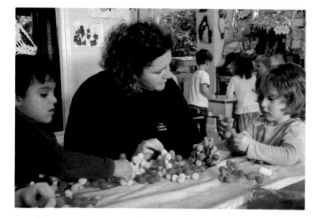

FIGURE 16.10 *Children may need adult support in play*

In other words, children who seem to lack certain skills when tested or working on their own may perform more effectively in the group situation where support is provided by someone with the necessary knowledge. This is an example of where skills shown in the social situation but not the isolated one fall within the zone of proximal development.

Jerome Bruner (born 1915)

Bruner suggested that children develop different types of thinking:

* enactive

* iconic

* symbolic.

He believed that children need to be able to move freely and be actively involved in their learning. Ideas and thinking are best developed through first-hand experiences. 'Enactive thinking' involves being able to remember and perform physical actions, for example, we can remember the feeling involved in floating on water or the feeling of balancing a bicycle but we may not be able to picture or explain these abilities using language.

Bruner demonstrated that children often need to be reminded of previous experiences as this helped them in their learning. This may be through pictures, books or interest tables. He called this 'iconic thinking' ('iconic' means 'in picture form'). We can remember events in pictures, for example,

we can recognise people's faces. We may have a picture memory of what a person looks like, but we cannot explain their face using words.

Symbolic thinking involves the use of language and other symbolic systems. Bruner described different ways of communicating such as language, dancing, painting, drawing and music. He saw these as types of 'codes'; children acquire more of these codes as they get older. In doing this, they acquire more modes of representation of the world.

Bruner also felt the role of the adult was important. Adults provide support as children develop their competence and confidence. He described this support as 'scaffolding'. In the early stages of learning, the adult has an important role in setting up experiences for the child, and in judging what the child needs next in order to develop cognitively. He likened this to scaffolding on a new building. As the child develops, the support from the adult would be reduced as the child gains confidence (Bruner 1974).

Language development

The study of language acquisition is also known as 'linguistics'. Language is defined as 'an organised system of symbols which humans use to communicate.' These symbols may be spoken, signed or written down. Spoken language is made up of basic sounds called 'phonemes' which combine to form more complex sounds called 'morphemes'. For example 'stop' is a morpheme made up of the phonemes 'st' and 'op'. Human beings use language to communicate.

> **Think it over**
>
> Identify other words in terms of the phonemes that make them up.

Communication is the transmission of something, usually a message or meaning, from one person to another. Human beings are the only species to have the ability to use language in this way. This sets humans apart from animals who may be able to communicate simple messages, such as being hungry or needing to go outside, but cannot use language.

Main stages of language development

Being able to talk requires control over breathing, face muscles and tongue muscles, as well as knowledge of words and their meanings. Therefore, babies take time to acquire these skills. All babies benefit from social interaction as this helps their language to develop. Quite a lot of language skills are acquired by imitation.

Language development occurs in three stages:

* pre-linguistic
* first words
* first sentences.

Children all over the world are thought to follow the same sequence in language acquisition. There are three broad stages to language development (see Table 16.5).

STAGE	FEATURES
Pre-linguistic stage (0–12 months)	From a few hours after birth, babies can distinguish speech from other sounds. Between 2–6 months, babies start to babble. At 10 months, babies start stringing sounds together, e.g. bababbaba. Babies enjoy babbling and seem to babble for their own pleasure.
First words (1–2 years)	Infants have now developed control over vocal cords, facial muscles, etc., and are cognitively mature enough to accept that sounds they hear or can make represent something they know. Initially, infants use sounds that mean something, e.g. kaa – juice, bottle. Infants learn first words which are most familiar to them – dada, mama, bath, drink, etc. They reduce words to the simplest sounds, e.g. spoon becomes 'poon' as they have not mastered all sounds. They will understand what some words mean long before they can use them and therefore have an 'active' vocabulary which they use and a 'passive' vocabulary which they understand. By two years, children have a vocabulary of about 50 words.
First sentences (18 months–2 years onwards)	Children start to combine words into simple two word sentences from 18 months onwards – this is known as 'telegraphic speech'. They start to use grammar or the rules of language. Several new words will be learned each day. Early speech has certain common themes – children talk about what has happened to what, e.g. 'me hit ball'; they are preoccupied with who owns what and possessions, e.g. 'teddy mine'; they have a concern about where things are, e.g. 'car in garage'. Some children are able to express feelings and say what they want. They understand non-existence, e.g. 'milk all gone'. They learn how to ask for a repeat of something, e.g. 'more milk, 'me go again'. By 30 months babbling will have disappeared. By 36 months, children have a vocabulary of about 1000 words and about 85 per cent of their utterances are understood, even by strangers.

TABLE 16.5 *The stages of language development*

Some theorists believe all babies are born with the ability to acquire any language but their skills are shaped by the language they hear most frequently. Table 16.5 represents what most two- and three-year-old children can achieve. However, not all children go through the stages at the same time. There have been examples of ten-month-old children using two-word sentences, but the average age for this is 18 months. However, it is not uncommon for children of two years not to have used two-word sentences.

Brown

Roger Brown conducted a ten-year study on the language development of three children he called Adam, Eve and Sarah. He taped each child speaking for an hour a week from about 27 months until they were five years old. He was specifically interested in how children learn the 14 most common morphemes and how they acquire grammar skills. From his research, Brown concluded that children went through the same sequences to acquire language even though the age at which they master the rules of grammar varied. He suggested that language developed in five stages.

Stage 1

Children use simple two- or three-word sentences, or telegraphic speech which describes actions or possessions. During this stage children will miss out unimportant words.

Stage 2

More complicated language is used as children learn the words for objects and events. They also start to use word endings.

Stage 3

Children ask a lot of questions using what, why, where and who.

Stage 4

Children start to join two short sentences together into a longer one.

Stage 5

Children start using more complex sentences which can include two subjects in the same sentence. At this stage children are ready for school, which relies on language that the children need to understand.

Brown suggested that children learn grammar one stage at a time. They concentrate on one stage, incorporate it into their 'schema', and then expand that basic idea, moving onto the next. By the time children go to school, they have usually acquired enough syntax or grammar to be able to communicate quite effectively.

Theories of language development

There have been several theories on language development. Skinner suggested language was learned through operant conditioning (see Unit 12). He felt that any speech, like sounds that babies make, would be reinforced and become words. Sounds that are not reinforced will eventually disappear and not be used. He did not refer to any mental structures in this process, such as schemas. He felt that a child's ability to name objects and ask questions would enable expansion of the vocabulary. This theory was discredited, as it did not really explain how children learn to combine all the words they use into different sentences. It was also felt that parents do not generally reinforce their children's speech. While they may correct speech if a child says something wrong, they are less likely to correct simple grammatical faults.

Chomsky

Noam Chomsky (born 1928), an American biologist, suggested that we are all born with an innate ability to communicate and have all the necessary attributes, including the left side of the brain which is linked to speech and language. He called this the 'language acquisition device' (LAD) through which we are able to understand the structure, vocabulary and grammar of the particular language we use. This theory explains why children sometimes make grammatical mistakes such as using 'ed' for all past tense words when they are learning (e.g. runned or goed). This is because the LAD will apply the rules of grammar – that the past tense generally has 'ed' attached to the word (Chomsky 1959).

Berko

Jean Berko Gleason, an American psycholinguist, was best known for developing the 'wug' test in 1958. The test aimed to assess how young children acquire an understanding of grammar, such as plurals. The test would involve the children being introduced to a 'wug' – a fictional character. They would be told, 'this is a wug'. They would then be introduced to two of them and be asked: 'Now there are two of them, there are two...?' Children who had acquired the rule would say 'wugs'; those that hadn't would say 'two wug'.

The test also explored children's ability to understand the agentive (er). For example, a man who builds is a 'builder'. The test asks, what is a man who zibs? Children who understand the concept would say 'zibber'; those that didn't would say a 'zibman'.

Berko also looked at a child's ability to understand compound words that they had in their vocabulary, for example, birthday. Some children would understand that birthday is the 'day' of your 'birth'; others would see birthday as meaning 'a day you get presents'.

The main finding of the test was that even very young children had internalised these grammar rules. This showed that children were able to acquire grammar rules by listening to the speech going on around them. This test has been proven very reliable, having been tried several times with similar results.

Work of other educational theorists and practitioners

Play is nowadays considered an important part of a child's development. It is widely recognised that play is a 'child's work' and it is through play that young children learn about the world in which they live.

Various theorists and practitioners have presented theories on the origin, function and pattern of play. Theories on play and children's learning have been put forward since the 1700s. Rousseau, a French philosopher (1712–1778) was a pioneer with his suggestion that children should be allowed to roam free and discover things for themselves. However, eighteenth century society was not impressed with his ideas, as at that time children were considered miniature adults and no special provision was made for them. The changing attitudes of society towards children and childhood through the centuries have influenced the type of care and activities provided for children.

Look up the following early theorists. Find out about their views on play and how they reflected the attitudes towards children in society.

* G. Stanley Hall

* Herbert Spencer

* Karl Groos.

Many of these early theories have been updated but nevertheless they have had a significant influence on the today's educational practice. All these theorists believed that care and education were inextricably linked and that when provided together, the best learning takes place. Many of the theorists who have had most influence on practices in the UK were born and developed their ideas in other countries. Some of these theorists and their work are outlined in Table 16.6.

THEORIST/ PRACTITIONER	COUNTRY	MAIN IDEAS AND THEORIES
Friedrich Froebel (1782–1852)	Germany	Children are born good and that to help them develop, adults need to provide the right environment and activities.
		Children can learn outdoors with other children as well as indoors.
		Outdoor activities encourage an interest in natural science.
		Children should be able to move around freely.
		Symbolic and imaginative play (such as children pretending that some counters in a pot are food and they are making breakfast) is important and shows a high level of learning.
		'Gifts' to play with would be an aid to children's learning, for example, a hard and a soft ball would develop awareness of the concepts of hardness and softness.
Maria Montessori (1869–1952)	Italy	Children under the age of six have the most powerful and receptive minds and this gives them a once-in-a-lifetime opportunity to learn.
		Developed a structured education programme based on the stages Montessori believed children have to go through to learn.
		Developed a number of specially devised pieces of equipment that encouraged children to develop certain skills. She called these 'didactic' materials – didactic means 'intended to instruct'. They have built-in control of error, so children can teach themselves in a non-competitive atmosphere.
		Encouraged children to learn about the world around them through exploration. They are given the freedom to move around, manipulate and touch.
		Placed limited emphasis on counting, reading and writing – these follow once the basic social and emotional development has taken place.
		Encouraged children's natural will to learn as this would foster a life-long motivation for learning.
		Encouraged children to work alone. Montessori felt the best learning occurred when children were focused, silent and completely absorbed in a task.
		All play needed to have a learning focus – free play was not encouraged.

continued on next page

THEORIST/ PRACTITIONER	COUNTRY	MAIN IDEAS AND THEORIES
Rudolph Steiner (1861–1925)	Austria	Developed ideas about teaching young children known as the Waldorf education system.
		Childhood was a separate period of life and his methods aimed to develop all aspects of the child.
		Designed a curriculum aimed to provide equal experience of the arts and sciences.
		Imaginative play, often with natural materials, is central to the Waldorf scheme, and manufactured toys are not allowed.
		Placed much emphasis on relationships and the community. Children in Steiner schools often stay with the same teacher for the whole of their primary education, and the teacher also gets to know the family well.
		Teacher makes up or retells stories, rather than reading from a book, as a way to encourage a child to think.
		Believed children have different temperaments, which affect their attitudes and behaviour:
		* sanguine (cheerful and confident)
		* choleric (bad tempered)
		* phlegmatic (stoic, unemotional)
		* melancholic (irritable).
		Steiner believed adults should work with these temperaments.
		Brighter children should be encouraged to support their weaker peers, for example, circle time where all children are encouraged to join in.
Susan Isaacs (1885–1948)	England	Play gave children the opportunity to think, develop their feelings and learn social skills.
		Children begin to understand the world in which they live through their play, as it allows them to move from fantasy into reality.
		Children should be allowed to roam freely, to explore the world around them – this is how they learn.
		Children need to be encouraged to express their feelings as keeping them bottled up can be damaging.
		Recognised the important role of parents in the education of the young child and promoted this through articles.
		Promoted the nursery as an extension of the home.
		Children were best educated in a nursery setting until the age of seven, as many children go backwards educationally at five when they enter school.

TABLE 16.6 *Influential theorists*

Summary

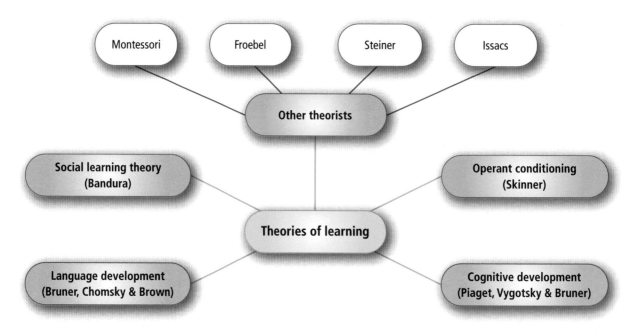

16.5 Assessment in early years education

Desirable learning outcomes

The current approach to the curriculum is based on *Desirable Learning Outcomes*, a major government document published in 1996, which set out minimum goals for children's learning. It reflected the way many other European countries organised their curriculum and therefore takes on many European ideas. The document set out what the government felt a child should be able to do on entering compulsory education at five years of age. They specified a curriculum which early years childcare providers needed to base their work on whether they were voluntary, statutory or private providers. Ofsted (the Office for Standards in Education), checks that providers have an appropriate curriculum to meet the demands of the 'desirable learning outcomes' and that children are being given a sound preparation for the National Curriculum, which starts with Key Stage 1 (Years 1 and 2, ages 5–7).

The National Curriculum

The National Curriculum is divided into four key stages for children aged 5–16. It sets out the areas of study in ten curriculum areas and the knowledge and skills which must be covered in each. Like the 'desirable learning outcomes', it leaves the method of delivery to the teacher and school. The curriculum areas are divided into core and foundation subjects. Core subjects are English, maths and science. Foundation subjects are design and technology, physical education, art, history, geography, music and information technology. Achievement in each of the areas can be measured at eight levels. At the end of Key Stage 1, most children in that phase will perform at level 2, with a few achieving either level 3 or level 1. Teachers often use level 1 as a measure of where children should be at the end of the first year in Key Stage 1. At the end of Key Stage 1, children take standard assessment tests (SATS) which are designed by the government and taken by almost all children. These provide a way of measuring children's achievement and the 'value' the school has added to that child's learning.

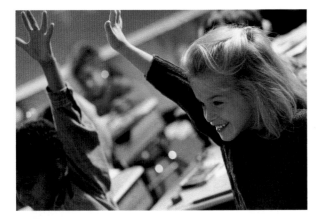

FIGURE 16.11 *Children in infant classes are aged 5–7*

In developing the curriculum proposals, particular attention was paid to literacy and numeracy, as the foundations for success are laid at an early stage. The emphasis on these skills has been strengthened recently with National Literacy and Numeracy Hours in primary schools. For further information on the foundation stage visit the Qualifications and Curriculum Authority's website (www.qca.org.uk).

The Foundation Stage

The Foundation Stage is a distinct phase of education for children aged 3–5. It sets out six areas of learning which form the basis of the Foundation Stage curriculum. These areas are:

* personal, social and emotional development
* communication, language and literacy
* mathematical development
* knowledge and understanding of the world
* physical development
* creative development.

Each area of learning has a set of related Early Learning Goals. The curriculum is designed to help early years practitioners plan to meet the diverse needs of all children so that most will achieve their potential. Some children, however, will go beyond the Early Learning Goals by the end of the Foundation Stage.

The Education Act (2002) extended the National Curriculum to include the Foundation Stage. It made the six areas of learning statutory. The act went further to establish a single national assessment system for the Foundation Stage called the Foundation Stage Profile. The profile has 13 summary scales, covering the six areas of learning, which need to be completed for each child receiving government-funded education by the end of their time in the Foundation Stage.

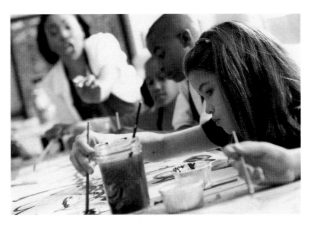

FIGURE 16.12 *Creative activities help children reach foundation goals*

As all children develop at different rates, individual achievement will vary. Not all children will fully achieve the Early Learning Goals by the time they start school, but some will achieve more than the minimum requirements. 'Extension statements' are provided for each of the six areas of learning to show how older or more able children might progress beyond the goals. Some special needs children may continue to work towards the outcomes throughout their time in education. Many early years providers already go beyond the minimum requirements, and they did so before Early Learning Goals came into existence.

Good practice in implementing the Early Learning Goals

The curriculum must cover all six areas of learning. Although the Early Learning Goals do not prescribe activities, guidelines are provided which identify good practice in planning how to deliver the goals. This has a great influence on early years providers, as many things contribute to a child successfully achieving the Early Learning Goals. The following list can act as a guide to creating a learning environment in which this will happen.

* The environment should be one in which children feel secure, valued and confident and can learn through enjoyable and rewarding experiences.

* Activities and the curriculum provided should encourage children to think and talk about their learning. It should recognise the value of first-hand experiences as a means of learning.

* Personal, social and emotional development is an essential part of the curriculum and should run through all the activities.

* Staff should be well trained, with a full understanding of the curriculum, the approach the setting uses and methods of assessment and recording being used.

* The setting should provide opportunities for a range of activities, including concentrated involvement in activities over longer periods of time.

* Staff recognise when it is appropriate to give help and the level of support that is needed. They only intervene if absolutely necessary. This helps develop independence in children.

* If a child is identified as having particular needs, appropriate support and intervention is provided. For example, a child with learning difficulties may be provided with extra one-to-one help.

* Progress and achievement are regularly recorded through accurate observations. This information is shared with parents.

* Parents are well informed about the curriculum and the approach to assessment the setting is using.

* The schools the children will progress to are also well informed of the approach of the setting and there are strong links.

* Adults in the setting should recognise the importance of training and actively undertake regular training.

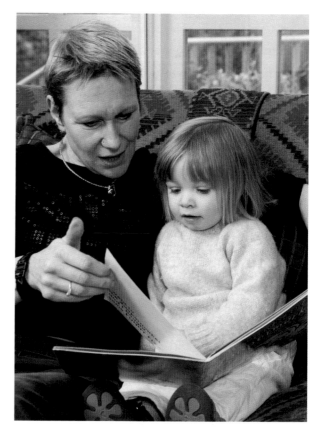

FIGURE 16.13 *Parents should be involved in their children's early learning activities*

Planning the curriculum

Any curriculum in settings for the rising fives must contain a full range of opportunities, activities and experiences to cover the learning goals. This requires detailed and thorough planning. Any plan must identify not only what the children should learn but also how they will learn it.

In order to ensure the children have opportunities to meet the Early Learning Goals, planning needs to be on various levels. There will need to be long-term, broad planning across the year; medium planning over a term; and short-term, more detailed planning on a day-to-day basis. This level of detail of planning will ensure that the children have a well-thought-out curriculum and that the Early Learning Goals are met in full.

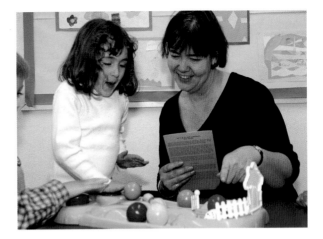

FIGURE 16.14 *Some children may need one-to-one attention*

Collecting evidence of children's learning

One of the aims of the Early Learning Goals is to enable a structured, systematic assessment of children as they enter school. Staff who are working with children are required to make a judgement on their skills and competence in relation to each of the six areas of learning. Assessments can, and should, happen throughout the foundation stage, not just at the end, although children are likely to achieve their best towards the end of the stage. Assessments will be recorded in 'assessment inventories'. Assessments must be based on evidence, which is collected in a number of ways, including:

* conversations between staff and children and between the children themselves
* observations carried out by staff
* assessment of the work children have produced
* conversations with parents.

Staff must be well trained and have a good knowledge of child development so that they know what they are looking for in children's work. Being able to observe objectively and record what is seen accurately takes tremendous skill. Poor interpretation, perhaps due to a lack of detailed understanding of child development, can mean important issues are missed.

To be reliable, evidence needs to be collected over a period of time, not based on just one example of performance. This will give a clearer indication of both achievement and development. Therefore, staff must observe and assess the children constantly. It is also important to use a combination of evidence in forming a judgement. For example, a lot more can be gained from talking to a child about a painting he or she has done, than from just looking at the finished product. The discussion of the process and ideas may show more complex thinking than is apparent from looking at the picture itself.

Foundation Stage Profile

The Foundation Stage Profile replaces the baseline assessment process which previously occurred halfway through a child's first term at school. It is the statutory assessment for children in the final year of the foundation stage. The word 'profile' has been carefully chosen – it reflects a new approach to assessment as one which is recording a picture of what a child has achieved, knows and can do. The profile is built up over a year, and there are no tests and no set tasks. The Foundation Stage Profile uses observations as a means of assessing learning. The foundation stage and the profile together support early years staff in providing a varied curriculum which is clearly linked to clear expectations as set out in the Early Learning Goals. The Foundation Stage

Profile provides both information on where the child is at the end of the reception year, as well as information to help further planning of learning for that child. It is therefore formative, summative and diagnostic.

The results of the Foundation Stage Profile not only identify a child's strengths and learning needs, allowing teachers to plan an appropriate curriculum, but also represent a point against which a child's progress through Key Stage 1 can be measured. It provides a benchmark which allows schools to show how a child has developed in a given period. Schools now have to show how they have made a positive contribution to a child's development or given 'added value'. The profiles should also:

* provide information for parents, which can inform discussions with teachers

* provide teachers with a range of information

* include the different achievements of children born in different months

* include achievements of children from different socio-economic groups

* help schools to plan to meet the differing needs of the children in their care.

Implications for early years groups

Early years settings are expected to carry out a number of tasks in relation to the Foundation Stage including:

* regular assessment of children to show how they are progressing towards the learning goals and achieving in terms of the Foundation Stage Profile

* planning, which should show how the activities provided are appropriate, build on these assessments and develop a child's skills and knowledge

* carry out assessments which are passed on to the child's first school.

This work is monitored through inspections by Ofsted. Children are not legally required to be in school until the term after their fifth birthday. Even if entry to school before the fifth birthday is possible in their area, some parents choose to keep their children at playgroup or nursery until this date. Many schools welcome information from early years groups, whatever the age of entry of the child.

How are children assessed?

The Foundation Stage Profile is compiled at intervals over the year as it assumes ongoing learning and development. The profile must be completed four weeks before the end of the reception class year. The profile measures a child's progress towards achieving the Early Learning Goals.

Each goal has nine points. The first three points describe a child who is still progressing towards achieving an early learning goal. The next five points record if a child has achieved a goal. They are ordered according to difficulty, but that does not prevent a child achieving one of the more difficult goals first. The final point is allocated to a child who has achieved all the goals and developed their understanding and skills further in terms of breadth and depth.

The profile aims to give a rounded view of the achievements of each child. As the results of the assessment are being used to compare achievements, it is important that all staff involved in assessing children do so in a consistent and fair way. This will help ensure comparability and confidence that the assessment judgments made of one child are comparable to those made for another. This is achieved by moderating judgments between practitioners, either within a setting or through a process supported by a local education authority moderator who will review the judgments made in different settings.

Think it over

What are the advantages and disadvantages of assessing children at such a young age?

Summary

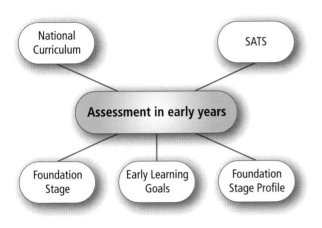

Imagine you have to plan an activity which could contribute to the assessment of early learning goals.

1. Choose the topic.

2. Outline five different activities you could use with that topic which would draw on different areas of learning, e.g. creative, language skills, reading skills.

3. Identify where the different Early Learning Goals might be covered.

16.6 Issues in early years learning and education

Education is an ever-developing and evolving area. There is often new thinking about how best to educate children. This brings issues which educational theorists discuss in an attempt to find the best way of developing education. Such issues can be contentious, as different theorists have different ideas; however, the debate helps move thinking forward. This section discusses three key issues.

Educating children by ability group

Some educational establishments choose to group children according to their ability for learning.

Many do this because they believe that children of similar ability will stimulate the others; particularly in groups of gifted and talented children where it is often suggested that they will stretch each other to achieve more. It has been suggested that, in mixed-ability groups, the teacher will aim for the middle ability and therefore not provide appropriate activities to move the less able forward or to stretch the more able children.

Others believe mixed-ability groupings are better as the more able children will support the less able, enabling the less able children to achieve more. Some believe mixed-ability groupings raise standards. Susan Hallam of the Institute of Education stated in 2002 that there was no evidence to suggest that teaching children in ability groups raises standards. She felt that in these cases the lower-ability groups were often repeatedly taught the same thing and that teaching was therefore monotonous. These children were often categorised by their teachers and school as slow and therefore they became demoralised and lacked motivation. The more able, on the other hand, continued to be motivated and the gap between the two groups became wider.

Think it over

Do you believe that mixed ability groupings are better for children's learning? How might this link to Piaget's theories on cognitive development?
List the advantages and disadvantages of this over streaming by ability. Think of this from the perspective of both the child and the teacher.

Testing children and setting targets

While everyone agrees that every child has the right to achieve their potential, there are many different views on the value of testing young children and setting targets. The current National Curriculum includes a significant amount of testing from an early age beginning with the Foundation Stage Profile and followed by regular SATs in primary and secondary school. The last SAT test takes place in Year 9, only to be followed by GCSEs, AS and A levels (A2s). Many believe that students following an English curriculum are among the most tested children in the world. Some believe that testing is unnecessary and puts undue pressure on young children. They feel that a good teacher can assess a child's achievement from their performance in class and that a test does not tell them anything more. Some children find the tests stressful with pressure from teachers and parents to achieve. School results are reported in league tables which are published and therefore, they will want their children to perform to the best of their ability.

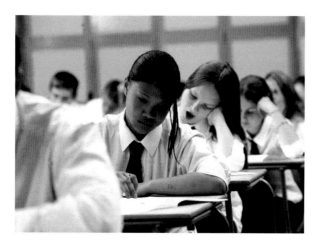

FIGURE 16.15 *There are varying views on the value of testing children*

There are others however, who feel that testing is an essential part of the curriculum and provides an unbiased view of a child's performance which can be matched against other children of the same age group across the country. Tests help schools to see how much 'value' they are adding to a child's development. They also provide teachers with crucial, objective details about how individual pupils are performing, helping them to tailor their teaching to meet pupils' needs. Some people believe that tests actually motivate children and encourage them to do well, in other words, tests can help children reach their full potential.

Think it over

How do you feel about tests?

Do you feel that young children should have to do tests in order to assess their ability or should the professional opinion of teachers count for more?

Having a set curriculum

Set curriculums, such as the National Curriculum, exist in many countries. They set out what children are expected to learn at particular ages and stages of education. In England there is a set curriculum from three years of age up to 16 years, first with the Foundation Stage and then the National Curriculum. All schools and early years providers who receive state funding must deliver the National Curriculum. The aim of the National Curriculum is to ensure all children receive the same basic grounding in their education. Curriculums are based on what the education department of the government at the time feels children should know, understand and do. Such curriculums also help planning, as teachers at each stage of education know what the children should have already studied. Set curriculums provide building blocks for learning and also help plan for assessment. However, there is freedom for early years providers, schools and teachers to decide how to deliver the content. Nevertheless, the compulsory tests or assessments which also form part of the curriculum impact on how much flexibility an establishment has, as organisations are judged on the children's results in national tests.

Some people believe that a set curriculum is too prescriptive and that children should be able to explore and learn to suit their interests. There are several theorists such as Steiner (see page 215), who believed this to be the case. Nevertheless, it could be argued that there are certain skills that all children should acquire as they are essential to being able to function in society and have the capacity to earn a decent salary – these include English and maths. Giving children complete freedom to explore what they please may not lead them to gain these skills and therefore may not equip them to function well in society.

How did the National Curriculum affect what you had to study in school?

Were there any restrictions on what you had to study, and did this mean you couldn't study areas you were more interested in?

In hindsight, which subjects do you think were most use to you and which would you make compulsory?

It has also been suggested that a set curriculum can disaffect children if they have to study areas they are not interested in or do not have an ability in (for example a foreign language) and that they are better focused on areas that interest them.

The government has changed the National Curriculum in a number of ways since its inception, including now allowing the curriculum to be 'disapplied' at Key Stage 4 to enable some young people to study an alternative curriculum more relevant to them and which may help to keep them interested in education.

Summary

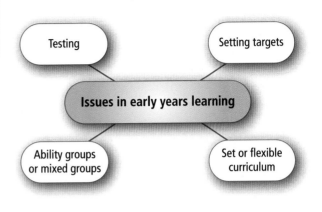

UNIT 16 ASSESSMENT

How you will be assessed

The assessment for this unit is based on a report which studies aspects of how children at a particular age learn. You have to choose an age group and two learning topics from a list given by the board. You then need to produce a report which contains a topic description, learning plans, an evaluation and source material.

To achieve the criteria, you need to carry out a research project which covers one age group and two learning topics. This section will help to guide you through this process.

Developing your project

1 Planning
Choose the age group you wish to work with from one of the following:

1 year, 2, 3, 4–5, 6–8 years.

Note that the first age group spans the time from the first birthday up to the second birthday and age group 4–5 should be understood to span the time from the fourth birthday up to the sixth birthday. You can either focus on learning for the majority group of children in that age group or looks at children with special educational needs – however, doing both will make the assignment too large.

Choose the learning topics you wish to focus on – you must choose two from the table below:

List 1 (choose one from this list)	List 2 (choose one from this list)
Language skills and how children learn: ٭ vocabulary ٭ sentence-construction skills ٭ to read ٭ handwriting ٭ to spell ٭ to punctuate ٭ comprehension skills. Numeracy skills and how children learn: ٭ to count ٭ to measure ٭ to add and subtract ٭ to multiply and divide ٭ about angles ٭ geometrical shapes and their properties.	Learning skills and how children learn: ٭ scientific concepts including: volume, mass, length, density, speed, acceleration, force, power ٭ scientific methods (experiment and observation) ٭ information technology skills ٭ construction skills ٭ about our planet including: the Earth, Sun and Moon in relation to the Universe and Solar System ٭ about natural and manufactured processes (e.g. weather, water cycle, erosion, food production, industry, transport and trade) ٭ about different cultures ٭ interpersonal skills and conventions ٭ moral rules and moral behaviour ٭ about work and occupations ٭ self-care, including hygiene, and caring for others, including pets ٭ about the human body (functions and processes) ٭ music skills ٭ creative skills (e.g. visual arts) ٭ physical co-ordination (e.g. game skills) ٭ acquiring an additional language ٭ about past times and past events.

Remember that some of the topics will be more appropriate to certain age groups because of the concepts involved. Therefore, you may need to research your age group briefly before you choose the topics.

It will be useful to be able to carry out the activities you plan as this will help you to effectively evaluate them. Therefore, the choice you make might be influenced by the age of children you easily have access to; for example in a playgroup, nursery or primary school, or a child in a family setting.

2 Research

You need to carry out some secondary research into the development of the age group you have chosen, focusing specifically on the area of literacy or numeracy and learning skills you have chosen.

Remember these are large topics so you do need to focus.

It will be worthwhile giving a synopsis of development in the area up to the stage you are specifically focusing on. Remember to use a wide range of sources for your research including books, the Internet and magazines.

3 Developing a learning plan

For each area you have chosen, you need to explore learning strategies and develop an activity or learning plan to show how you might work with a child on this area.

One way of doing this is to produce a 'detailed activity plan'. This helps you think through the activity and plan it effectively. There is no set layout for a learning activity plan; however, a good plan should always contain certain pieced of information within it.

Learning activity plans should usually include:

* title or name of the activity

* number of children it is for (maximum and minimum may be given)

* age range the activity is aimed at

* time needed to prepare for the activity

* estimated time the activity will take to carry out

* reason or rationale for doing the activity – this may link to a theme which a setting is following if you are in a nursery for example or a skill or experience you want the children to develop.

This section may also include:

Aims and objectives

Aims outline the broad intentions of the activity – what it hopes to achieve overall. The objectives should explain exactly how the activity will achieve its aims.

For example an aim might be:

* to develop an appreciation of colour.

The objective could therefore be:

* to provide opportunity for colour mixing of primary colours.

Learning opportunities that arise from the activity

This will cover a comment on developmental potential as well as how it will cover the Early Learning Goals. A good detailed plan will include references to textbooks to highlight how the comments made about the learning benefits are backed up by theory.

Resources and equipment required

This acts as a checklist and ensures that all equipment is available before the start of the activity.

Implementation

This sets out a step-by-step approach to the activity. It may include timings of each stage as well as what the adult might be doing to support the children. This section is like a list of instructions, e.g.

9.00: introduce the children to the activity – talk about favourite colours

9.05: explain the activity to the children – demonstrate an example – talk about primary colours and what happens when they are mixed

9.15: children have a go at the activity – help them where necessary.

Extension possibilities

A learning activity plan may outline how the activity might be adapted to meet individual needs such as a child with a disability or a child who is particularly gifted.

Once you have planned your activities you need to carry them out with children if at all possible.

4 Evaluation

You must carry out an evaluation of your learning plans. The evaluation should refer to relevant educational issues, theory and/or empirical evidence, which can be used to justify and/or criticise what you did and the outcomes.

The evaluation should also reflect on how appropriate your activity was for the age group chosen and if it achieved your aims. You should also consider what the child gained from doing the activity from both a learning and enjoyment point of view.

Good activity plans will also have references and a bibliography – if theorists have been referred to in the plan.

5 References

It is important that you include references to any sources of information you have used in your project. This may be for the research section or in the development of your learning plans. Good referencing and a clear bibliography are useful as they allow the reader to check the source of a reference if they wish to. The Harvard method of referencing is usually used.

Harvard method

When writing other authors ideas in your own words, you must acknowledge this by giving their name and the date of the publication in which you have read their ideas, e.g. 'Brain (1999) suggested that the links between social and language development in infants…'.

If you are directly quoting something that has appeared in another text, you must give author, date and page number. Directly quoted material usually appears indented in the text.

As Brain states:

'Social and language development . . .' (1999, page 14)

References must be supported by a bibliography which lists all the texts you have used. The Harvard method for a bibliography has the following headings:

Author (Surname, initial); date published; Title (italics); Place where published; Publisher.

Brain, A. (1999) *Development in infants* London: Educational Publishers

Tassoni, P. and Hucker, K. (1999) *Planning Play and the Early* Years Oxford: Heinemann

References and further reading

Bandura, A., Ross, D. and Ross, S.A. (1963), 'Imitation of film-mediated aggressive models' *Journal of Abnormal and Social Psychology*, 66, 3–11 (1996) *Desirable Learning Outcomes* London: HMSO

Bee, H. et al (2003) *The Developing Child* Allyn and Bacon

Bee, H. et al (2005) *Lifespan Development* Allyn and Bacon

Bruce, T. and Meggitt, C. (2002) *Childcare and Education* London: Hodder and Stoughton

Bruner, J. S. (1974) *Beyond the Information given* London: George Allen & Unwin

Chomsky, N. (1959) 'Review of Skinner's Verbal Behaviour *Language*, 35, 26–58

Hucker, K. (2001) Research Methods in *Health, Care and Early Years* Oxford: Heinemann

Sheridan, M. et al (1997) *From Birth to Five Years: Children's Developmental Progress* Routledge

Tassoni, P. Hucker, K. (2005) *Planning Play and the Early Years* Oxford: Heinemann

Useful websites

www.qca.gov.uk

www.surestart.gov.uk
Outlines the first Sure Start programme introduced in 2002

www.dfes.gov.uk

www.under5s.co.uk

www.preschool.org.uk

http://en.wikipedia.org/wiki/Wug_test

Physiological aspects of health

This unit covers the following sections:

19.1 Physiological measurements of service users

19.2 Control mechanisms

19.3 Structure and functions

Introduction

This unit builds on your understanding of health and disease gained from AS Unit 2 Effective communication, Unit 3 Health, illness and disease, Unit 5 Nutrients and Dietetics, Unit 6 Common diseases and disorders, Unit 9 Complementary therapies, Unit 10 Psychological perspectives and A2 Unit 12 Human development and Unit 21 Research methods and perspectives.

You will learn about the routine monitoring of individuals and how the information gained provides insight into their health status by comparing normal values to those representing dysfunction. Learning about the control mechanisms behind routine measurements and how the process of homeostasis operates is fundamental to understanding. This is further supported by learning about the structure and function of the respiratory, cardiovascular and nervous systems.

Unit assessment

This unit is internally assessed. You must produce a report of the practical results of monitoring and compare the physiological status of three individuals. The report should include:

* a description of how to perform physiological measurements
* the health risks involved
* potential errors and ways of reducing them
* presentation of results, analysis and evaluation
* descriptions of the relevant control mechanisms
* understanding of negative feedback in both rising and falling contexts in relation to homeostasis
* descriptions and explanations of the relevant structures and functions of the body systems involved
* a sound understanding of the interrelationships between the body systems.

The work should be wholly your own and cannot be shared or part of a group exercise.

19.1 Physiological measurements of service users

You will learn how the following routine measurements are made:

* pulse rate
* body temperature
* blood pressure
* lung function, such as tidal volume, vital capacity and peak flow.

Pulse rate measurements

A pulse can be detected when an artery is close to the surface of the body and runs over a firm structure such as bone. The pulse is the elastic expansion and recoil of an artery caused by the left ventricle of the heart contracting to drive blood around the body. When you feel your pulse, you are feeling the 'shock' wave of the contraction as it travels rapidly down the arteries.

You may wish to repeat the measurement twice more, and then calculate the mean pulse rate. An average resting pulse, in a healthy individual, ranges from 60 to 80 beats per minute. As well as the pulse rate, professional health care workers will also monitor the rhythm of the pulse noting any irregularities and the quality of the pulse – some of the terms used are 'full', 'bounding', 'normal' and 'weak'.

They will also take note of the character of the blood vessel; in a young person it feels straight, flexible and elastic, but in an elderly person it might feel much firmer, or even hard, and it may take a winding course due to **arteriosclerosis.** This condition might mean that the pulse is harder to count.

Variations in pulse rate

A pulse taken in babies or young children is much faster than in adults. Exercise, or even just moving about before or during the pulse-taking will cause an increase in rate, as will an increased body temperature. Hypothermia will produce a slow pulse rate.

Once you have familiarised yourself with taking pulse rate measurements at rest, practice taking them at different levels of activity. You could team up with another student and take each other's pulses.

Think about the different activities that you might use and at this point make your practice measurements fit the individuals on whom you might carry out the assessment task. For example, if you want to be able to take the pulse after a hot bath or shower, or after or during sleep, you will probably need to choose a family member for your assessment rather than a fellow student.

You might take the pulse rate after:

* light, medium or intense exercise

* eating and drinking

* a hot bath or shower.

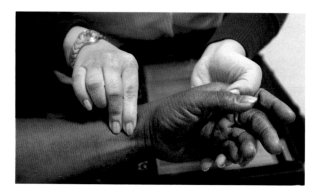

FIGURE 19.1 *Taking a radial pulse*

Potential health and safety risks

You must not compress the artery over the bone when taking measurements or you may stop the blood flow to part of the hand, causing pain and cramp. This is more likely to occur in babies and older people when the pulse is more difficult to detect and count.

Did you know?

The radial pulse is difficult to detect in a baby so the preferred location is the brachial artery on the inner side of the upper arm.

Ensure that the individual under assessment is suitably healthy to undertake any physical exercise involved in your assessment task – for example, you might not ask your grandmother to run up and down the stairs several times or do a 'step test', for this might trigger **angina** or a heart attack. The individual must be accustomed to participating in and compliant with the exercise you devise. There must be no risk to health in carrying out the activities. Ensure that hands are washed before and after the procedure to prevent cross-infection.

Using electronic recorders

Many establishments use electronic digital recorders for measuring pulse rates, blood pressure, body temperature and other physiological features. You should be familiar with the manufacturer's instructions for safe practice, potential risks and levels of accuracy. In addition, you must be trained by an appropriately qualified person to use this type of equipment. Different pieces of equipment may operate in different ways.

All items of electrical equipment are potentially hazardous, both to the client and the carer operating the devices. The major hazards are burns and electric shock. You should be constantly on the alert for:

* malfunction of the equipment

* frayed electric flexes and trapped wires

* loose connections, plugs and sockets.

Any fault must be reported immediately, verbally and in writing: most establishments have standard forms for reporting faults or damaged equipment. The device must be clearly identified with a notice 'Faulty, Do Not Use' and taken out of use. No one should be asked to use faulty equipment in his or her job role. Only suitably qualified personnel should investigate, modify, repair or scrap equipment belonging to the establishment.

Sources of error in practical measuring systems and ways of reducing them

Many carers measure the pulse rate for 10 or 15 second periods and multiply by 6 or 4 respectively to gain the pulse rate per minute. Any error in counting will thus be magnified six- or four-fold. However, a single error is still unlikely to be significant in terms of results for monitoring purposes. Counting for the whole 60 seconds is not a long time and reduces these errors.

Irregular pulses (patients with heart disease or ectopic beats) and fast pulses (patients with tachycardia, or babies and young children) can prove difficult to count. Arteriosclerotic arteries are also more difficult to count. Multiple counting errors are more likely to occur and when multiplied these could be significant.

What if?

Imagine you used a pulse meter to measure a friend's pulse rate and found it to be 80 beats per minute. The manufacturer's instructions quote accuracy at ± 2.5 per cent. This means that the rate might range from 78 to 82 beats per minute.

Explanation: Accuracy $= 2.5\% = \frac{5}{200}$

$$\frac{80 \times 5}{200} = \frac{400}{200} = \pm 2$$

Range $= 80 - 2$ to $80 + 2$

$= 78 - 82$ beats per minute

When you are taking a resting pulse, ensure that the individual is not disturbed or anxious and has been resting for at least ten minutes or you might get a false reading.

Body temperature measurements

Body temperature must be kept within a narrow range in order for the physiological processes of the body to function at their maximum efficiency. However, body temperature varies between individuals even when they are in the same environment. Body temperature can vary in the same person, at different times of day, during different activity levels and whether food and drink has been consumed or not. In women, body temperature is affected by the stages of the menstrual cycle – being highest at ovulation and lowest during menstruation. Most people experience their lowest temperature around 3.00 am and their highest around 6.00 pm.

In addition to all these influences, body temperature varies according to the location of the measurement, e.g. mouth, axilla (armpit), ear canal and rectum. Rectal measurement is only used in patients where the other sites are unavailable, and in unconscious and very seriously ill patients, as the procedure causes raised anxiety and stress levels. Rectal temperatures are nearer to actual body core temperatures, but slower to change. Mouth or oral temperatures are about 0.5 °C higher than axillary temperatures. Normal body temperatures range from 36.5–37.2 °C. Normal body temperature is usually quoted as 37 °C but, given the range of influencing factors, this is rather too precise.

Temperatures are often taken once or twice daily as a routine, but the frequency can be varied according to need. A patient suffering from or at risk of developing an infection, recovering from hypothermia or post-operatively may have temperatures taken hourly or every four hours. Since mercury-filled thermometers were banned in care establishments, several types of non-mercury thermometers are now available. These are:

* disposable thermometers
* calibrated electronic probes
* tympanic (ear canal) thermometers.

However, you must remember that in many private homes in the country, mercury-filled, clinical thermometers are still in existence.

Temperatures used to be measured in degrees Fahrenheit, but now degrees Celsius are used. In a

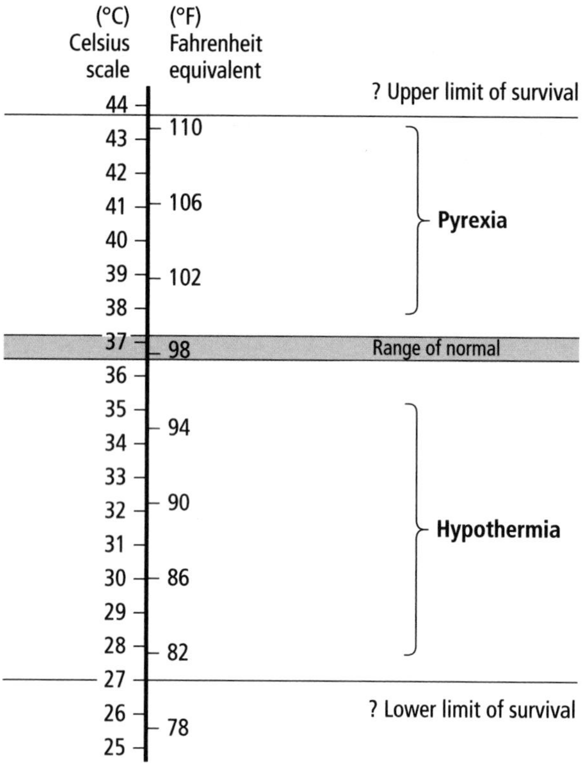
(°C)
Celsius
scale
(°F)
Fahrenheit
equivalent
? Upper limit of survival
44
43
110
42
41
106
Pyrexia
40
39
102
38
37
98
Range of normal
36
35
94
34
33
32
90
Hypothermia
31
30
86
29
28
82
27
? Lower limit of survival
26
78
25

FIGURE 19.2 *Body temperature range*

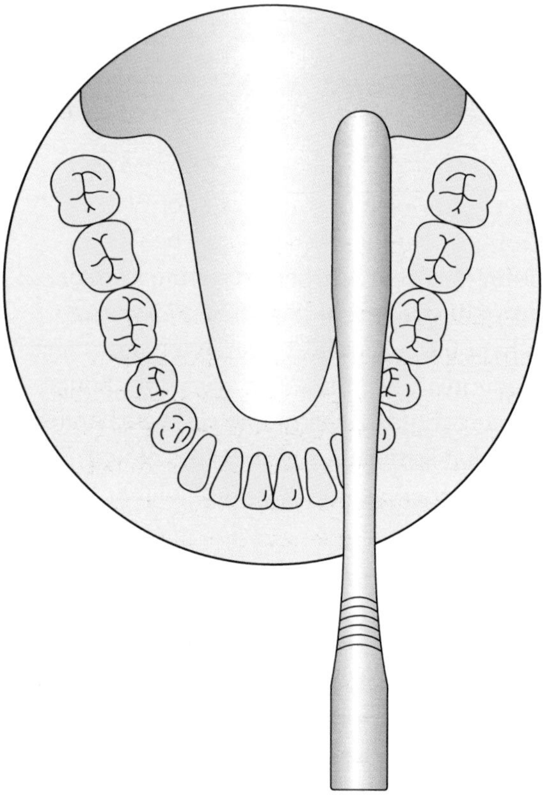

FIGURE 19.3 *Oral pouch for the location of an oral thermometer*

Try it out

You are most likely to take temperatures in the **axilla** (the armpit).

Wash your hands first to prevent cross-infection.

Explain what you are going to do to the individual and obtain their consent and co-operation.

Make sure that the individual is sitting or lying comfortably and can keep that position for a few minutes.

Respect privacy and help to remove clothing from one axilla.

Dry the axilla with a disposable tissue.

Place the temperature probe in the axilla so that it is surrounded by skin.

Observe the individual throughout the process to check for signs of distress.

Ask the individual to hold his or her arm across the chest to hold the probe in position.

Leave for the correct time (as per manufacturer's instructions).

Stay with the individual to ensure position is maintained.

After the appropriate time has elapsed, remove the thermometer, read and record the temperature with date and time.

Safely dispose of or clean and store the thermometer as appropriate for the establishment. Wash your hands again.

Check that the individual is still comfortable and, if relevant, compare with previous readings.

Notify any significant change in the temperature to a supervisor.

This procedure can be adapted to any type of axillary thermometer.

private home, you must observe the thermometer closely to see the measuring scale as old ones must still exist.

Disposable oral and oral probe thermometers should be placed under the tongue. There are right and left pouches on either side of the fold of membrane (the frenulum) on the underside of the tongue. Either one of these is a suitable place for the thermometer. The individual should not bite or chew on the probe and should close his or her lips around it for the prescribed length of time. The rest of the procedure is the same as for axillary temperature-taking.

Rectal thermometry should not be carried out by unqualified individuals and thus will not be described here.

Tympanic thermometers measure the temperature of the ear drum (tympanic membrane) and this is very near to the body core temperature. A probe with a disposable cover is inserted into the ear canal while gently pulling the ear lobe downwards. When the ear drum cannot be seen because of the position of the probe, hold the thermometer still and take the recording. Remove the probe and dispose of the cover before storing the equipment safely. Otherwise, use the same procedure as for axillary recordings. This is the preferred method for taking temperatures in children as it is fast and children find this method quite acceptable.

LCD (liquid crystal display) strip thermometers are cheap, disposable, safe and easy to use. They are also available in high street pharmacies and parents of young children are encouraged to keep a supply at home. They are single-use only and the manufacturer's instructions must be followed to obtain correct results.

Try it out

Purchase an LCD strip thermometer and try it out for yourself. If you can, immediately take your temperature with another type of thermometer and compare the results.

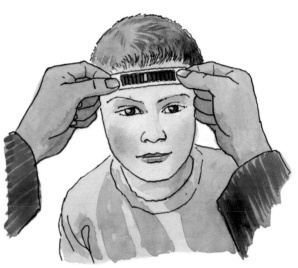

FIGURE 19.5 *Using an LCD strip*

Potential health and safety risks

Refer to page 234 for dealing with electrical equipment. Oral temperatures should only be taken with attentive, co-operative adults, to ensure that the probe is not bitten or chewed with accompanying risks to safety. All equipment should have disposable covers or sheaths or be thoroughly cleaned after use to prevent cross-infection.

Even with the use of disposable covers, tympanic thermometers have been found to transmit ear infections (often with drug-resistant bacteria) between individuals. Extra care should be taken with personal and equipment hygiene.

Mercury and glass thermometers are now considered obsolete and even domestic settings

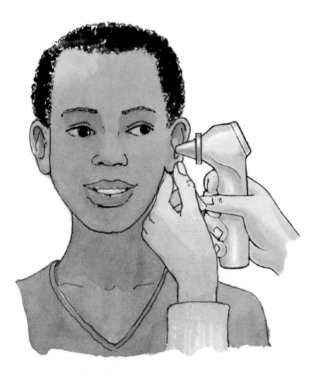

FIGURE 19.4 *Taking a tympanic temperature*

should be encouraged to substitute LCD thermometers. The danger is from mercury poisoning and inhalation or glass ingestion.

Sources of error in practical measuring systems and ways of reducing them

Ensure that you know how to use the temperature measuring device and know both the correct location of the sensitive probe, strip or bulb and the length of time for the measuring. Failure to comply with the manufacturer's instructions may lead to inacurate readings and errors. Prepare the equipment correctly and make sure that it is calibrated where this is appropriate.

> **What if?**
>
> How would you take a temperature if your client had had a hot or cold drink or a bath or shower in the last few minutes, or had been engaged in a form of exercise?
>
> Normally you should delay the temperature recording, unless you are interested in the ensuing variation in temperature for study purposes (e.g. in the context of this unit assessment).

The accuracy of a thermometer depends on fully-functioning equipment and your skill in carrying out the measurements. When taking oral temperatures do not ask the individual questions or allow them to converse as the colder air flowing over the thermometer will cause inaccuracies.

There have been several studies relating to the accuracy of temperatures taken with tympanic thermometers but, over time, carers are becoming more experienced with using these devices.

LCD strips, while valuable in domestic and community settings, are not absolutely accurate, but provide useful guidance when the temperature is raised. Consult the manufacturer's instructions for accuracy levels.

Blood pressure

The force blood exerts on the walls of the blood vessels it is passing through is known as the blood pressure (BP). It can be measured using a special piece of equipment called a **sphygmomanometer**, often abbreviated to 'sphygmo' (pronounced *sfigmo*). There are three types of sphygmo in current use. The traditional device, still used in some places but being phased out, is a mercury sphygmo. This should have been replaced by aneroid or electronic sphygmos. Operation of the mercury sphygmo will not be described, although essentially it is similar to the aneroid sphygmo.

Principles of taking blood pressure

An inflatable cuff is pumped up to flatten the artery near to the surface of the body and slowly released until blood can just force its way through during ventricular contraction, producing intermittent pulses heard as sound taps through the stethoscope placed over the artery. The reading at the first sounds is taken to be the systolic blood pressure. Further slow deflation leads to the sounds continuing loud and clear, then they suddenly become soft and muffled. This change in sound is the diastolic reading and represents the stage when blood is flowing freely through the artery.

An aneroid sphygmomanometer is used with a stethoscope so that sounds of tapping pulses can be heard. The cuff contains an inflatable bladder connected by rubber tubing to the aneroid scale and rubber hand pump. There is a screw valve attached to the scale/pump apparatus for controlling deflation. This should be closed when inflating and slowly unscrewed to deflate. A second tube may run from the cuff to an integral stethoscope so that a bell or diaphragm end of a stethoscope is not required.

> **Did you know?**
>
> **Systolic** BP corresponds to the pressure of the blood when the ventricles are contracting. **Diastolic** BP represents blood pressure when the ventricles are relaxed and filling. BP is usually written as systolic/diastolic, e.g. 120/80 and the units are still mmHg (millimetres of mercury). Systeme Internationale (SI) units are kPa (kilopascals), but few establishments have converted.
>
> 120/80 mmHg is taken as standard young healthy adult BP, (15.79/10.53 kPa).

You must know how to take a blood pressure properly before you can assess whether or not a patient's BP is raised, hypertensive etc.

As usual, best practice is to explain the procedure to the individual being measured and gain consent and co-operation. Reduce any anxiety and make the individual comfortable; ensure privacy and remove clothing to expose the arm. Hands should be washed before and after the procedure.

Feel for the pulse of the brachial artery (artery to the arm) around the inner bend of the elbow. (When doing this for the first few times on a friend or fellow student, you might find it helpful to mark this point with a small dot in washable ink). Place the cuff smoothly and firmly around the arm about 4 cm above the pulse. The inflatable bladder must be over the artery and you can feel this through the cloth of the cuff. Most cuffs now have 'Velcro' fastening. The arm should rest on a firm surface and remain still. Feel for the radial pulse at the base of the thumb and inflate the cuff until the pulse disappears – slowly deflate until the pulse returns and note the reading. Deflate fully.

Inflate the cuff again to approximately 20 mmHg above your previous reading with the stethoscope over the brachial artery.

Slowly deflate once again and note the reading when the first tap begins – the systolic reading. Continue deflating until the sharp tapping sounds are replaced by softer, muffled sounds – the diastolic reading. Deflate fully and record the two figures with the systolic reading first.

Most carers do not take an initial reading using the radial pulse, but this gives guidance about the systolic blood pressure figure and so stops carers making the error of not inflating the cuff high enough. When the cuff is inflated above 150–175 mmHg, many individuals feel pain and this raises anxiety levels. When using a mercury sphygmo, the procedure is virtually the same, but the manometer (the mercury-filled tube and scale) should be placed on a firm surface at the height of the heart.

Electronic sphygmomanometers are easy to use and do not require a stethoscope. The cuff is similar to that described for aneroid sphygmos, but one tubing runs to the electronic device and the other to an inflatable bulb with screw or push button valve. There is a microphone or transducer built into the cuff. Using the hand pump to inflate the cuff is the same but deflation and read out are automatic. Many electronic sphygmos also measure pulse rate (see Figure 19.6).

Potential health and safety risks

See page 234 for information on handling electrical equipment.

* Handwashing before and after the procedure reduces the risk of cross-infection.

* Stethoscope ear pieces should be cleaned before and after use with alcohol-saturated swabs and all equipment kept clean and stored safely.

* An inexperienced sphygmomanometer user should be supervised by a qualified person during the procedure.

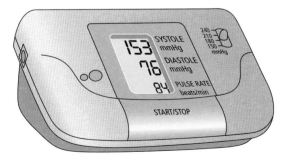
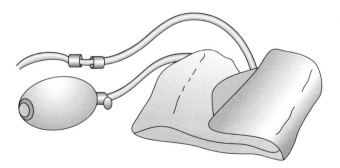

FIGURE 19.6 *An electronic sphygmomanometer*

Sources of error in practical measuring systems and ways of reducing them

Many people become anxious during a BP measurement and this can increase the systolic figure, particularly. Pain from an over-inflated cuff may do likewise. Exercise and smoking just before the measurement will result in a higher BP. A suitable time interval will reduce this error. Arteriosclerosis of the blood vessel will also affect readings as the vessel wall is not as flexible; however, you can only note this as there is no remedy.

The size of the inflatable bladder must be appropriate to the individual's size as a bladder that is too small or too large will result in a higher or lower reading respectively. The bladder should cover around four-fifths of the arm width. Arm movements may lead to inaccurate measurements and this should be explained to the individual.

A busy carer may under-inflate the cuff and deflate too quickly, pre-judging the BP from previous readings or recordings. Few carers carry out a preliminary assessment via the radial artery to eliminate this error.

A valve that is hard to manipulate can increase errors, and kinks or blockages in the tubing of sphygmos or stethoscopes may interfere with results. Studies have shown that in many establishments, sphygmos in constant use are poorly maintained. Some electronic sphygmos use a wrist band rather than an arm cuff; these are far less reliable and less accurate.

Partial hearing loss or slow reaction times experienced by the carer may lead to lower results. BP measurements repeated quickly may result in inaccurate readings due to the venous congestion produced by the inflatable cuff. Well-maintained equipment and experienced, qualified users will provide results with a small margin of error that is of no significance.

Lung function

Pulmonary function tests are a group of tests carried out to evaluate the function of the lungs in an individual and to confirm a diagnosis of disorder. Respiratory rate is a routine measurement similar to a pulse rate but counting the number of breaths in one minute. **Spirometry** and measurement of lung volumes are used to determine whether there is obstruction to air-flow or lung expansion, and **peak-flow** monitoring examines the degree of narrowing of the air-flow. Other tests included in this category but beyond the scope of this unit and assessment involve blood gas measurements.

You will need to observe the rise and fall of the individual's chest in order to count the respiratory rate. It is best to do this after pulse-taking. The problem encountered is that as soon as the individual is aware of the count, voluntary control takes over and the rate may alter. Many carers continue to keep the fingers on the pulse for an extra 60 seconds to distract the individual while counting the respirations. One rise and one fall counts as one respiration. You can then record both pulse and respiration rates. Normal respiratory rate is said to be 12–20 breaths per minute. Exercise, fever and infection will cause the breathing rate to rise and hypothermia will cause it to slow down.

Tidal volume is the volume of air passing in and out of the lungs at each breath and at rest is approximately $0.5\,dm^3$ ($500\,cm^3$ or half a litre). During activity, the demand for air (oxygen) by the muscular activity is much greater and tidal volume increases with activity levels.

Vital capacity is the volume of air that can be expelled after a maximum inspiration and clearly will vary according to the size of the chest and the health status of the individual. Males tend to have larger vital capacities than females and adults greater than children. The normal range for adults is between 4.5 and 6 dm^3.

Any disease process resulting in reduced air intake or output will affect vital capacity, such as asthma, chronic obstructive lung disorders, cancer or skeletal deformity of the chest.

Did you know?

$1\,dm^3$ is the same as 1 litre, and stands for a decimetre cubed, i.e. $10 \times 10 \times 10 = 1000\,cm^3$

Vital capacity is often used to determine lung function in patients with asthma and **chronic** obstructive pulmonary disease (COPD). There are three ways to measure these volumes depending on the equipment available.

1. Using a biological spirometer such as those found in a biology laboratory at school or college. There are many types available depending on the time of purchase; sophisticated spirometers can be linked to computers or have their own printout or display. Essentially, a spirometer consists of a box and tubing connected to a mouthpiece. The tubing has valves for one-way flow of air, there being one for blowing in and another for the exit of air. Some types have boxes suspended over water and others have a piston-like arrangement. There is a marker pen attached to mimic the movements of the box if there is no integral arrangement for printout or graphical display. A container filled with soda lime is placed on the route for absorption of carbon dioxide, for after a few exhalations the box would have a high concentration of carbon dioxide within. This would interfere with breathing rate and depth and be dangerous. A typical spirometer chart might look like the one in Figure 19.7.

2. In the absence of any specialised equipment, a bucket or large water trough, rubber tubing and a plastic container over 5 dm³ in capacity can be used. First, the container

must be calibrated in 100 cm³ intervals. You will eventually be using the container upside down so, when you mark the scale using a water-resistant pen, write the figures upside down to enable you to read them easily. Fill the container with 100 cm³ of water and place a neat horizontal mark on a previously drawn vertical line at the water level.

Continue repeating this until you have placed 1000 cm³ in the container and mark this with a longer line and numeral 1 to represent 1 dm³. Repeat the procedure until the container is fully marked or calibrated. Half fill the trough, and completely fill the container with water. Using a stopper in the neck of the container or your hand, invert the container into the trough. Then remove the stopper or hand. Although some water will flow out, most of it will stay – held by the atmospheric pressure pressing on the water in the trough. Your apparatus should look like that shown in Figure 19.8. Read and record the level of the water in the container. Place a length of rubber tubing through the container into the air space above its water. After breathing out normally, take as big a breath as possible and blow out all the air you can through the rubber tubing. This expired air will force water out of the container into the trough or bucket – you may get wet! To avoid this, the trough should be capable of taking an extra 5 or 6 dm³ of water, so don't

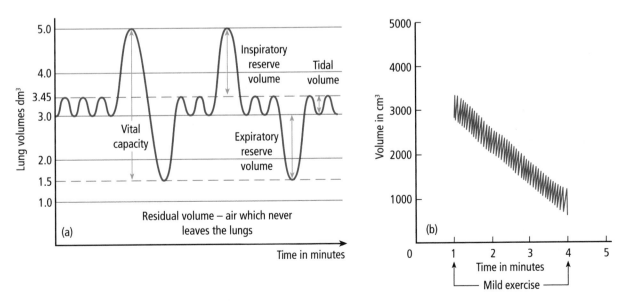

FIGURE 19.7 *A biological spirometer chart*

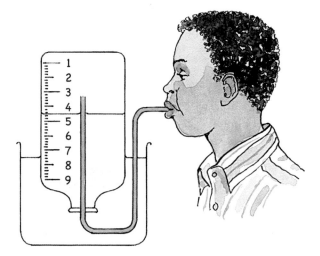

FIGURE 19.8 *A simple spirometer to calculate vital capacity*

overfill it in the first instance. Read and record the water level now. The difference in the two volumes is roughly equal to the vital capacity.

You can repeat this experiment by quietly breathing in and out of the tubing and getting a partner to record the different levels for tidal volume. You can also repeat these experiments after a variety of different activities.

3. You can also measure these lung volumes using a medical spirometer of which there are many types. Similar to the biological machines, some are linked to computers and many have integrated graphic displays.

Special training is needed to operate and interpret the recordings from medical spirometers. Vital capacity measurement is often called slow vital capacity or VC for short. Another useful recording is that of a forced expiratory volume, or the quantity of air expelled in the first second of a forced expiration (FEV1). Skilled operators can distinguish lung dysfunction between chronic asthma and COPD from a ratio of VC and FEV1.

Peak-flow measurement

Peak-flow measurement is important in lung function and is quite easy to take. This measures the maximum speed of expiration and is associated with the calibre of the subject's main airways. A baseline is often obtained using a medical spirometer with a skilled operator, and then a simple

You will need to be familiar with the type of spirometer and the manufacturer's instructions, and you must only carry out this procedure under the supervision of a suitably qualified person.

General guidelines for obtaining vital capacity:

* Explain the procedure to the subject and obtain their consent and co-operation.

* Set up the equipment correctly and according to instructions.

* Wash your hands

* Attach a clean disposable mouthpiece to the spirometer.

* Ask the subject to breathe in as deeply as possible (maximum inspiration).

* Ask the subject to hold the breath while sealing lips around the mouthpiece

* Ask them to breathe out steadily until no more air can be expelled.

* Print out or record the result.

* Best practice is to take three readings.

* Remove mouthpiece and dispose of safely.

* Clean and store the equipment safely.

* You may also record quiet breathing (tidal volume) at rest and under other conditions of activity.

peak flow meter is used, particularly in domestic settings, for monitoring. Special sizes are available for children. Electronic peak-flow meters are available but expensive. Many children and adults with asthma use peak-flow meters twice daily, to monitor their condition and modify their therapy. They are asked to record the readings and take the records with them on visits to clinics or hospitals. Patients with chronic **bronchitis** and **emphysema** will also monitor their lung function in the same way. Athletes in training and patients requiring physiotherapy of the chest may also find peak-flow readings useful.

The normal range of PEF for men is 500–700 dm^3 per minute and 380–500 for women. Children will vary according to height and chest size. When a personal best has been recorded by spirometry, subsequent readings are expressed as a percentage of this figure:

$$\frac{\text{observed reading}}{\text{personal best reading}} \times 100$$

Patients with readings of 50 per cent or less are classed as severely asthmatic, moderate **asthma** is 50–80 per cent and mild asthmatics 80–100 per cent. PEF recordings vary with age, sex, height, race, muscle strength, etc. and a new personal best should be obtained annually.

Potential health and safety risks

For guidance on using electrical equipment, see page 234. There is a potential for fungal infection of portable peak-flow devices and spirometers even with disposable mouthpieces, and equipment must be cleaned regularly either with soap and

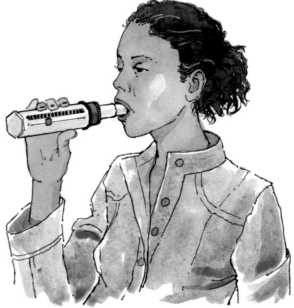

FIGURE 19.9 *Using a peak-flow meter*

water or as per the manufacturer's instructions. Rubber tubing used for simple lung volume measurments must be cleaned between each user, preferably with alcohol-saturated swabs.

Forced expirations into equipment, such as spirometers or peak-flow devices, can initiate an asthmatic attack for some asthma sufferers, and such patients should not use these types of equipment.

Peak-flow meters should be replaced every 1–2 years and may fail before that. When a client misreads a scale, this can lead to over-medication. Failure to obtain new base-line spirometer measurements may lead to errors of judgement, and children will need to have peak-flow meters replaced as they grow.

Soda lime containers must be changed regularly to prevent non-absorption of carbon dioxide in biological spirometers of this type.

All measuring equipment used in these ways by unqualified people must be supervised by a suitably qualified individual to prevent misuse.

Sources of error in practical measuring systems and ways of reducing them

All peak-flow meters should meet specified guidelines for accuracy and precision, but variation between devices made by different manufacturers is unpredictable and the same device should be used for serial monitoring. Most devices monitor up to a 2 per cent change in peak flow and this is considered to be a satisfactory margin of error for serial monitoring. As previously stated, peak-flow meters need to be changed regularly to prevent malfunction.

The most common reason for inaccurate results in measuring lung volumes is patient technique, and subjects should be observed throughout the procedures. The source of problems can be:

* insufficient or incomplete inspiration
* failure to exhale adequately or completely
* an extra breath taken during the procedure
* lips not sealed around the mouthpiece
* coughing
* air flowing out through the nasal passages (nose clips should not be worn with most devices).

Equipment must be regularly calibrated; some types can be calibrated *in situ* while others need to be sent back to the manufacturer for recalibration. Equipment must be kept clean and well-maintained to achieve accurate results.

Summary

Did you know?

If the manufacturer's instructions have been lost over time, you can contact your supplier for another copy and make several copies for future use. Suppliers usually keep instruction booklets for a very long time.

Consider this

Angus, aged 55 years, started smoking in his early teens and has smoked 30–40 cigarettes a day since. He knows that he is not as fit as he should be and over the last two or three years he has had difficulty loading and unloading his lorry. When he had a check-up recently, his doctor measured his resting BP at 170/100 mmHg and pulse rate at 75 beats/min. Angus complained of breathlessness when he walked his dog up an incline and the doctor decided to send him for a chest X-ray.

1. Can you identify the alternative ways to check BP without using a mercury sphygmomanometer?

2. Can you identify whether Angus's BP was in the normal range? Justify your answer.

3. Justify the doctor's decision to send Angus for a chest X-ray.

4. The chest X-ray appeared normal. Using the background information supplied, evaluate the options available to the doctor now.

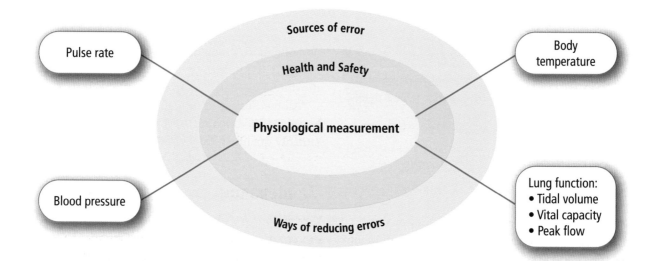

19.2 Control mechanisms

General principles of homeostasis

As external changes occur, the body needs to detect these changes. This detection is carried out by receptors capable of informing a central control (usually found in the nervous system, particularly the brain) to receive the information from the receptors and activate change by effectors. Effectors will then do something to bring the system back to normal. This is known as the negative feedback effect.

In maintaining **homeostasis** we will be dealing with negative feedback systems to dampen down external changes.

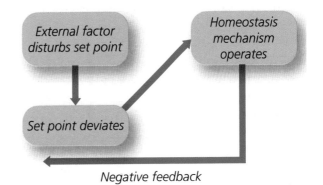

FIGURE 19.10 *Principles of negative feedback*

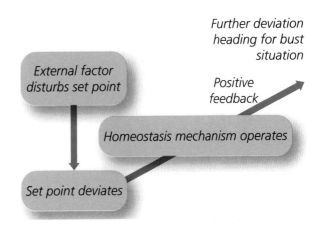

FIGURE 19.11 *Principles of positive feedback*

The flow chart in Figure 19.12 illustrates how the receptors, control centre and effectors operate to restore normal activity. Important homeostatic mechanisms within the body are the maintenance of:

* body temperature
* heart rate
* respiratory rate
* water balance
* blood glucose levels
* pH (acid/base balance).

In this section, you will be learning about the maintenance of body temperature, heart rate and respiratory rate.

Maintenance of body temperature

Human beings are the only animals that can survive in both tropical and polar regions of the planet. This is largely due to thermo-regulatory

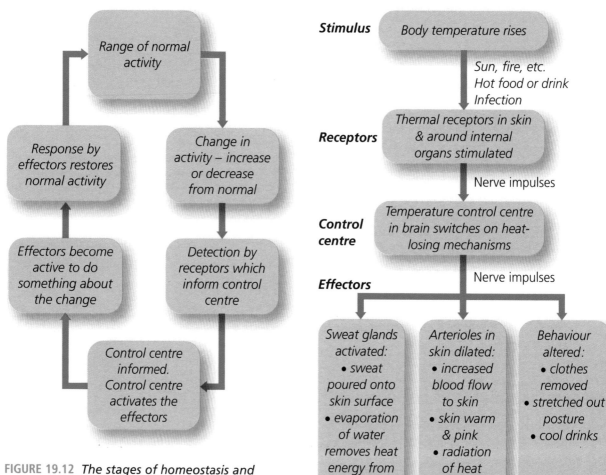

FIGURE 19.12 *The stages of homeostasis and negative feedback*

homeostatic processes and intelligence (which enables us to provide shelter and clothing). This means that body temperature varies only minimally.

The fundamental precept is to keep the inner core of the body (containing the vital organs) at normal temperatures while allowing the periphery (skin, limbs etc.) to adapt to changing conditions of external temperature.

The receptors for temperature, both heat and cold, are located in the peripheral skin and around internal organs. These are specially adapted cells with nerve fibres that run up the spinal cord to the temperature control centre in the hypothalamus of the brain. The hypothalamus sends nerve impulses to muscles,

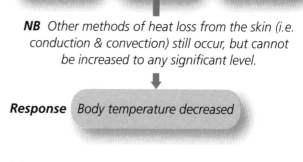

FIGURE 19.13 *The homeostatic mechanism for a rising body temperature*

sweat glands and skin blood vessels to cause changes that counteract the external changes. You can see the precise effects of a rising and falling external temperature in the flow charts in Figures 19.13 and 19.14.

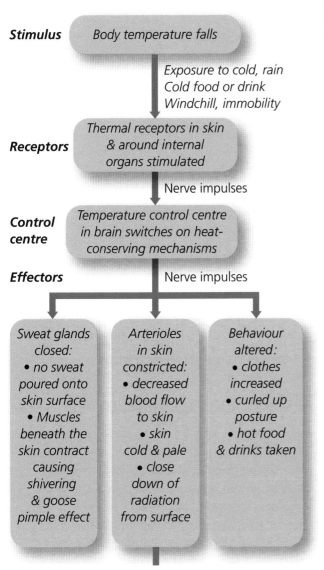

Stimulus — Body temperature falls

Exposure to cold, rain
Cold food or drink
Windchill, immobility

Receptors — Thermal receptors in skin & around internal organs stimulated

Nerve impulses

Control centre — Temperature control centre in brain switches on heat-conserving mechanisms

Effectors — Nerve impulses

Sweat glands closed:
• no sweat poured onto skin surface
• Muscles beneath the skin contract causing shivering & goose pimple effect

Arterioles in skin constricted:
• decreased blood flow to skin
• skin cold & pale
• close down of radiation from surface

Behaviour altered:
• clothes increased
• curled up posture
• hot food & drinks taken

NB *Other methods of heat loss from the skin (i.e. conduction & convection) still occur, but cannot be decreased to any significant level.*

Response — Body temperature increased

FIGURE 19.14 *The homeostatic mechanism for regulating a falling body temperature*

Skin capillaries form networks just below the outer layer or epidermis. When you are hot, you need to lose heat from the skin surface to cool yourself down by a process known as radiation. There are four ways of losing heat from the skin:

✳ *conduction:* warming up anything that you are in contact with, like clothes or seats. Even a

pen becomes warm from your hand when you are writing!

✳ *convection:* this is when you warm up the layer of air next to your skin and it moves upwards (because hot air is less dense and rises) to be replaced by colder air from the ground.

✳ *radiation:* you can think of this as rather like diffusion but of heat temperature. In other words, heat will pass from your skin to warm up any colder objects around you and conversely, you will warm up by radiation from any object hotter than yourself, like a fire.

✳ *evaporation of sweat:* when liquid water is converted into water vapour (evaporation) it requires heat energy to do so. When you are hot, sweating will only cool the skin if it can take heat energy from the skin surface to convert to water vapour and evaporate.

What if?

What if you are in a very hot climate in the monsoon season when the air is saturated with water vapour and sweat cannot evaporate? You will be very uncomfortable and at risk of heatstroke. This is why people tend to avoid travelling in the monsoon seasons.

Although conduction and convection still take place when you are hot, they cannot be changed significantly to alter body temperature. The main methods of regulating temperature are by changing radiation and sweat evaporation processes. The liver and skeletal muscles are the main heat generators in the body and heat is distributed around the whole body by the bloodstream.

The temperature of the skin is crucial to the quantity of heat lost or gained via radiation. When skin capillaries are full of blood from dilated arterioles, the skin is warm and radiation is increased, thereby losing body heat to the surroundings. When arterioles are constricted, capillaries contain very little blood (and heat), and the skin is cold to touch. Radiation then is minimal, conserving the heat in the body for the inner core containing the vital organs. The muscle wall of the arterioles supplying the capillaries is controlled by the sympathetic nervous system. Figure 19.15 illustrates the changes in skin radiation.

Did you know?

If there is continuous, long-lasting extreme cold, the skin begins to break down from lack of oxygen and nutrients – a condition called frostbite. Fingers and toes, because they are furthest from the core, are particularly vulnerable. Many polar explorers have lost fingers and toes from frostbite.

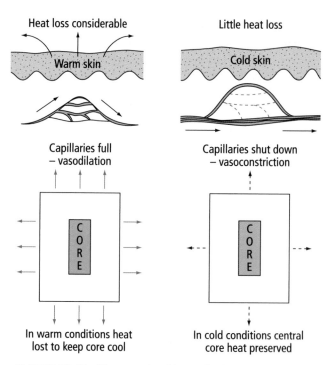

FIGURE 19.15 *Changes in skin radiation*

Homeostatic regulation of heart rate

The heart pumps blood around the body to vital organs, skeletal muscles, skin and other less vital organs. The blood contains key raw materials, such as oxygen, glucose, lipids, hormones and enzymes, for energy-releasing chemical reactions and for building up more complex substances. Blood also plays a vital role in the excretion of waste materials, such as carbon dioxide and urea. It is extremely important that the rate at which blood is pumped around the body can adapt to changing circumstances within seconds, particularly in emergency situations when life might be threatened, and during physical and mental stress. Heart rate is, therefore, controlled by homeostatic control mechanisms.

The heart rate is controlled by a special area of excitable cells (cells capable of responding to stimuli like muscle and nerve cells) located in the upper right atrium of the heart. The common term for this is the 'pacemaker' but technically it is the sino-atrial node (abbreviated to S–A node).

The S–A node is the beginning of the heart conduction system (see Figure 19.16) that spreads stimuli through the heart to enable the cardiac muscle to contract and drive the blood through the circulation. The S–A node alone will cause the heart to beat around 100 beats per minute, but it is influenced by a variety of factors. The main factors are:

* sympathetic nervous system
* parasympathetic nervous system
* **adrenaline**
* **noradrenaline.**

The **autonomic nervous system** has two main branches, the **sympathetic** and **parasympathetic** nervous sytems, which send nerves to all major internal organs. The autonomic nervous system can be thought of as the internal nervous system as opposed to the **somatic nervous system** that responds to voluntary action (i.e. under the conscious will) and external stimuli. It would be very convenient to state that the sympathetic always excites and the parasympathetic always damps down organ activity, but regrettably this is not so. However, this is true for the heart – the sympathetic speeds up the heart rate and increases the strength of the beat, which in turn increases cardiac output during physical and mental stress, while the parasympathetic is active in calming the heart down to a resting level.

In everyday activity, interplay between the 'accelerator' of the sympathetic and the 'brake' of the parasympathetic nervous systems occurs, thus fine-tuning the heart rate to suit the level of activity.

During physical and mental stress, the body becomes prepared for action. Actions such as running away, becoming aggressive and showing fear may not always be appropriate in modern society, but this is a primitive response designed to respond to enemies and predators of man that still exists today.

The activity of the sympathetic nervous system and the outpouring of the hormones adrenaline and noradrenaline from the adrenal gland cause the rapid changes responsible for preparing the body for action. During sympathetic nerve activity, impulses pass automatically to the adrenal gland, causing the secretion of adrenaline and noradrenaline into the bloodstream.

The main role of adrenaline, which comprises 80 per cent of the adrenal secretions, is to increase the heart rate and strength of ventricular contraction. It is said to boost the sympathetic action by up to ten times.

The main role of noradrenaline (20 per cent of adrenal secretions) is to maintain blood pressure by narrowing muscular arterioles in a process called vasoconstriction. This smaller volume of adrenal noradrenaline is augmented by the secretion of noradrenaline at the ends of sympathetic nerves when impulses arrive. This noradrenaline is called a neurotransmitter, for it allows the impulses to cross over the **synapses** to the involuntary muscles or glands involved in sympathetic activity. Figure 19.16 summarises the influence of the sympathetic nervous system and associated hormones.

Parasympathetic nerve fibres ending on the S–A node cause a decrease in its excitability, and so the heart rate is lower than 100 beats per

Try it out

Sit quietly for at least 10 minutes and take the average of three resting radial pulse measurements. Still sitting, wave your arms up and down ten times, and take your pulse again. You will notice a rise in pulse rate, although you could hardly be said to have carried out energetic, stressful work. This is an example of the fine-tuning. The sympathetic has slightly increased impulses to the S–A node while the parasympathetic has decreased slightly. After a few minutes' rest, take your pulse again, and you will find that it has returned to normal. This is why the average pulse rate is a range between 60 and 80 beats per minute. It simply is not rational to state that the average pulse rate is 72 beats per minute.

Did you know?

The swollen end or synaptic knob of a nerve fibre or axon is not continuous with the muscle or gland it supplies. The impulses can only pass over the minute gap or synapse if a neurotransmitter substance fills the space. Nerve impulses have to be sufficiently close together in time or space to pass on. This prevents over-stimulation by a constant bombardment of single impulses. Synapses act rather like gates opening up routes through the nervous systems.

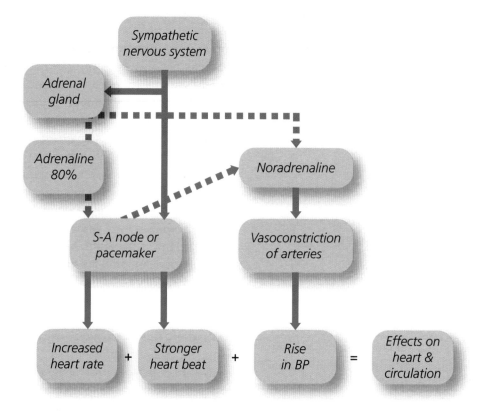

FIGURE 19.16 *The S–A node and the sympathetic nervous system*

minute. There are hardly any parasympathetic fibres to ventricular muscle so there is no effect on strength of contraction. As well as influencing the S–A node, the autonomic nervous system also exerts effects on the A–V node (see page 264).

These cardiac changes are important to deliver huge increases of oxygen and glucose-enriched blood to the skeletal muscles and to the heart muscle for the 'flight, fright or fight' response. At the same time, circulation to non-essential organs, mainly the digestive system and the skin, is drastically reduced to conserve blood for the vital responses. When the emergency has passed, the parasympathetic becomes active again, reducing heart rate.

What if?

What if an individual works in a mentally stressful job every day for long hours for many years? That person might suffer from **palpitations** and **hypertension** and may be a candidate for coronary heart disease.

Homeostatic control of respiratory rate

The diaphragm and intercostal muscles are skeletal muscles, which cannot contract unless stimulated to do so by nerve impulses passing down the nerves to those muscles. They are responsible for inspiration, which is a cyclical process. Nerve impulses stop abruptly, thus promoting the elastic recoil of the lungs and expiration. Automatic control of this nervous activity resides in the medulla of the brain that also contains the major cardiovascular centres. There are many influences impacting on the brain's respiratory centre, and you will learn about one of these: carbon dioxide levels.

The brain's respiratory centre is believed to contain two sets of nerve cells, each responsible for either inspiration or expiraton. It is thought that these two sets of neurones (nerve cells) have an intrinsic rhythmicity, rather like the S–A node, and that this is fine-tuned by higher centres in the pons of the brain, the apneustic and pneumotaxic centres. The inspiratory and expiratory centres are mutually exclusive: this means that when one is actively firing nerve impulses, the other is inhibited, and vice versa. Respiratory rate and tidal volume are not fixed and can be changed over a wide range.

One of the most important influences on the inspiratory centre is the input from **chemoreceptors,** and once again there are peripheral and central chemoreceptors. The peripheral receptors, unlike those for temperature, are located inside the body, in the neck and thorax close to major arteries, while the central receptors are in the medulla itself. The peripheral receptors are grouped into clusters called the aortic and carotid bodies. The carotid and aortic bodies respond to chemical changes in the arterial blood, namely:

* decreased oxygen levels
* decreased hydrogen ion concentration (acidity)
* increased carbon dioxide levels.

The central receptors in the medulla respond to changes in the composition of tissue fluid surrounding the brain cells, and to increased carbon dioxide (CO_2) levels. A tiny rise in CO_2 levels in arterial blood has a marked effect on respiratory rate, increasing it until the extra CO_2 is removed in gaseous exchange. In fact, not only the rate is changed, depth of breathing increases too. CO_2 and hydrogen ion (H^+) concentrations are closely linked because dissolved CO_2 forms carbonic acid (H_3CO_2) and this ionises into hydrogen carbonate ions (HCO_3^-) and hydrogen ions (H^+). It is rare for only one of the three chemicals (oxygen, carbon dioxide and hydrogen ions) to drive changes in respiratory rate as changes in the rate usually affect all three. However, the response to CO_2 changes is much stronger and tends to dominate and may obscure other influences.

A rise in plasma CO_2 increases the rise in tissue fluid, thus stimulating the central and peripheral receptors and reflexly increasing respiratory rate and depth. This 'blows off' the extra carbon dioxide returning levels to normal.

You would expect that exercise would increase CO_2 levels through increased metabolism in the muscles, and that this would be responsible for increased respiration. In fact, this does not happen – it seems that oxygen (O_2) and CO_2 levels remain more or less the same because the increase in

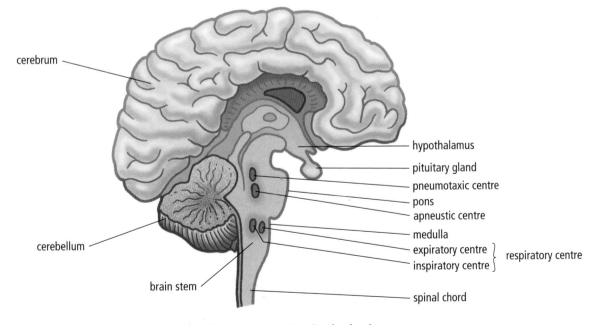

FIGURE 19.17 *The centres concerned with respiration in the brain*

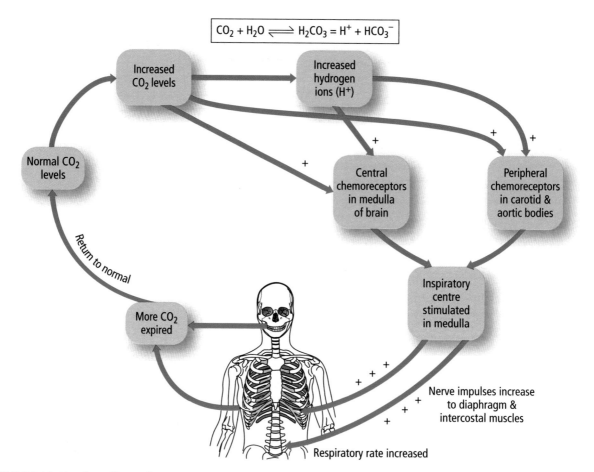

$$CO_2 + H_2O \rightleftharpoons H_2CO_3 = H^+ + HCO_3^-$$

FIGURE 19.18 *The effect of increased carbon dioxide (CO_2) and hydrogen ion (H^+) levels in arterial blood*

metabolism matches the increased respiratory rate. It would seem that lactic acid produced by muscles in the initial anaerobic respiration increases the H^+ concentration and that this is largely responsible for the increased respiratory rate.

Try it out

Ask a friend to count your respiratory rate at rest when you are distracted by something else so that you are not aware of the measuring. When the figure is revealed to you in breaths per minute, calculate how long the interval is between breaths. For example, if your respiratory rate is 15 breaths/min, then 60 divided by 15 is the time between breaths – in this case, you are breathing once every 4 seconds. Now, with a stop clock handy, try panting for about 3 minutes, stop and take the time interval before the next breath. The panting has washed out too much carbon dioxide; the apneustic centre has inhibited the inspiratory centre until levels return to normal.

Summary

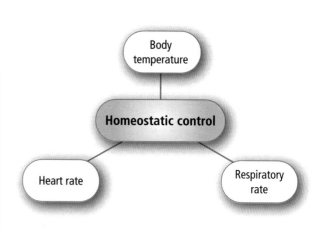

19.3 Structure and functions

In order to have a sound understanding of the methods of monitoring measurements, health and safety risks to individuals, errors and ways of reducing them and the complex control systems involved in homeostasis, you will need a thorough knowledge of some of the body systems and this section will lead you through the structure and function of the respiratory system, the cardiovascular system and the nervous system. You will also explore the links or interconnections between these systems.

The respiratory system

The respiratory system comprises the anatomical structures and the physiological processes that take oxygen from the air into the body, and uses the blood to transport oxygen to the body cells. Inside the body cells, internal respiration uses dissolved oxygen to release the energy from food and enable essential metabolic processes to be carried out.

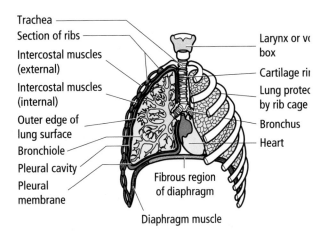

Trachea
Section of ribs
Intercostal muscles (external)
Intercostal muscles (internal)
Outer edge of lung surface
Bronchiole
Pleural cavity
Pleural membrane
Larynx or voice box
Cartilage ring
Lung protected by rib cage
Bronchus
Heart
Fibrous region of diaphragm
Diaphragm muscle

FIGURE 19.19 *Section through the thorax showing the respiratory organs*

Respiration can be artificially subdivided into four sections to facilitate study; these are:

* breathing
* gaseous exchange
* blood transport
* internal or cell respiration.

Breathing

The thorax, or chest, is an airtight box containing the lungs and their associated tubes, the bronchi and the heart. The trachea commences at the back of the throat or pharynx and divides into two main bronchi each serving one lung on each side of the heart. The first part of the trachea is specially adapted to produce sound and is called the larynx or voice box. It is protected by a moveable cartilage flap, the epiglottis, which prevents food entering during swallowing.

The trachea (or windpipe) and the bronchi have rings of cartilage to prevent them collapsing; those in the trachea are C-shaped with the gap at the back against the main food tube, the oesophagus. This is because when food is chewed in the mouth, it is made into a ball shape (called a bolus) before swallowing. The bolus stretches the oesophagus as it passes down to the stomach, and whole rings of cartilage in the trachea would hamper its progress. The gap is filled with soft muscle tissue that stretches easily, allowing the bolus to pass down the oesophagus.

On entering the lung, each bronchus divides and sub-divides repeatedly, spreading to each part of the lung. The tiniest sub-divisions supplying air sacs in the lung are called bronchioles, and even these are held open by minute areas of cartilage.

The inner lining of the trachea and bronchi is composed of mucus-secreting and ciliated, columnar epithelium cells. Mucus is the sticky white gel which traps dust particles that may enter with the air, and cilia are microscopic filaments on the outer edges of cells. Cilia 'beat' towards the nearest external orifice, causing the flow of mucus (with its trapped dirt particles) to leave via the nose or the throat.

The lungs themselves are pink and have a spongy feel to them. They are lined on the outside by a thin, moist membrane known as the pleura.

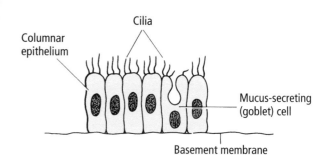

FIGURE 19.20 *Mucus-secreting cells (goblet cells) and ciliated cells lining the trachea and bronchi*

The pleura continues around the inner thoracic cavity so that the two pleural layers slide over one another with ease and without friction. The surface tension of the thin film of moisture between the pleural layers does not allow the two layers to pull apart, but does allow them to slide. This means that when the chest wall moves in breathing, the lungs move with it.

Forming the thoracic wall outside the pleura are the bones of the rib cage and two sets of oblique muscles joining them together. These are the external and internal intercostal muscles (inter means between and costal means ribs). The action of these muscles enables the rib cage to move upwards and outwards on inspiration and downwards and inwards when the air moves out of the chest. A sheet of muscle called the diaphragm forms the floor and lower boundary of the thorax. The diaphragm is dome-shaped, with the highest, more fibrous, part in the centre and the muscular, fleshy fringes firmly attached to the lower ribs. The only way that air can enter or leave the thorax is by the trachea, and the air-tight

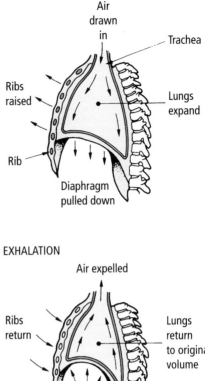

INHALATION

Air drawn in

Trachea

Ribs raised

Lungs expand

Rib

Diaphragm pulled down

EXHALATION

Air expelled

Ribs return

Lungs return to original volume

Diaphragm relaxes

FIGURE 19.22 *Changes in the thorax during inspiration and expiration*

cavity of the thorax is vital for breathing. Rhythmic breathing is controlled by the respiratory centre in the brain, as shown in the Figures 19.21 and 19.22.

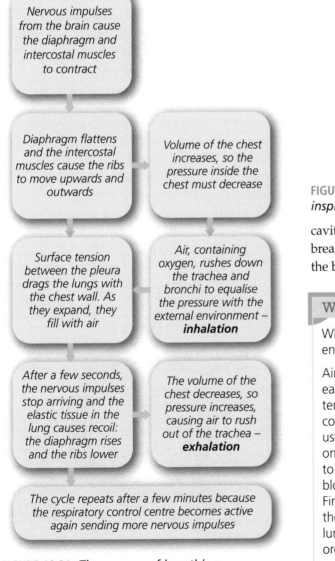

Nervous impulses from the brain cause the diaphragm and intercostal muscles to contract

Diaphragm flattens and the intercostal muscles cause the ribs to move upwards and outwards

Volume of the chest increases, so the pressure inside the chest must decrease

Surface tension between the pleura drags the lungs with the chest wall. As they expand, they fill with air

Air, containing oxygen, rushes down the trachea and bronchi to equalise the pressure with the external environment – **inhalation**

After a few seconds, the nervous impulses stop arriving and the elastic tissue in the lung causes recoil: the diaphragm rises and the ribs lower

The volume of the chest decreases, so pressure increases, causing air to rush out of the trachea – **exhalation**

The cycle repeats after a few minutes because the respiratory control centre becomes active again sending more nervous impulses

FIGURE 19.21 *The process of breathing*

What if?

What happens if a gunshot or stab wound enters the chest wall?

Air can now enter through the wound more easily than through the trachea and the surface tension of the pleura is destroyed. The lung collapses to a much smaller size and is virtually useless. Individuals can live quite well with only one lung – but in this type of injury there is likely to be shock and loss of vital oxygen-carrying blood as well. The individual's life is threatened. First aid treatment is to place a large pad over the wound as quickly as possible to prevent the lung collapsing and send for emergency aid in order to get the patient to hospital quickly.

The composition of inspired (also called inhaled) air, which is the air around us, and that of expired (or exhaled) air is shown in Table 19.1

COMPONENT	INSPIRED AIR	EXPIRED AIR
Oxygen	20%	16%
Nitrogen	80%	80%
Carbon dioxide	Virtually 0% (0.04)%	4%
Water vapour	Depends on climate	Saturated

TABLE 19.1 *Composition of inhaled and exhaled air*

Try it out

Study Table 19.1 and write down the differences that you can see. These are the changes that must have happened in the lungs by gaseous exchange.

Gaseous exchange

The bronchioles end in thousands of tiny air sacs each of which contains a cluster of single-layered alveoli, rather like a bunch of grapes on a stem. The walls of the alveoli consist of very thin, flat simple squamous epithelium, and each alveolus is surrounded by the smallest blood vessels known as capillaries. The walls of the capillaries are also composed of simple squamous epithelium, in a single layer. This means that the air entering the alveoli during breathing is separated from the blood by only two single-layered, very thin walls. There are elastic fibres round the alveoli enabling them to expand and recoil with inspiration and expiration respectively. A film of moisture lines the inside of each alveolus to enable the air gases to pass into solution. As the two layers of epithelium are so thin and semi-permeable, the dissolved gases can easily and rapidly pass

Key concept

Diffusion: the passage of molecules from a high concentration of molecules to a low concentration of molecules.

through. Although the largest component of air is nitrogen and this too passes into solution, it takes no part in the process of respiration. The gases exchange through the process of **diffusion.**

Diffusion occurs in liquids or gases because the molecules are in constant random motion, and diffusion is an overall 'equalling up' of a situation where you have a lot of molecules meeting a few molecules. Diffusion will stop in time, as the numbers of molecules become more evenly distributed. This is said to be **equilibrium.** (Note: this does not mean the molecules stop moving, only that there are equal numbers of molecules passing in each direction, so there is no overall gain or loss).

In the human body, where diffusion is a common method of transport, the state of equilibrium is not desirable as overall transport will cease. To prevent equilibrium being attained, the high concentration must be continually kept high and the low concentration must also be maintained.

Breathing in fresh air replenishes the high concentration of dissolved oxygen molecules, and the removal of diffused oxygen by the bloodstream maintains the low concentration. With carbon dioxide, the situation is reversed; the high concentration is in the blood and the low concentration in the refreshed air, so diffusion removes dissolved carbon dioxide from the blood into the expired air from the lungs. Carbon dioxide and water are waste products from internal respiration in cells.

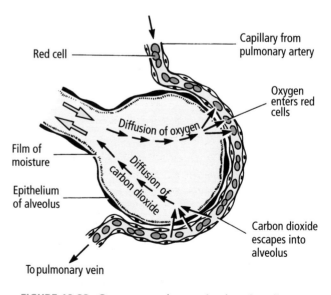

FIGURE 19.23 *Gaseous exchange in the alveoli*

Blood transport

Although not required in detail for this unit, you should know that the dissolved oxygen forms a chemical bond with the haemoglobin of the red blood cells when in a high oxygen concentration such as the lungs, and this is called oxyhaemoglobin. Oxygen is thus 'anchored' to the haemoglobin as it is transported to the tissues. The surrounding environment of the tissues is much lower in oxygen concentration (because the oxygen is continually used up in tissue respiration) and the haemoglobin releases its oxygen which passes by diffusion to the tissue cells.

Tissue or internal respiration

Once inside the cell, the oxygen is used up in the chemical process of respiration.

The respiratory centres in the brain alternately excite and suppress the activity of the neurones supplying the respiratory nerves (mainly the phrenic nerve to the diaphragm) causing inspiration and expiration. Nervous receptors, sensitive to chemicals dissolved in the blood (particularly oxygen, carbon dioxide and hydrogen ions) are located both centrally and peripherally in the body. These chemical receptors, known as chemoreceptors, initiate reflexes when they are stimulated and send nerve impulses to the respiratory centre to change breathing activity to restore the concentrations of the chemicals. This is part of homeostasis in the body.

Factors affecting breathing

The main factors affecting breathing and respiration are:

* exercise

* emotion

* altitude

* adrenaline (released in e.g. frightening circumstances).

All these increase the rate of ventilation or breathing to an appropriate level, and when the stimulating factor is removed, ventilation returns to normal.

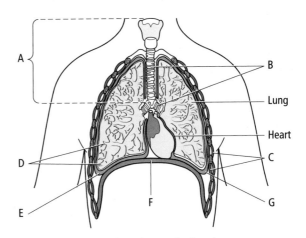

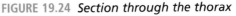

FIGURE 19.24 *Section through the thorax*

Function of the respiratory system

1. To provide a supply of oxygen for carriage by the blood to body cells.

2. To remove waste products (i.e. carbon dioxide and water) from the blood to the exterior.

3. To help maintain acid-base balance in body tissues.

4. To assist in homeostasis.

The cardiovascular system

The cardiovascular system is the main transport system of the body, carrying oxygen, carbon dioxide, nutrients such as amino acids, glucose, and digested fats, hormones, antibodies and urea.

The heart

The heart is a muscular pump which forces blood around the body through a system of blood vessels, namely arteries, veins and capillaries. Blood carries dissolved oxygen to the body cells and at the same time removes the waste products of respiration (carbon dioxide and water). However, blood is also important in distributing the following around the body:

* heat

* hormones

* nutrients

* salts

* enzymes

* urea.

The adult heart is the size of a closed fist, located in the thoracic cavity between the lungs and protected by the rib cage. It is surrounded by a tough membrane, the pericardium, which contains a thin film of fluid to prevent friction.

The heart is a double pump, each side consisting of an upper chamber (the atrium) and lower chamber (the ventricle). The right side of the heart pumps deoxygenated blood from the veins to the lungs for oxygenation. The left side pumps oxygenated blood from the lungs to the body, and the two sides are completely separated by a septum. The blood passes twice through the heart in any one cycle and this is often termed a double circulation. Figure 19.25 is a schematic diagram showing the double circulation with the heart artificially separated.

Each of the four heart chambers has a major blood vessel entering or leaving it. Veins enter the atria and arteries leave the ventricles.

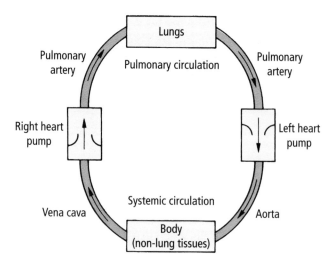

FIGURE 19.25 *Schematic diagram showing double circulation*

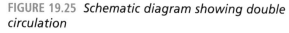

Did you know?

It is useful to remember that atria have veins entering and ventricles have arteries leaving – in each case, A and V, never two As or two Vs.

The circulation to and from the lungs is known as the pulmonary circulation and the circulation around the body is the systemic circulation.

Arteries are blood vessels that leave the heart while veins take blood towards the heart. In the pulmonary circulation, the pulmonary artery carrying deoxygenated blood leaves the right ventricle to go to the lungs – you will realise that it must divide fairly soon after leaving the heart because there are two lungs to be supplied – hence the right and left pulmonary arteries. The pulmonary veins (there are four of them) now carrying oxygenated blood, must enter the left atrium.

Did you know?

The pulmonary artery and vein are the exception to the rule that arteries carry oxygenated blood and veins carry deoxygenated blood.

The main artery to the body leaving the left ventricle is the aorta and the main vein bringing blood back to the heart from the body is the vena cava, which enters the right atrium. The vena cava has two branches, the superior vena cava returning blood from the head and neck and the inferior vena cava returning blood from the rest of the body. In many diagrams of the heart, these are treated as one vessel.

It is important that the blood flows in only one direction through the heart, so it is supplied with special valves to ensure that this happens. There are two sets of valves between the atria and the ventricles, one on each side. Sometimes these are called the right and left atrio-ventricular valves, but the older names are also used – the bicuspid (left side) and tricuspid valves. These names refer to the number of 'flaps' known as cusps that make up the valve, the bicuspid having two and the tricuspid having three cusps. Each cusp is fairly thin, so to prevent them turning inside out with the force of the blood flowing by, they have tendinous cords attached to their free ends and these are tethered to the heart muscles of the ventricles by small papillary muscles. The papillary muscles tense just before the full force of the muscle in the ventricles contracts so the tendinous cords act like guy ropes holding the valves in place.

The two large arteries, the pulmonary and the aorta, also have exits guarded by valves called semi-lunar valves (so-called because the three cusps forming each valve are half-moon shaped). These valves are needed because when the blood has been forced into the arteries by the ventricular muscle contractions, the blood must not be allowed to fall back into the ventricles when they relax. These valves can also be called the pulmonary and aortic valves.

Did you know?

It is easy to remember the names of the valves between the atria and the ventricles because **tri**cuspid fits **ri**ght, so the left must be the bicuspid valve.

You should also understand that when you view a heart diagram or picture in front of you, you are looking at it the opposite way round i.e. the right side of the heart diagram is on your left side and vice versa. If you get confused, pick up the diagram and place it over your heart facing outwards. Now it corresponds to your left and right hands.

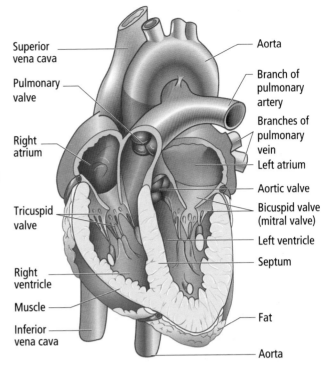

FIGURE 19.26 *A section through the heart*

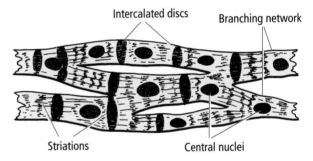

FIGURE 19.27 *Microscopic diagram of heart muscle*

Heart muscle is cardiac muscle composed of partially striped, interlocking, branched cells. It is myogenic, which means 'capable of rhythmic contractions without a nerve supply'. However, the atrial muscle beats at a different pace from the ventricular muscle, so it needs a nerve supply to organise and co-ordinate the contractions to make the heart an efficient pump. The heart muscle has its own blood supply through the coronary arteries and veins.

The muscular walls of the atria are much thinner than the ventricular walls, as the flow of blood from the atria is aided by gravity and the distance travelled by the blood here is very short – just from the atria to the ventricles. The ventricles are much thicker than the atria, but there are differences between the two ventricles. The right ventricle is about one third the thickness of the left ventricle because the left ventricle has to drive oxygenated blood around the whole of the body, including the head and neck, which involves pushing the blood upwards against the force of gravity.

Try it out

From your knowledge gained so far, estimate the distance that blood from the right ventricle has to travel, and compare this to the effort that the left ventricle has to exert to drive blood as far as your toes. This is the reason for the difference in thickness between the two ventricles.

Did you know?

Valves make a noise when they close, but not when they open – rather like clapping your hands. These noises are often called heart sounds and can be heard through a stethoscope placed over the heart.

The noises sound rather like 'lubb, dup, lubb, dup'. Lubb is the atrio-ventricular valves closing and dup is the semi-lunar valves closing.

In some people, there may be a swishing sound between heart sounds; this is called a murmur. Some murmurs are significant while others are not; they are due to disturbed blood flow.

Try it out

In pairs, using a stethoscope, listen to each other's heart sounds and identify the lubb and dupp. Try to count the exact heart rate using this method remembering that one pair of sounds equals one beat. Carry out some mild exercise and listen again.

Arteries and veins

Arteries leave the heart and supply smaller vessels known as arterioles which, in turn, supply the smallest blood vessels, the capillaries. Arteries usually carry oxygenated blood.

Veins carry blood towards the heart, picking up blood from capillaries and smaller veins known as venules. Veins usually carry deoxygenated blood. Each type of blood vessel has structural and functional differences outlined in Table 19.2 and Figure 19.28.

Each organ has an arterial and venous supply bringing blood to the organ tissues and draining blood away respectively. The link vessels supplying the cells of the organ tissues are the capillaries. A protein-free plasma filtrate is driven

ARTERIES	VEINS	CAPILLARIES
Carry blood away from heart to organs	Carry blood to heart from the organs	Connects arteries to veins
Carry blood under high pressure	Carry blood under low pressure	Arterioles and capillaries cause greatest drop in pressure due to overcoming the friction of blood passing through small vessels
Usually contain blood high in oxygen, low in carbon dioxide and water	Usually contain blood low in oxygen, high in carbon dioxide and water	Delivers protein-free plasma filtrate high in oxygen to cells and collects up respiratory waste products of carbon dioxide and water
What are the exceptions? Large arteries close to the heart help the intermittent flow from the ventricles become a continuous flow through the circulation		

TABLE 19.2 *The functional differences of blood vessels*

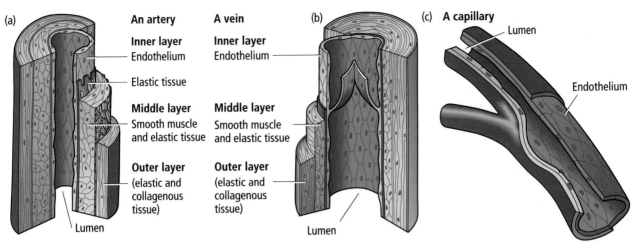

FIGURE 19.28 *Sections through blood vessels to show their structure*

out of the capillaries to supply the cells with oxygen and nutrients. Figure 19.29 shows a simple diagram of the blood circulation to the body organs.

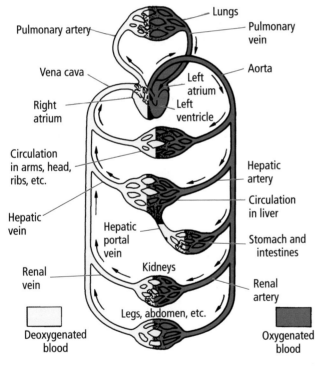

FIGURE 19.29 *The human circulatory system*

Type and general function of blood cells

Blood consists of straw-coloured plasma in which several types of blood cells are carried. Plasma is mainly water in which various substances are carried, such as dissolved gases like oxygen and carbon dioxide, nutrients like glucose and amino acids, salts, enzymes and hormones. There is also

a combination of important proteins, collectively known as the plasma proteins, which have roles in blood clotting, transport, defence and osmotic regulation.

The most common cells by far in the plasma are red blood cells, also known as erythrocytes. These are very small cells with a bi-concave shape and elastic membrane (as they often have to distort to travel through the smallest capillaries). Erythrocytes have no nucleus in their mature state (the loss produces a depression in the top and bottom of the cell, hence their shape) to provide a larger surface area for exposure to oxygen. They are packed with haemoglobin which gives them a red colour – this is why blood is red. In oxygenated blood, the oxyhaemoglobin (in arterial blood) is bright red, but after the dissolved oxygen

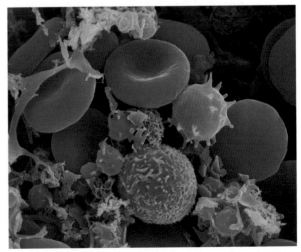

FIGURE 19.30 *Human blood*

is delivered to body cells the reduced haemoglobin (in venous blood) is dark red in colour. Due to the absence of nuclei, erythrocytes cannot divide and have a limited lifespan of around 120 days.

White blood cells, or leucocytes, are larger, nucleated and less numerous than red blood cells. There are several types, but the most common are the granulocytes (also termed polymorphs, neutrophils and phagocytes), so-called because they contain granules in their cytoplasm as well as lobed nuclei. They are capable of changing their shape and engulfing foreign material such as bacteria and carbon particles. This process is known as phagocytosis. A granulocyte acts rather like an **amoeba** and is sometimes said to be amoeboid. Granulocytes, because of their ability to engulf microbes and foreign material, are very important in the defence of the body.

Smaller white blood cells are the lymphocytes with round nuclei and clear cytoplasm – they assist in the production of **antibodies. Antigens** are found on the surface coats of disease-causing microbes or pathogens and act as identity markers for different types of pathogens (rather like name tags on school uniform). Antibodies neutralise antigens and prevent the microbes from multiplying. They can then be phagocytosed by granulocytes and monocytes. Antibodies are classed as globulins, types of plasma protein carried in the plasma. In a completely different way from granulocytes, lymphocytes also contribute to the defence of the body because of their role in the production of antibodies.

Monocytes are another type of white blood cell, larger than the lymphocytes. They also have large round nuclei and clear cytoplasm. They are very efficient at phagocytosis of foreign material and, like granulocytes, can leave the circulatory blood vessels to travel to the site of an infection and begin phagocytosing pathogens very rapidly.

Thrombocytes are not true cells, but are usually classed with the white blood cells. They are more commonly called platelets. They are products of much larger cells which have broken up. They have an important role in blood clotting.

The function of the cardiovascular system and the cardiac cycle

The cardiac cycle comprises the events taking place in the heart during one heart beat. Taking the average number of beats in a minute or 60 seconds at rest to be 70, then the time for one beat or one cardiac cycle is 60 divided by 70 seconds, which works out at 0.8 seconds. You must remember that this is based on an average resting heart rate. When the heart rate rises to, say, 120 beats during moderate activity, the cardiac cycle will reduce to 0.5 seconds. As we can see, the higher the heart rate, the smaller the cardiac cycle until a limit is reached, when the heart would not have time to fill between successive cycles.

Using the resting figures above, we can show the cardiac cycle in a series of boxes representing 0.1 second each, to study the events occurring in the heart. This is shown in Figure 19.31.

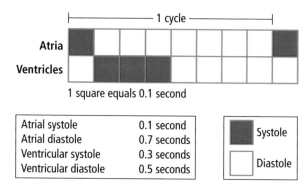

FIGURE 19.31 *Timed events in the cardiac cycle; systole and diastole*

The shaded boxes signify when contraction is occurring, and relaxation time is left blank. The technical term for contraction is systole and for relaxation, diastole. The atrial and ventricular activity is shown on separate lines.

The events in the cardiac cycle can be described in stages as follows:

✳ both atria contract forcing blood under pressure into the ventricles

* ventricles are bulging with blood and the increased pressure forces the atrio-ventricular valves shut (giving rise to the first heart sound – lubb)

* muscle in the ventricular walls begins to contract, pressure on blood inside rises and forces open the semi-lunar valves in the aorta and pulmonary artery

* ventricular systole forces blood into the aorta (left side) and pulmonary artery (right side). These arteries have elastic walls and begin to expand

* as the blood leaves the ventricles, the muscle starts to relax. For a fraction of a second blood falls backwards, catching the pockets of the semi-lunar valves and making them close (giving the second heart sound – dup)

* with the ventricles in diastole, the atrio-ventricular valves are pushed open with the blood that has been filling the atria. When the ventricles are about 70 per cent full, the atria contract to push the remaining blood in rapidly and the next cycle has begun.

You can see that when the chambers are in diastole and relaxed, they are still filling. The cycle is continuous and with a high heart rate it is the filling time which has shortened.

The cardiac output is the quantity of blood expelled from the heart in one minute. To calculate this, you need to know the quantity of blood expelled from the left ventricle in one beat

Try it out

1. Construct another diagram similar to Figure 19.31 but this time with an enhanced heart rate of 120 beats per minute. Notice how little time the heart has to fill in diastole. This is why the heart rate has an upper limit, which is different between individuals.

2. Trace the route of blood through the heart. Start at the right atrium, right ventricle, pulmonary artery, lungs, pulmonary veins, left atrium, left ventricle and aorta.

Never forget that, in a healthy heart, both atria and both ventricles contract at the same time.

(known as the stroke volume) and the number of beats in one minute (or the heart rate) The average individual has a stroke volume of $70\,cm^3$ and a heart rate between 60 and 80 beats per minute. An individual who trains regularly might have a lower heart rate but a higher stroke volume.

Try it out

Heather is a sprinter and has trained every day since she entered her teens, while Samantha enjoys watching TV and only occasionally goes clubbing. Explain the figures in the table below with respect to their lifestyle and calculate their cardiac outputs.

Heart statistics	Heather	Samantha
Stroke volume (cm^3)	95	72
Resting heart rate (beats/minute)	62	72
Cardiac output (cm^3/min)		

Control of the cardiac cycle

The heart is controlled by the autonomic nervous system, which has two branches – namely the sympathetic nervous system and the parasympathetic nervous system. These two systems act rather like an accelerator and a brake on the heart. The sympathetic nervous system is active during muscular work, fear and stress, causing each heartbeat to be increased in strength and an increased heart rate. The parasympathetic nervous system calms the heart output and is active during peace and contentment. The sympathetic nervous system is boosted by the hormone adrenaline during periods of fright, flight and fight!

Did you know?

Palpitations are forceful, often rapid heart beats that an individual becomes aware of – most commonly due to an active sympathetic nervous system combined with adrenaline secretion as a consequence of fright, flight or fight.

The sympathetic and parasympathetic nervous systems supply a special cluster of excitable cells in the upper part of the right atrium, this is called the sino-atrial node (S–A node) or in general terms 'the pacemaker'. An interplay of impulses from the sympathetic and parasympathetic nerves acting on the S–A node regulate the activity of the heart to suit circumstances from minute to minute, hour to hour and day to day.

Every few seconds, the S–A node sends out a cluster of nerve impulses across the branching network of atrial muscle fibres to cause contraction. The impulses are caught by another group of cells forming the atrio-ventricular node (A–V node) and relayed to a band of conducting tissue made of large, modified muscle cells called Purkinje fibres. The transmission of impulses is delayed slightly in the A–V node to enable the atria to complete their contractions and the atrio-ventricular valves to start to close.

Heart valves are located on a fibrous figure of eight between the atrial and ventricular muscle masses, and the first part of the conducting tissue (the bundle of His) enables the excitatory impulses to cross to the ventricles. The bundle of His then splits into the right and left bundle branches which run down either side of the ventricular septum before spreading out into the ventricle muscle masses. Impulses now pass very rapidly so that the two ventricles contract together forcing blood around the body organs.

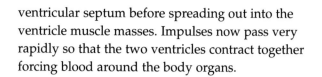

Did you know?

Any interference in the conducting system, possibly as a result of a blocked coronary artery causing tissue death, can result in a condition called heart block which can mean some parts of the heart beat at a different rhythm.

The nervous system

The nervous system (NS) is responsible for receiving and interpreting sensation, activating muscles and many glands, and regulating activities of the internal organs. Although it is really one single system, for study purposes it is often split into the somatic NS and the autonomic NS. The somatic NS is further broken down into the central and the peripheral nervous systems. You have already met the two branches of the autonomic NS, the sympathetic and parasympathetic nervous systems. Figure 19.33 demonstrates these divisions.

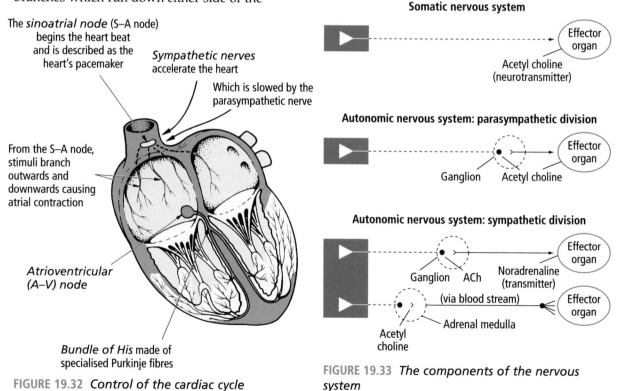

The *sinoatrial node* (S–A node) begins the heart beat and is described as the heart's pacemaker

Sympathetic nerves accelerate the heart

Which is slowed by the parasympathetic nerve

From the S–A node, stimuli branch outwards and downwards causing atrial contraction

Atrioventricular (A–V) node

Bundle of His made of specialised Purkinje fibres

FIGURE 19.32 *Control of the cardiac cycle*

Somatic nervous system

Effector organ

Acetyl choline (neurotransmitter)

Autonomic nervous system: parasympathetic division

Ganglion   Acetyl choline   Effector organ

Autonomic nervous system: sympathetic division

Ganglion   ACh   Noradrenaline (transmitter)   Effector organ

(via blood stream)   Effector organ

Acetyl choline   Adrenal medulla

FIGURE 19.33 *The components of the nervous system*

The functions of the NS can be summed up in two words:

* communication
* co-ordination.

To function efficiently, the various regions and organs of the body must transfer information from one source to another and enable events to work in a co-ordinated way. For instance, there is no point in preparing to pour digestive juices into the alimentary canal if there is no food in the tract for it to act upon. Generally speaking, communication and co-ordination are the functions of the **endocrine** (or hormonal) system, but the nervous system tends to react more quickly than the hormonal system. Hormones travel via the circulating blood so there might be over a minute between production of a hormone and its effect. In a life-threatening emergency this method of communication is too slow, and considerable damage might be sustained. Travelling via nerve fibres, however, is much faster and is therefore preferred in actions requiring almost immediate effect. For example, reproductive processes such as menstruation and childbirth can

be controlled by hormones, but preparing to run from an aggressive dog needs an instant response and is controlled by nervous pathways.

The autonomic NS mainly acts involuntarily; i.e. the system is not controlled by will or conscious thought. Heart rate, peristalsis of the muscles in the alimentary tract moving food, and outpouring of adrenaline are not events you can control; they happen automatically. The somatic NS acts mainly under your control and is said to be voluntary. When you need to move skeletal muscles to brush off a fly, lift a spoon to your mouth or clean your teeth – you are in control.

The sympathetic and parasympathetic nervous systems both send branches to many organs, but not all. For example, the sympathetic NS sends a branch to the adrenal medulla and the kidneys, but the parasympathetic NS does not. As you learned in the section on the heart (see page 248), the sympathetic NS can be usefully thought of as the system preparing the body for emergency. However, this is not always so, as the sympathetic stimulation of the skin arterioles is a response to changes in body temperature.

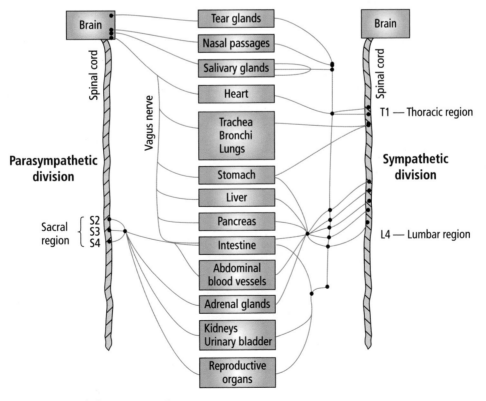

FIGURE 19.34 *Structure of the autonomic nervous system*

Autonomic nerves differ from somatic nerves in that they do not pass directly to the organ concerned, instead they synapse with another neurone that travels direct to the organ. In the sympathetic branch, these synapses lie in a chain of ganglia which lies close to the spinal cord, whereas in the parasympathetic, the synapses are usually in the wall of the organ concerned.

You will notice the different distribution of the two branches – the sympathetic NS emanates from the thoracic and upper lumbar spinal cord sections, whereas the parasympathetic NS emerges from the underside of the brain via the cranial nerves and the sacral sections of the cord. All the **neurotransmitters** are **acetyl choline** (a common transmitter) apart from the postganglionic sympathetic synapses that use noradrenaline (see section on the heart rate on page 248).

Voluntary movement

Running transversely across the outer wrinkled surface of the brain is a noticeable cleavage, or central sulcus, dividing two important areas of the cerebral cortex. In front of the sulcus, on each side, is the centre for motor or muscle control, and behind it is the centre for receiving sensation, the sensory cortex.

Voluntary movement begins in the motor cortex where the body image is represented upside down with the legs nearest the central sulcus and the head and speech area is the lowest part. The right cerebral hemisphere controls the left side of the body and vice versa. The muscles requiring very precise control, such as the face, tongue and hands, have much larger areas allocated on the cortex surface than those controlling less precise movements such as the back muscles, despite the fact that the muscles associated with less precise movements are mainly larger muscles.

The nerve fibres, or axons, leaving the motor neurones in the motor cortex form a thick nerve fibre pathway that crosses over to the other side in the medulla. This passes down the white matter of the spinal cord to the appropriate level for the spinal nerve to emerge and supply the relevant muscles.

At this level, the appropriate fibres pass into the H-shaped grey matter of the spinal cord to synapse with the lower motor neurones and pass to the muscles.

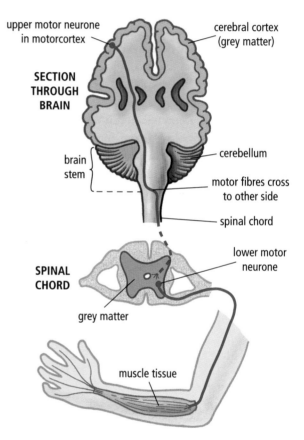

upper motor neurone in motorcortex

cerebral cortex (grey matter)

SECTION THROUGH BRAIN

brain stem

cerebellum

motor fibres cross to other side

spinal chord

lower motor neurone

SPINAL CHORD

grey matter

muscle tissue

FIGURE 19.35 *Motor pathways*

Although we use the term voluntary movement freely, there is a massive input from other neurones at the unconscious level – from different areas such as the cerebellum, where muscle co-ordination, information about the position of the body and balance are controlled and the sensory cortex, where information is received from receptors in joints and muscles.

Inter-relationships between the respiratory, cardiovascular and nervous systems

You have learned about the relationship between the cardiac cycle and the autonomic control of the S–A node (see page 264). The cardiac and vasomotor (control of the muscular walls of blood vessels) centres also lie in the medulla of the brain close to the respiratory centre, which exerts an influence on both of them. You have also learned how the oxygen and carbon dioxide in circulating blood influences respiratory rate, and how voluntary muscular activity demands more oxygen and exerts its influence on heart and respiratory rates.

Summary

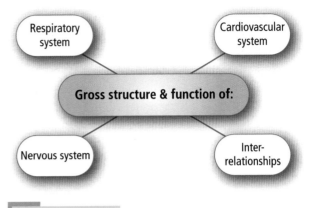

Consider this

Sadie Johnson is the general manager of a large manufacturing organisation that is about to make a loss for the second year running. She is very worried about having to make workers redundant, especially at the end of the year. She has been having palpitations, night sweats and acute anxiety attacks for the last three years.

1. Identify the factors that might have contributed to these symptoms.

2. Explain the term 'palpitations'.

3. Explain the links between the autonomic system and Sadie's symptoms.

4. Explain the role of hormones in producing these symptoms.

5. Evaluate the consequences of such symptoms for Sadie's future health.

UNIT ASSESSMENT

How you will be assessed

The assessment of this unit will consist of a report of the results of a practical investigation monitoring and comparing the physiological status of at least **three** individuals. Your investigation will be internally assessed by the teachers in your centre.

Your report should include:

* A description of how you will perform physiological measurements of pulse rate, body temperature, blood pressure and lung volumes.

* The health risks involved, potential sources of error and ways of minimising these.

* A presentation of results, together with analysis and evaluation.

* Indication of the normal range for a typical individual.
* A detailed account of the relevant control systems in each case for both rising and falling contexts.
* Descriptions of the structures and explanations of functions of the respiratory, cardiovascular and nervous sytems.
* An explanation of the interrelationships between the different body systems named above.

Grading of assessment

In order to achieve a high grade you need to include the details given in the table below.

ASSESSMENT OBJECTIVE	DETAILS
AO1 Descriptions of how to perform physiological measurements Control mechanisms and system structure	This should include monitoring and comparing the results of a practical investigation of at least three individuals for pulse rate, body temperature, blood pressure and lung volumes. There should be a clear, detailed account of the relevant control structure in each case, explaining how the body responds to different activity levels. A description of the relevant structures of each system and an accurate explanation of function is required.
AO2 Health risks and results data Interrelationship between systems and functions	A description of the health risks involved and evaluation of the results data is required. This should demonstrate an understanding of the interrelationships of the different systems and their functions.
AO3 Health risks and results data Control mechanisms and system structure Interrelationship between systems and functions	Health risks to individuals should be explained, possible errors described and ways to minimise them. A results data presentation is required togethers with analysis and evaluation. Clear indication of the normal range for typical individuals. This should demonstrate an understanding of the interrelationships of the different systems and their functions.
AO4 Health risks and results data Interrelationship between systems and functions	Evaluation of results data must be included. This should demonstrate an understanding of the interrelationships of the different systems and their functions.

Assessment preparation

For this unit you need to demonstrate your understanding of the structure and function of selected body systems including homeostatic control mechanisms. Using non-invasive techniques (this means not puncturing the body surface), you will monitor the physiological status of at least three individuals at different levels of activity.

One of the earliest tasks will be to investigate the type of equipment that is available for your use, whether this is portable and whether you can obtain permission to remove it from the premises. For example, if you have only one or two bulky biological spirometers available to investigate lung volumes, it is no use deciding to monitor your grandfather who is disabled. Your tutor will explain the availability of equipment and provide time and supervision for you to become confident and competent. When this is clear, the best way to start is to make a plan of what you are going to do and when. You will need to consider the different types of activities that you will ask the individuals to perform. Allow your tutor to give feedback on your plan and act on the comments received. You will not have the experience to know if you are being over-ambitious or not reaching the higher mark bands of the assessment objectives (AOs), whereas your tutor will know. There are up to 80 marks available for assessment of your portfolio and you should be very familiar with the assessment criteria for each assessment objective. Mark credit is available for written work of good quality using specialist vocabulary.

A Description of how to perfom physiological measurements

You will need to describe how you will use or have used your equipment to monitor your individuals' measurements. This must be in your own words; the information in this or other textbooks or instruction manuals must not be copied and is for information and guidance.

Being mindful of the need for confidentiality, you can provide faked names or letters for your chosen individuals and describe precisely how the measurement is carried out in the first person, e.g. I asked individual A for permission to count her pulse rate under various conditions of activity. Having explained fully the procedure that I have planned, A agreed to assist in my assessment of her physiological status. . .

Writing your description before you carry out the monitoring will provide you with a micro-plan for that procedure on A and the other individuals, and you will then ensure that the same process is applied to each person. You will also need to note any variations due to the different activities that you have planned, for example taking pulse rate every 1 minute after exercise until it returns to normal, but taking blood pressure every 3 minutes until it reaches the resting measurement.

You may be able to access information, equipment and a wider range of clients if you have placement or part-time work in a care setting, but permission must always be sought from the individual, your tutor and your workplace supervisor. When you are completing your assessment in school or college, your equipment might be more limited and your clients might be your peers or friends.

When you have decided on the activities to be performed, construct charts for recording the results. You will need to print out or photocopy the charts for the number of individuals under monitoring.

You will need to show that you have an understanding of the structure and function of the relevant body systems in this work.

B The health risks involved, evaluation of results data

In this section, you will need to explain fully the health risks to individuals involved in carrying out the procedure and any potential errors of measurement and ways to reduce these.

Read all instruction manuals and standard operating procedures provided for your use.

Never take measurements without supervision unless you have permission from your tutor. Carry out a 'practice' set of measurements on a willing peer to check out the results chart you have made and make any necessary adjustments before you begin the real assessment tasks.

You will need to state the normal range for the physiological measurement and this can be identified on the relevant results chart. You might decide to monitor pulse rate at rest, during mild exercise (perhaps a set walk or climbing stairs) and moderate/severe exercise (running for x minutes around a defined area) and repeat the activities say, after a meal to see if there are any differences. You might repeat this on two further days. A chart might look like the one below:

Individual A

Date/time	Pulse rate (beats per minute)					
	At rest	Mild exercise	Moderate exercise	At rest 15 mins after a meal	Mild exercise 15 mins after a meal	Moderate exercise 15 mins after a meal

After collecting the data, you will have to analyse the results depending on the activities and evaluate the individual's physiological status. Evaluation involves selecting the strengths and weaknesses of your method or results and then forming a conclusion. For example: Individual A had a higher resting pulse than B or C at the first monitoring, this was just outside normal range but was not reflected in significantly higher results during mild or moderate exercise. Individual A admitted some anxiety before the initial measurement. The subsequent periods of monitoring demonstrated a lower resting pulse than at first. I have concluded that A's pulse rate is within the normal range. You will also need to evaluate the risks to different individuals at different levels of activity.

You may quote secondary sources (with acknowledgement in your bibliography) for comparison.

C A description of the control mechanisms and structures of each system
In your own words, you should explain how each relevant control system responds to different activity levels including understanding the concept of negative feedback in both rising and falling contexts. You might prefer to use diagrams to support your explanations, these must be full and detailed and to your own design.

D An explanation of the functions performed and the interrelationship between systems and functions
You must provide sound evidence in good detail of the relationship between different body systems and their functions.

References and further reading

You will have access to a variety of textbooks on human biology, the following references represent several of the latest texts at various levels of learning.

Baker, M. et. al. (2001) *Further studies in Human Biology* (AQA) London: Hodder Murray

Boyle, M. et al. (2002) *Human Biology* London: Collins Educational

Givens, P. and Reiss, M. (2002) *Human Biology and Health Studies* Cheltenham: Nelson Thornes

Indge, B. et al (2000) *A New Introduction to Human Biology* (AQA) London: Hodder Murray

Jones, M. Jones, G. (2004) *Human Biology for AS Level* Cambridge: Cambridge University Press

Moonie, N. et. al. (2000) *Advanced Health and Social Care* Oxford: Heinemann

Pickering, W.R. (2001) *Advanced Human Biology through Diagrams* Oxford: Oxford University Press

Stretch, B. et. al. (2002) *BTEC National Health Studies* Oxford: Heinemann

Vander, A.J. (2003) *Human Physiology: The Mechanisms of Body Function* Maidenhead: McGraw Hill.

Wright, D. (2000) *Human Physiology and Health for GCSE* Oxford: Heinemann

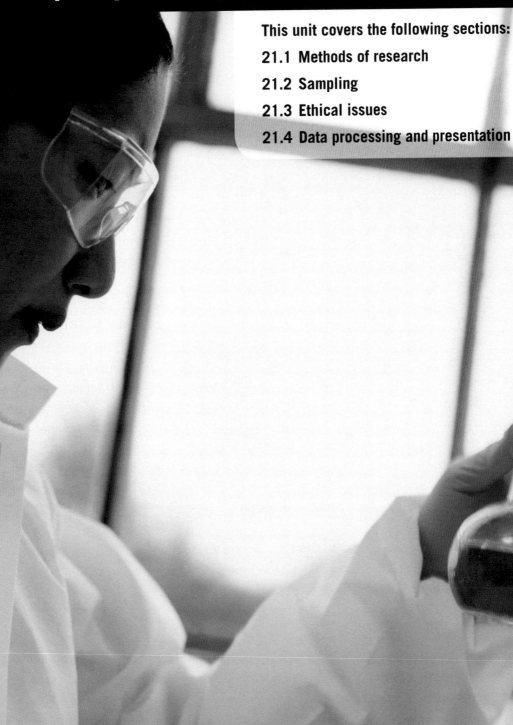

Research methods and perspectives

This unit covers the following sections:

21.1 **Methods of research**

21.2 **Sampling**

21.3 **Ethical issues**

21.4 **Data processing and presentation**

Unit
21

Introduction

This unit looks at the different types of research methods used by researchers in the field of health and social care including the experiment, the quasi-experiment, the correlation method, systematic observation, interview survey methods and questionnaires. The unit will increase your understanding of research methods and will help you to choose, design and carry out your own study.

A good research project is dependent on the way the research is carried out. This unit is all about how to carry out research effectively. It explains the different methods of research and helps to identify where mistakes can be easily made. Research is the way we find out new things. In all types of work, people use different methods of research to find new information or to analyse how they might do something better or more efficiently.

Research is an organised activity carried out in a systematic manner to find out information and gain knowledge. It can range from scientific experiments which are trying to find a cure for an illness to a local health centre carrying out a questionnaire with its patients to see how the service of the centre might be improved. Research provides evidence about published statements. There are many assumptions made about things which happen in society. This means that people draw conclusions about issues but may not have any 'evidence' that their views are true. The research may prove or disprove these statements. The results of research can make people change their minds, or help them to decide what action to take to improve or change something.

Research is carried out by many different groups of people for many different reasons. This includes local and central government, service providers such as the health service, voluntary organisations and individuals.

Unit assessment

This unit is assessed through a research project. You will need to select a topic in the field of health and social care, research into previously published studies in the area, then design, carry out and report on your own empirical study. The research project should allow for the collection of numerical data. A full explanation of the research project is at the end of this unit.

21.1 Methods of research

Types of research methods

There are two main ways of gathering the information for a research project:

* finding out information for yourself
* looking at information that others have produced.

Finding things out for yourself is known as **primary research.** Using material that others have produced is called **secondary research** and this is often the starting point for any research topic.

Secondary research

Carrying out secondary research means looking at material that has already been produced on the topic you are researching. This research should always be done at the beginning of any study, as it will give you an idea of the issues linked to your topic area and any previous research that has been carried out. It may also give you some idea of the focus of the work, as well as the research methods you should be using for your primary research. It will also give you information to compare with your own findings.

Key concept

Secondary research: material that has already been written on the topic you are researching.

There are several sources of secondary information. These include:

* text books
* journals
* the Internet
* media sources, e.g. newspapers, magazines, government publications (including statistics).

The topic chosen will determine which of these is relevant for your study. There will usually be some secondary source material, whatever your topic. However, for more up-to-date or current topics, the sources are likely to be professional journals or the Internet and specialist journals rather than text books. It can take up to a year for new information to be published.

It is also worth remembering that information can be distorted, so read it carefully. Researchers sometimes use statistics to distort information. For example, a researcher may report that 70 per cent of parents use a particular nursery school, which sounds like a lot and a major finding. However, if the sample was just ten parents and the 70 per cent was in fact seven out of ten, it isn't quite so credible.

Assessing secondary sources of information is not always easy. When looking at any secondary research, think about the way in which the information has been collected. If the research methods have not been carried out thoroughly and accurately, then the results and conclusions will not be valid.

Key concepts

Valid: this means the research produces information that is relevant to the topic you are looking at.

Reliable: this means that your research methods produce information which could be replicated by someone else doing the same survey with a similar sample of people.

Primary research

Primary research methods include questionnaires, interviews, observations, surveys and experiments. All primary research methods need careful planning if they are to produce information which is valid and reliable. The primary research methods chosen will depend on the focus of the topic and the outcomes the researcher hopes to find.

Key concept

Primary research: where you collect your own original data using one of the primary research techniques.

Did you know?

Primary research methods can either be qualitative or quantitative.

Quantitative research methods

Quantative research methods produce data which can be analysed statistically. They generate large amounts of information as samples sizes are usually big. The most effective way to handle and make sense of the information is through mathematical manipulation or statistics. The use of statistics to analyse the information means that a lot of information can be presented in a manageable format, usually graphs, charts and diagrams. This way the reader can get an overview of the findings easily and can quickly see patterns.

Questionnaires and surveys are generally considered quantitative research methods as they seek information from large numbers of people. In order to handle the large amount of data, most researchers would design questionnaires and surveys with questions that have a choice of specified answers. The responses are most effectively analysed in the form of statistics.

Qualitative research methods

Qualitative research methods tend to be aiming for depth of response rather than large numbers of respondents. Therefore, this method of research is interested in attitudes, opinions and thoughts on issues. The methods allow the researcher to understand the situation in more detail. This type of information cannot be easily analysed in a mathematical way and therefore qualitative data are not usually converted into statistics: much of the quality and meaning of responses would be lost through this process. Therefore, the information is used to support arguments, and is often quoted as it has been said (verbatim). Good examples of qualitative research methods are interviews and observations.

> ### Key concept
>
> *Triangulation:* an important concept in research. It means that a researcher uses at least three methods to collect data on a topic – such as secondary research, questionnaires and interviews in a single research project. The reason for this is to try to show similar findings across a range of research methods to support the validity and reliability of the work.

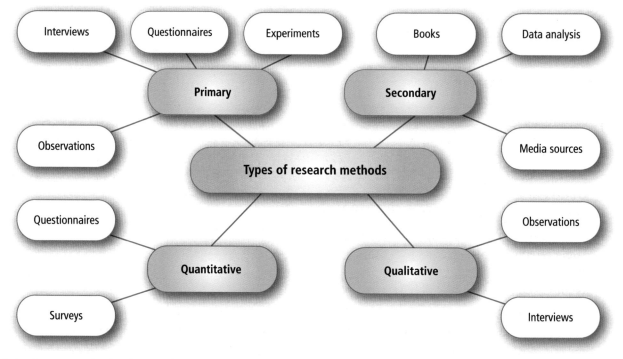

FIGURE 21.1 *Methods of research*

Other research methods

Look at Figure 21.1 to get an overview of the various methods used in research. Then read on for information about these methods.

The experiment

In the English language, the word experiment can have two meanings. Firstly, it can mean trying out something new or a new way of doing something – people can see this as an 'experiment'. The other definition, more commonly linked to research, relates to testing an idea or hypothesis through a carefully controlled experiment. In this situation an experiment is defined as 'systematic observation and measurement of a number of variables and influences on those variables within a controlled environment'.

> **Key concept**
>
> *Variable:* something that changes. It is an element, feature or factor in the experiment that is liable to vary or change. Variables need to be clearly defined and understood, in order to follow the experiment and what it proves.

This type of experiment has its basis in the scientific experimental process, although social experiments are also carried out which are based on the scientific approach.

Scientific experiments

A scientific experiment is a carefully designed procedure which aims to discover, demonstrate or test significant truths about reality. It takes place under controlled conditions and is carried out in such a way that it can be repeated by other people who, if they did so, would obtain similar results.

An experiment often has two or more groups:

* a test or experimental group which is subject to some intervention depending on the nature of the experiment – this might be a treatment, or being given some information

* a control group, which does not receive the experimental intervention, the aim being to record responses without intervention which can be compared to the test or experimental group.

Double-blind techniques

Sometimes it is necessary to use double-blind techniques. These are a way of ensuring any outcomes of the experiment can be attributed directly to the experiment and not influenced by the beliefs and behaviours of either researchers or participants. It is believed that if the participants did know they were part of the experimental group, they might report back in a way that they thought would please the researcher (demand characteristics). This is why participants have to remain 'blind' or unaware as to which group they are in. It is also possible that the researcher may treat the control group less enthusiastically than the experimental group. Therefore, to ensure all participants are treated in exactly the same way, the researcher may not be told which participants are in the control group and which are in the experimental group. Experiments like this are known as double-blind experiments.

> **Key concept**
>
> *Demand characteristics:* the name given to the way participants respond to an experiment when they appear to be trying to 'help' the experimenter by giving the answers or behaving in the manner they think the experimenter wants.

Demand characteristics are a major threat to the validity of any experiment, as the experimenter will find it difficult to claim that the behaviour observed is valid. If participants behave in ways which reflect their beliefs about what they think they should do rather than behaving 'naturally' it will be difficult to claim that observed differences in the dependent variable are due to the independent variable.

Stages of an experiment

Stage 1
Develop the theory that specifies the effect of one variable upon another.

For example, in an experiment relating to the testing of a new drug for blood pressure the theory may be that a particular dosage of the drug will reduce high blood pressure.

Stage 2

Define the dependent and independent variables – the independent variable being the aspect of the experiment that the experimenter is changing and the dependent variable being the aspect that may change as a result of the changes in the independent variable.

For example, in an experiment to test a new drug, the new drug being given to the participants will be the independent variable, as it is being changed by the experimenter; the reaction to the drug by the participants will be the dependent variable.

Stage 3

Define how the variables will be measured – if appropriate.

For example, this may include specifying both observations and specific measurements to take at specific times, such as blood pressure or temperature.

Stage 4

Express the experiment in terms of a hypothesis. A hypothesis is an idea or theory that predicts what might happen. An experimental hypothesis is a prediction, made to be tested, that one variable will affect another.

For example, drug X, when taken once per day, will reduce high blood pressure. In this hypothesis, drug X is the independent variable and the blood pressure is the dependent variable. The hypothesis clearly states that one variable will change as a result of a change in the other variable.

Stage 5

Decide on the sample – in this case, people with high blood pressure – and sample size (the number of people needed to conduct the experiment). Divide the sample size in two – one half will be the control group.

For example, in the above experiment the sample are those people with high blood pressure and the sample size is the number.

Stage 6

Carry out the experiment and record the results. There will be two sets of results, one for the experimental group and one for the control group.

They should show how the dependent variable has altered as the independent variable was altered.

Stage 7

Analyse the results – this may result in a 'null hypothesis' which means that there was no significant difference between the two groups.

Stage 8

Draw a conclusion stating if the original hypothesis was proven or not.

Aspects of experimental design

Specifically repeated measures

Specifically repeated measures occur when the same participant is tested under the various conditions of the independent variable. For example, if you were carrying out an experiment to compare the effect of age (dependant variable) on reading speed (independent variable), you might also look at how the time of day affects this (another independent variable). In this case you would ask participants to read the passage several times at different times of the day. In doing this you will be comparing two or more performances by the same participants.

Independent group designs

This is used where you are comparing performance between groups and therefore more than one group will be required for the experiment. For example, in an experiment which compares performance by age or by condition such as bilingualism. In this situation, you cannot use the same person to test all variables and therefore more groups are required.

Social experiments

Although carried out by social scientists, these have their roots in the natural and physical sciences and involve the formal testing of hypotheses about causation. A woman smoking a pipe in public could be an example of a social experiment. It could be an experiment to test the reaction of others – testing by experiment. Such an approach would follow similar stages to that of a scientific experiment but the analysis may not be so statistical.

Advantages of experiments

* potential causal relationships can be tested

* independent variables can be controlled

* participants can be randomly assigned to various experimental conditions.

* relatively convenient to organise.

Difficulties with experiments

* must have clear measures for comparing during experiment

* time interval is critical

* selecting comparable groups for control and experimental group can be difficult

* people react differently to the experimental situation

* ethical issues including deception, causing disadvantage and dealing with ill-health (refer to page 282 for more information on ethical issues)

* laboratory experiments may be questioned in terms of how accurately they may reflect what is happening in 'real life'

* there can be a tendency to use subjects who are easily accessible and this may not truly reflect the population. This then affects the conclusion which can be drawn as a result of the experiment.

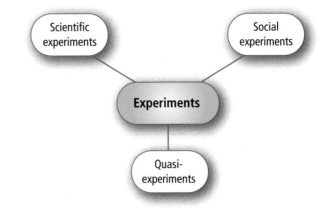

FIGURE 21.2 *Types of experiment*

> **What if?**
>
> Imagine a sample of participants all of whom suffer from a chronic health problem, for example high blood pressure or heart disease. A pharmaceutical company has a drug which it believes may significantly help improve the illness and therefore an individual's life expectancy.

Is it ethical to carry out an experiment where half the group (the control) will be using a placebo (a dummy drug) and therefore not offering them the same opportunity as the half using the active drug.

Quasi-experiments

Quasi-experiments are those in which the experimenter has no control over the 'independent variable'. An example of this may be how people react to a natural disaster – the natural disaster being the independent variable. The researcher can, however, choose who, how, and when 'dependent variables' are measured. For example, the researcher can decide the structure of the sample chosen and what aspects are being researched. Quasi-experiments are a useful method of research as they allow the study of variables which cannot be changed. Some phenomena can only be studied this way.

However, as a researcher, you have no control over the participants as you cannot predict who will experience the situation or 'independent variable' and therefore the random allocation of participants to conditions is more difficult. Also as they often relate to unpredictable phenomena, there is a limit on preparation time to set up the experiment and the way results are being recorded. This means that the interpretation of results has to be more cautious.

The correlation method

The correlation method is a softer approach than the experimental method. Experiments focus on specific variables and how one variable is affected by another. The correlation method collects data on two variables to see if there is any relationship between them that can be identified. It focuses on the strength and nature of the relationship. It then uses that relationship to predict future outcomes. The method establishes a statistical relationship.

An example of a correlation would be the link between smoking and lung cancer. It can clearly be stated that people who smoke are more likely to develop lung cancer, as there is a correlation between the two variables – smoking and cancer. However, it cannot be stated that all smokers will get lung cancer, as this is not the case. Therefore, only a correlation can be concluded. A correlation method is often used when experiment is ethically impossible.

Systematic observation

Systematic observations can be used in research as a way of analysing and finding meaning in a range of situations. Observations are commonly used when working in health and social care settings in a range of ways, including as a way of monitoring aspects of health, such as blood pressure, or as a method of identifying the developmental stages of children.

Developing a scientific approach

When carrying out observations, it is important that you develop a scientific approach to your work. This means that you need to carry out the process in an ordered, systematic way to make sure what you do is accurate. You need to be objective, which means you observe with an open mind. Knowing someone can reduce the objectivity; if you know the person you are observing, it is easy to allow what you already know to affect what you see them doing and how you record it. This is known as having pre-conceived ideas. If you are not totally objective, the whole observation will be invalid. The findings will not be accurate and therefore they will be meaningless. It is very important that you are objective from the start.

Being objective also means that you do not become personally involved with your subject or subjects. The word 'subject' can be used to describe the person or people you are observing. It can be very easy to become emotionally involved, especially if working with children, and this can affect how objective you are. You need to be able to stand back and write what you see, not what you think you see because you are influenced by other information you already have.

Why observe?

Observations are used in a number of research situations. They can be used as a way of looking at social relationships. A researcher may observe people to see how they react in certain situations or to certain stimuli, for example, how they respond to advertisements.

You might also observe people on a particular type of medication to see if or how it affects behaviour. Observations can also be used to look at interaction between people in a range of settings such as residential care or in public places. Observations can be used to study all aspects of development including physical, social, emotional and intellectual development. They can be used as the main method of research as part of a longitudinal study: that is, a study which takes place over a longer period of time, perhaps six months or more, to chart developments over the period. They may also be used as one research method to support others used, or as one off pieces of work.

Participant and non-participant observations

There are two different types of observation which basically are dependent on whether the observer chooses to get involved in what they are observing.

Participant observation

This is where the observer becomes part of the group they are observing. Being part of a group and observing at the same time can make recording detail difficult. It is also worth considering that the observer may also influence the outcome by being involved. However, this type of observation can result in a more reflective picture of what goes on as the observer is part of the group.

Non-participant observation

In this type of observations, the observer is an onlooker who is not involved in the action in any way. They purely record what they see and have no interaction with the person(s) being observed at all. The observer can record a lot of detail in this way as they can concentrate on this rather than getting involved. They can also see things which are not immediately obvious when part of the group. The main disadvantage with this type of observation is that the observer may have an effect on what happens as those involved know they are being watched. This can make the situation seem false, as those being observed feel intimidated or self-conscious and this may result in an inaccurate picture. The same problem can also be found in health care observations as people react differently if they know they are being observed or measured. For example, often blood pressure may rise as people are anxious about having their blood pressure tested.

> **Key concepts**
>
> *Participant observation:* where the observer becomes part of the group they are observing.
>
> *Non-participant observation:* where the observer has no interaction with the group being observed.

Covert or overt?

In both participant and non-participant observations the observer can be overt or covert. Overt observation is where the observer does not hide that they are observing or why they are observing. In covert observation, on the other hand, the observer does not inform those being observed that this is what they are doing, or why they are doing it. This may raise ethical issues as those being observed may feel they have been deceived when they find out.

> **Try it out**
>
> Make a list of the advantages and disadvantages of covert and overt observations.
>
> Do they differ for participant and non-participant observations?
>
> Is there any situation where you feel a particular type of observation is best used?

Main types of observations

There are many different types of observations that can be used in a health and social care research project, depending on the focus of the work.

Checklists

What is it?
A checklist is a list of skills, attributes or signs being looked for or assessed during an observation. These can be used to assess against norms or expectations. This method can also be used to compare skill levels across different groups, e.g. by gender, age or developmental stage.

When may it be used?
A checklist may be used to assess physical development; gross and fine motor skills, social skills, levels of ability, e.g. in reading levels, key health indicators such as blood pressure, heart rate, etc.

Advantages and disadvantages
A checklist is very quick to compile and produces clear results which are easily interpreted. However, to be really effective, the checklist needs to be well-prepared and thought through. It is also important that the observer only records what they see. There may be a risk of not getting true results if the person being observed feels under pressure to perform.

Event samples

What is it?
Event samples may be used to record how often a particular 'event' happens. An 'event' may include inappropriate behaviour, such as hitting out, biting or swearing, or loss of concentration or other action. It can be a useful way to explore any factors which may be causing such actions to happen, including what happens immediately before an event.

When may it be used?
Event samples can be used in any situation where there is a need to observe how often something happens and why.

Advantages and disadvantages
This type of observation produces detailed information on the behaviour being observed and will clearly show if there is a pattern, indicate events that may trigger the behaviour and confirm if there is a need for concern. The disadvantage is that the method does require the observer to

concentrate on one person for a long period of time. It is also possible that the person being observed will know they are being observed and this could affect the outcome.

Time samples

What is it?
A time sample involves recording activity over a long period of time. It is often used when carrying out child studies to record what a child might do over the period of an hour. It is often carried out over a number of days to establish patterns. This could also be applied to observing patterns of behaviour in residential care or health settings.

When may it be used?
It may be used to record how an individual fills their time. It may also be used to see if the person being observed joins in activities provided for them, or the extent of social interaction they participate in over a certain period of time.

Advantages and disadvantages
This method of observation records what is happening in detail and therefore provides a lot of information. However, it is time consuming.

Sociograms

What is it?
A sociogram is used as a way of looking at social interaction and friendship groups.

When may it be used?
One way of doing this is to ask members of the group you are studying to list their three best friends and then to plot against all the members of the group as a way of assessing popularity.

Advantages and disadvantages
This type of observation is relatively quick to carry out and produces clear results.

Limitations on observations

Observation as a method of research can have its limitations and these affect the quality of the results gained. The objectivity of observation can be affected by the actions of the observer. Other factors can also affect the situation and the person being observed so that they behave in a way which is out of the ordinary. It is worth being aware of some of these factors.

* Familiarity with the environment – if the person being observed is in a familiar environment, they will be more relaxed and feel more comfortable. The observation which takes place in this situation is likely to give a more accurate impression than one which takes place in unfamiliar surroundings.

* Timing of the observation – observing an adult who is waiting for an appointment, who perhaps is anxious, is likely to produce an observation which shows non-typical behaviour. This is not the best situation in which to carry out a straightforward observation. It may be that observing in this situation is done deliberately to look at how the unknown or stressful situations affect behaviour.

* Environmental factors such as the weather – windy or stormy weather is known to have an effect on behaviour. Therefore observations that are out of the norm may be obtained if observing is done in these conditions.

* Time of the year – there are certain times of the year when traditionally people act out of character because they are excited, such as Christmas, and this is likely to affect the observation results.

* Changes in the immediate environment – changes in noise levels, changes in the organisation of the immediate environment or changes in the people who are usually in an area (e.g. a new carer or new colleague) can all trigger changes in behaviour which will be reflected in any observation that is carried out.

An observation needs to be a true record, which is not adversely affected by anything, as this makes it easier to interpret. It also gives a fairer analysis of what is going on. However, due to the nature of observations, you cannot use observations to prove causation.

Ethical issues in observation

Ethical issues need to be carefully considered when carrying out observations. People who are being observed have a right to access the information which is being collected about them. Permission will be needed before information about them can be given out. This may be from the person themselves if an adult, or the parent, guardian or carer if a child or a vulnerable adult.

Confidentiality must also be considered as all the information which is collected is confidential. Therefore, it is important that any information gained is not discussed in any situation, and particularly not with family or friends. In order to maintain confidentiality, it is important that the participants – the people you are observing – remain anonymous. This can be achieved by using first names, a false name if the first name is unusual and easily recognisable, or each participant can be give a code – usually a number or a letter.

All observations should show an awareness of culture, race, family circumstance, gender, disability age and sexual orientation. Respect for others includes respect for their customs and beliefs. It can be useful to include photographs or videos of the person being observed as part of the evidence. Photographs or videos can be a way of illuminating the area of study but they should not be used to decorate or pad out the work. They should only be used as a way of making the information clearer or if they actually demonstrate something. Any photograph or video which is used must be commented on or explained. This is a good test of the usefulness of a photograph. If there is nothing to say about it, then it shouldn't be there and it should be removed.

Interview survey methods

An interview survey is a qualitative method because it provides more detailed information than questionnaires. Interviews take longer to carry out than questionnaires, but they make it possible to explore issues in more depth. Interviews can be a more responsive method of research as it may be possible to adapt the questions to the answers the interviewee gives. This means that an interviewer can obtain more information. Interviews also have better response rates than questionnaires. If asked directly, people are more likely to agree to answer questions, whereas a questionnaire can be easily discarded or forgotten.

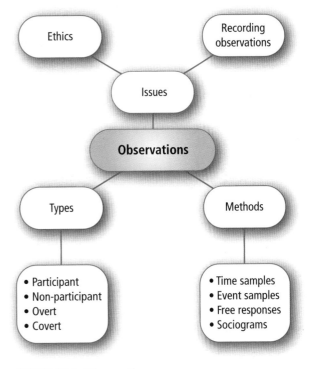

FIGURE 21.3 *Observations*

Interviews can be recorded on tape. This means that the researcher can replay an interview as many times as needed to accurately collect the information. However, it is important to be aware of how the interaction between the interviewer and the participant can affect the response. Factors such as the interviewer's appearance, gender, age and even accent can affect the answers you may get. Interviewers can also influence responses without knowing they are doing so, through normal mannerisms such as nodding or smiling. Uttering 'mmm' or even 'yes' when someone speaks can influence the relationship.

Why are interviews chosen?

An interview is a research method which allows the researcher to explore issues in more depth and collect more detail. This is particularly useful when researching beliefs, attitudes and feelings, as these cannot be fully explored through experiments, observations or questionnaires. In an interview situation a researcher can capture more personal views and experiences. Interviews have the capacity to draw out reasons and explanations in a way that questionnaires cannot, due to their very structured nature and the fact that,

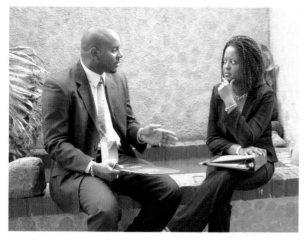

FIGURE 21.4 *Interviews are a type of research method*

for analysis purposes, questionnaires often have a limited possible response. In addition, when completing questionnaires, even when a free response question is asked, people often write as little as possible.

Advantages of interviews

✳ Interviews are based on communication and interaction between two people. If a good rapport develops, they result in the interviewer getting detailed information. This relationship will allow the interviewer to ask questions of a personal and sensitive nature.

✳ Interviews allow researchers to find out reasons and understand people's thinking, and allow people to speak directly and at length in a way that questionnaires do not.

✳ Many interviews allow researchers to follow up responses and this makes them more flexible and reactive to the answers given by the interviewee. It allows more detailed information to be obtained.

Disadvantages of interviews

✳ The success of the interview is directly influenced by the skill of the interviewer.

✳ Interviews are generally one-to-one and are therefore expensive in terms of man-power. They are also quite time consuming and therefore are generally used for smaller samples.

✳ Interviewers need to be aware that interviewees may respond to questions with what they feel

the interviewer wants to hear rather than their true feelings or behaviour.

✳ Interviewers can be unconsciously affecting the responses. Non-verbal communication such as frowning, smiling or nodding can influence what an interviewee says or discloses. If they feel the interviewer disapproves of their views, interviewees may not be as open as they could be.

✳ It is easy to introduce inconsistency in informal interviews, where the interviewer can follow up responses. Interviewers may only follow up what they personally consider to be important and valuable information may be missed.

✳ The nature of the data collected during interviews makes it more difficult to draw overall conclusions or generalisations. Such qualitative data is not generally used to produce detailed statistics.

Types of interviews

There are several different approaches to using interviews as a method of research.

Formal interviews

A formal interview is one where there is a standard set of questions which are put to each participant. The interviewer can only ask these questions, despite the responses given, and cannot adapt the wording of the questions or change them in any way. It is a very rigid form of interviewing and therefore it is similar to a questionnaire.

Designing the questions for a formal interview follows a process which is very similar to that of designing a questionnaire as it:

✳ uses standardised questions which allow generalisations to be made

✳ has less chance of an interviewer introducing any bias as he or she has to ask a specific set of questions.

However, being so rigid may mean that opportunities for developing information are lost as interviewers cannot follow up answers which may be of interest.

Informal interviews

These are interviews where the interviewer has much more control and influence over the questions that are asked. Interviewers have the freedom to develop the questions as they feel appropriate. The interview process often resembles a discussion more than a question and answer session, and therefore is more unpredictable.

An interviewer usually has a list of areas or issues they wish to cover during the interview. These are often called 'trigger questions'. They are also able to follow up responses and develop the interview more fully. This type of interview has the advantage that it can produce richer information as interviewers can probe for thoughts and develop what might appear to be off-the-cuff comments into fuller answers. It is therefore a good source of detailed qualitative data.

Semi-structured interviews

Semi-structured interviews are a combination of the structured and unstructured approaches. They have the advantage of collecting some specific information from set questions but also allowing the interviewer to follow leads and develop interesting responses more fully.

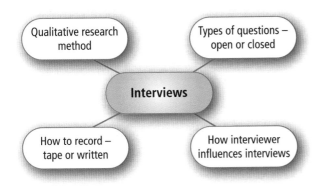

FIGURE 21.5 *Interviews*

Questionnaire survey methods

A questionnaire is a list of questions designed by the researcher, which are given to potential respondents in a written format. They are not usually completed with a researcher present and therefore, as a research method, they are not as expensive as interviews. Questionnaires are often used because they give breadth of information about a subject. However, they do not generally provide any depth; depth of information is best gained through interviews.

A questionnaire is a piece of quantitative research in that it can provide lots of responses relatively easily and responses can be directly compared, collated and analysed. It is a good way of asking straightforward questions to a large number of people. However, it does take time to collate and analyse the large number of responses that are gained.

Devising a good questionnaire

To design a good questionnaire, there are a number of stages which you will need to go through. It is important that you do go through each stage to ensure you design the questionnaire that gets you the information you need. If you miss or rush through any stage, it is likely that the finished result will not be useful or will yield results which are neither reliable nor valid.

Pre-construction issues (Stage 1)

Before you start to design the questionnaire, consider the following:

The length of the questionnaire

It is wise to keep the questionnaire brief as long questionnaires tend to put potential respondents off and they are less likely to complete it. Therefore, keep it as short as possible by only asking what really needs to be asked.

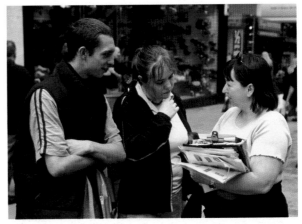

FIGURE 21.6 *It is wise to keep your questionnaire brief*

The presentation of the questionnaire

A questionnaire which looks complicated and wordy is more likely to be discarded by the respondent. People are put off by a lot of words on things they see as 'non-essential'. Therefore, when designing the questionnaire, it is important to:

* make the layout attractive

* leave plenty of space around each question as this gives the appearance of fewer words

* position of boxes for responses on the right, as most people are right handed.

> **Example**
> How many pieces of fruit do you eat in a day? [ ]
>
> [ ] How many pieces of fruit do you eat in a day?

The question above is far easier for the respondent to complete with the boxes on the right.

Designing the questionnaire

It is essential that you have a very clear idea about what you want the questionnaire to find out from the beginning, as this will ensure that you get information that will be genuinely useful in your research. To do this effectively it is important that you have researched your topic well. A good questionnaire often comes from thorough research of secondary source material, such as text books and media articles. The research should help direct you towards the results you want and will also give you something to compare your results with when you analyse them.

Sometimes the area you wish to investigate has no previously published material available. If this is the case, you will have to consider your line of enquiry even more carefully to ensure you are clear about the purpose of your questionnaire.

Decide on your sample (Stage 2)

To ensure your questionnaire is valid and reliable, it is important that you consider who you will give the questionnaire to, and how many people you will ask. This is called your sample frame. There are many different types of sample, as outlined in the section on sampling (page 292). The choice you make will vary according to the aim of the questionnaire within the scope of the overall research. Remember, however, that a small sample, especially a sample of less than 20, is not likely to be representative regardless of how the sample has been chosen.

Whichever method you choose to select your sample, it is important to identify your reason for choosing the method when you write up the research. Most samples will be a balance between the ideal sample and that which is practical and available. The choice is likely to be affected by cost, time and resource limitations, but as long as this is recognised in the analysis of the results and the evaluation, then this is acceptable.

Preamble (Stage 3)

A clear, concise preamble is important as it explains the purpose of any questionnaire. It should outline what the questionnaire is trying to do and why, as well as how the results will be used. Confidentiality should also be mentioned as this will encourage more people to complete it. It may be useful to explain how long it should take to complete the questionnaire. The preamble should aim to encourage the potential respondent, so they can see there is a use or value in completing it.

It should also outline how to complete the questionnaire, any deadline dates and how to return it. This is particularly important as response rates to questionnaires are typically below 30 per cent so it is important to make the questionnaire as easy to return as possible. Some people include a stamped addressed envelope as a way of increasing the return rate.

> **Try it out**
>
> Devise a preamble for a questionnaire on eating habits in pregnancy.
>
> How might you choose your sample for such a questionnaire?

Devising questions (Stage 4)

Writing good questions for a questionnaire is a challenge. Questions need to be clear to ensure that the respondents understand what is being asked. It is easy to write a question that you believe will gain information in a specific way, but those completing the questionnaire may interpret it completely differently. Therefore, it is worth spending some time considering your questions to ensure they are right. There are several points to bear in mind when designing a questionnaire. These will help you avoid the potential pitfalls.

Relevance

Questions must be relevant. Questions on age, gender and occupation are often included on questionnaires but you need to consider whether this information is relevant to your study. The rule is, if the question is not relevant to the study, leave it out. Respondents give up their own time to answer questionnaires and irrelevant questions are likely to put them off.

Language

Think carefully about the language you are using and who you are hoping will complete the questionnaire. Choose words that are straightforward and that people will understand. People are less likely to answer a question if it looks complicated or contains jargon.

Open versus closed questions

Open questions are questions which require more than a yes or no answer. They will a get wide range of responses and therefore are more difficult to analyse.

> **Example**
>
> 'What do you feel is the most effective way of improving health care in the UK?'

The responses to open questions give a more personal insight into the respondents' thoughts. Closed questions are more limiting in their possible responses. They generally have a yes or no answer, or there are a number of predetermined responses for the respondent to choose from.

> **Example**
>
> Do you take vitamin pills on a daily basis?
>
> Yes/No

This type of question is useful if you are covering facts, or where it is reasonable to guess the range of possible responses. Closed questions are also used where you need to categorise age or time into sections. When using pre-selected responses, it is important to think about these to ensure that they have clear meaning and are sufficiently different for the respondent to be able to make a definite choice. Don't use words such as poor, adequate or good, as each respondent will have a different interpretation of these words. Try a grading scale instead, such as 1–5, as this may bring a better response for analysis. Closed questions are easy to analyse and also easy for the respondent to complete as often they only involve ticking a box.

> **Example**
>
> Oranges are a good source of
>
> a) protein [ ]
> b) iron [ ]
> c) vitamin C [ ]
> d) fat [ ]

Remember when classifying age groups there shouldn't be any cross over in the categories. For example, under 20, 21–35, 36–50, and so on, not 20, 20–35, 35–50, etc., as those who are 20, 35 or 50 will not know which category to tick.

Sometimes closed questions are pre-coded to make analysis easier and quicker. Each potential response is given a code so that it is not necessary to record the answers in full every time an individual responds.

Personal information

Respondents do not usually like giving personal information, so only ask if it is necessary and relevant to the questionnaire. If personal information is needed respondents are more likely to give their age or income if there is a range to complete rather than requesting exact information.

Therefore, closed questions are best for this type of question.

Example

Is your gross income bracket, per annum:

<£10,000	[ ]
£10,001–£20,000	[ ]
£20,001–£30,000	[ ]
£30,000+	[ ]

Questions requesting personal information can be placed at the end of the questionnaire, as the respondent is more likely to have completed most of the questionnaire before reaching that section and will probably complete it. If the respondent chooses not to give personal data, then you still have the information from the rest of the completed questionnaire.

Multiple questions

It is easy to write a question which really asks more than one question. An example would be:

Example

How many times a week do you exercise for more than half an hour and which sport do you do?

With such questions, some respondents will only answer the second part of the question and this will reduce the reliability of your results. If both parts of the question are important, it is better to break the question into parts (a) and (b), or make them two very separate questions.

Example

1(a) How many times a week do you exercise for 30 minutes?

Once	[ ]
Twice	[ ]
Three times +	[ ]
Never	[ ]

(b) What sports do you do?

....

....

....

Breaking up a question into separate parts will ensure that all respondents are clearly directed into answering all questions.

Assumptions

Always avoid questions that assume something about the opinions or actions of the respondent. This also applies to knowledge and experiences. A question such as 'How long have you been married?' assumes all respondents are married. Every question asked must be one that the respondent can reasonably answer.

Memory

Most people may be expected to remember up to one year before with relative accuracy. However, it is not wise to ask people for information about things which happened five or ten years ago. If you need information from the past, you are likely to need memory joggers, such as prompts about special events at the time. In most situations where detailed information from the past is needed, interviews are probably a better research method.

Try it out

Note down your diet over the last fortnight. Write down everything you ate and drank.

How accurately do you remember?

When does your memory get hazy?

How would you manage if you had to note down everything eaten over the last month?

Leading questions

It is important to devise questions which do not suggest a preferred response to the respondent. This trap can be easy to fall into if you have a particular view yourself. This can lead to bias in the answers you receive.

Example

Should the cruel and heartless sport of boxing be banned?　　Yes　[ ]

No　[ ]

Organising the questionnaire and testing the questions (Stage 5)

Questions need to be grouped in an ordered manner so that, where appropriate, one question leads to another. Once all the questions have been drafted, they can be written on small pieces of card or sticky notes and ordered and reordered until they flow well. This avoids having to rewrite the questions every time. It is a better way of assessing the way the questionnaire will finally look rather than just renumbering the questions. Once you are happy with the layout, the questionnaire can be typed up and reproduced as many times as is necessary.

Piloting the questionnaire (Stage 6)

A questionnaire needs to be piloted by a small number of people to identify any areas you have missed. It is always better to have objective people looking at the work to comment on it with a fresh eye. The designer doesn't always see the errors, mistakes or confusing sections because they are so close to the work. It is worth testing the questionnaire on five to ten people to ensure you get a fair view of the quality of the questionnaire.

When you give the questionnaires to the people who are piloting it, ask them to comment on such things as the clarity of the instructions and layout, time for completion, any ambiguities, as well as any questions they feel are irrelevant or offensive, or any additional relevant questions that have been missed. Analyse these results and adjust the original questionnaire accordingly before it is sent out to your main sample. Keep a record of these changes to include in your write-up.

Carry out the questionnaire (Stage 7)

The next stage is to carry out the actual questionnaire and wait for the responses to come back.

Collating and analysing the results (Stage 8)

Questionnaires generally produce large amounts of data which need analysing. The method of analysis chosen will depend on the way the questions have been asked. Closed questions lend themselves to graphical presentation, as the data will be quantitative, whereas open questions will produce qualitative information which will be best presented in a written format. Information on presenting results can be found in the section on data processing and presentation on page 298.

Questionnaires – a summary

* plan the interview – what are you trying to find out
* decide on the sample
* construct a preamble to the questionnaire
* devise questions – consider relevance at all times
* order the questions in a logical order
* pilot or test the questionnaire
* adjust the questionnaire after piloting
* carry out the questionnaire
* collate and analyse the results.

Data collection surveys

Data collection surveys are a method of quantitative research used to collect information in a general or detailed way. They can produce a lot of data in a numerical format. They may involve direct questioning of participants (e.g. in an on-street survey) and can therefore be similar to questionnaires. Some surveys involve observation only, such as traffic surveys. Therefore, data collection surveys are often designed in one of two formats – either as a list of questions which the researcher asks people, or as a chart to record relevant information as it is observed. Generally, participants are not required to complete any paperwork themselves with this type of research method. Surveys which involve asking questions tend to be quite brief, as generally people do not like spending a lot of time answering questions when stopped at random.

A survey to find out how far people have travelled to a health centre.

Is this your usual health centre?

Yes   [ ]
No   [ ]

Have you made the trip to see the doctor or for another reason?

Doctor   [ ]
Nurse   [ ]
Get repeat prescription   [ ]
Make appointment   [ ]
Other   [ ]

Have you made the trip just to come to the health centre or are you combining it with something else?

Just health centre   [ ]
With shopping   [ ]
On way to work   [ ]
Other   [ ]

How far have you travelled to this centre?

Under 1 mile   [ ]
1–2 miles   [ ]
2–4 miles   [ ]
Over 4 miles   [ ]

With this type of survey, many of the questionnaire-design guidelines (see page 286) apply. Therefore, it is again important that the researcher considers what they want to find out when designing the survey, especially as people are reluctant to spend a long time answering questions. A well thought out survey can produce a lot of data in a short period of time.

Tips for designing a survey

✳ Research your topic thoroughly – a well researched topic will lead to a relevant, well designed survey.

✳ Be clear about your focus and exactly what you want to find out from the survey.

✳ Think carefully about the questions you want to ask.

✳ Keep it brief – make sure the questions are relevant and focus on the issues you want to cover – this way you will get good value from the limited time people are willing to spend answering questions 'on the street'.

✳ Place the response boxes on the right hand side of the response sheet as most people are right handed, and therefore the answers can be recorded quickly.

✳ Consider the sample you will use – the most likely methods will be the quota sample, cluster sample or opportunity sample (see page 293). Be clear about which you are choosing and why.

Preamble

The preamble at the start of the survey, which tells participants what you are doing, will be very important. This should explain the purpose of the survey and approximately how long it will take. It will help a potential participant decide if they want to take part. It is also usual to explain how the results will be used.

Example
I am conducting a survey into the use of the health centre for the practice. It will take about five minutes. All responses are confidential and names are not needed. The information gained will be written up in a report for the partners of the practice.

Devising questions

Consider all the issues relevant to designing questionnaires (page 286). Make sure you trial or pilot the questions to ensure they make sense, are relevant and cover the categories needed.

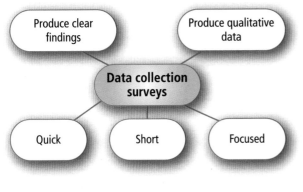

FIGURE 21.7 *Data collection surveys*

Example

Title: A survey of the way children arrive at Mountfield Nursery School

Day: Tuesday 25 November

Time: 8.30–9.00 am

Car	IIII
Walk	IIII
Taxi	II
School bus	II
Public transport (bus)	III

Surveys which record observed information

Surveys which just record observations need to be designed carefully. They will not require input from individuals in the form of questions, but nevertheless need careful planning to ensure the required information is collected. It is possible to record too little information and then the survey won't tell you anything. An example of a simple tally survey is given below.

Survey results are best presented in a way which shows the overall responses, such as a tally chart or a results table. A graph or other pictorial format could also be used depending on the results gained. The important consideration is to ensure the format presents the findings to the reader in a clear manner.

Summary

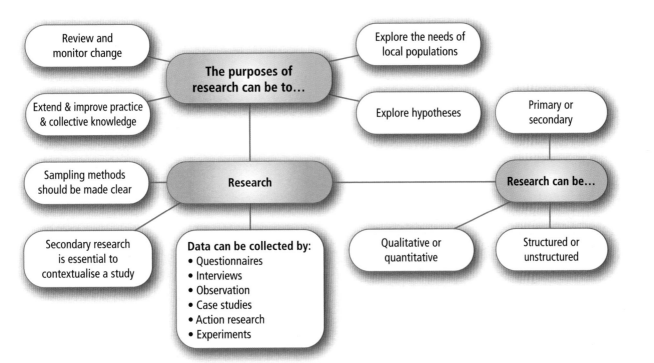

Consider this

A health centre wants to consider how it can improve its services to its clients. It wants to find out what they like about the centre and what they would like to see improved. It has asked you to develop a research plan.

1. Which research methods would not be suitable for this and why?

2. Which different research methods could you use for this project and why?

3. Design a questionnaire for clients using the service to find out what they like about the centre.

4. Develop some interview questions for a structured interview to find out what other services clients may like to see.

21.2 Sampling

Sampling is the name given to the way in which you decide who is going to be involved in your research. There are many different types of sampling methods and the one you choose will depend on what you are researching and the potential number of people who could be involved.

Random samples

In this sample, respondents are chosen at random – almost as a lottery, out of a hat. Everyone from the list of people has an equal chance of being chosen.

The size of the list of potential respondents (the 'population') will vary according to the topic. It could be everyone in a class, all clients at a surgery, all the parents who use a nursery, the electoral role in a town, etc.

Try it out

Make a list of other 'populations' who may be used for a random sample.

Stratified samples

This is a sample which reflects the age and culture of the group. Therefore, you need to analyse the age and cultural groups of the potential respondents and then ensure your sample reflects this. For example, imagine you were researching the views of elderly people who attended day centre facilities and there were 360 who attended over three days of a week. The elderly people were all from the same cultural group and their gender and year groups were divided up as shown in Table 21.1.

If you were going to take a 33 per cent sample (120 participants), you would divide the allocation of the questionnaires as shown in Table 21.2.

Table 21.2 shows the sample frame. By using this, the researcher can ensure that every group is represented in the appropriate proportions. This sample reflects the structure of the full numbers of elderly using the facility. It can then be assumed that any findings could reflect

DAY	NUMBERS	NUMBER OF MALES (%)	NUMBER OF FEMALES (%)	% OF TOTAL NUMBER IN COHORT
Monday	180	100 (56)	80 (44)	50
Wednesday	140	70 (50)	70 (50)	39
Friday	40	31 (75)	10 (10)	11

TABLE 21.1 *Numbers attending day centres*

DAY	% OF SAMPLE	NO OF QUESTIONNAIRES	NUMBER OF MALES	NUMBER OF FEMALES
Monday	50	60	34	26
Wednesday	39	46	23	23
Friday	11	14	10	4

TABLE 21.2 *Sample frame*

the views of all users. This careful calculation takes time, but it is useful in that any results can be seen as representative of the group being investigated. It becomes even more complicated if you consider ethnic origin or culture as categories as well.

Quota samples

This type of sampling is where you choose the number of respondents you want from each category you have identified before the start. Questionnaires are then given out at random until the stated number has been reached. This is less precise than a stratified sample and the researcher may be told to stop when a certain number of people have been questioned; for example 50 women over 30 years, or 100 males.

Cluster samples

This is a type of sampling where the researcher chooses a particular group of people who are located in a particular area for a specific reason. An example may be people who live in a specific street, or all of a particular group, e.g. people who use a specific health centre. In cluster sampling you may question all the people within the cluster, or a sample of them.

Such a sample is generally chosen because there is a specific reason for doing so, such as work specifically focusing on that area. In this type of sampling frame, you are likely to question the whole target group.

Opportunity samples

This sample consists of anyone who passes by a particular point when the research is being carried out. There is no selecting done by the researcher; all who happen to pass by are given a questionnaire and included in the sample.

Systematic samples

This is a structured sample where the researcher chooses respondents in an organised manner. They generally have a list of people such as an electoral role or a register. They then choose every so many people on the list, e.g. every sixth person. This method can also be used in the street, where a researcher may give a questionnaire, for example, to every fifth person who passes by.

Self-selected samples

This type of sampling method is one where people volunteer to take part. Sometimes, incentives such as prizes are offered to encourage people to do this. This does mean, however, that you will attract a particular type of person so your results may be affected.

Snowball samples

This is another form of natural selection whereby the sample selects itself through word of mouth. Respondents put themselves forward to take part in the questionnaire. For example, companies may put out an advert asking for volunteers to take part in some research, or people may see a researcher in the street and approach them to take part.

Summary

TYPE OF SAMPLE	EXPLANATION	ADVANTAGES	DISADVANTAGES
Random sample	Respondents chosen at random	Good cross-section of respondents All have an equal chance of being chosen	People may not take part May not get a true cross-section of the population being researched due to the random way the sample is taken
Stratified sample	Respondents are a carefully chosen cross-section of the sample	Should be a true cross-section of the sample Results can be analysed in sub-sections as well as the whole group	Can be complicated to develop the sample frame
Quota sample	Set number of respondents identified by category	Sample clearly set out	May not be able to find the required number in each group easily
Cluster sample	A specific cohort is chosen to respond	Cohort is easily identified Cohort may be located in one place so access is easy	No use for a research project which wants to draw broad conclusions Narrow focus
Opportunity sample	Anyone who passes by	Easy to administer as anyone can be a respondent	May have a bias in the profile of the respondents due to the random nature of the sample
Systematic sample	Respondents chosen in a systematic way	Logical way to structure sample Sample should be a good cross-section	Sample may be biased due to where the choice falls
Self-selected sample	Respondents choose to take part themselves	Respondents are willing to take part No persuasion is needed	May not get enough respondents May get a bias in the respondents as a result of the topic of the research
Snowball sample	Self-selected sample via word of mouth	No persuasion needed People want to take part	If a prize is offered as an incentive, the respondents may only be involved due to this May get a bias as a result of the sample

TABLE 21.3 *Summary of the sampling method*

21.3 Ethical issues

Research usually involves finding out information from people – often the information is about themselves and their decisions or thoughts. Therefore, it is essential that the rights of the person involved in the research are considered before it is carried out. This means thinking about the need to maintain confidentiality and ensuring the people you use in your research remain anonymous. This important consideration is known as **ethics.** Ethics is all about human behaviour and if the way something is carried out is right or wrong. This includes behaviour that is morally right or wrong as well as the way in which any actions may affect others.

Ethics are used as guidelines when making decisions. Every individual has a set of ethics. They may differ from person to person but will broadly be the same in any society and define what individuals believe is right and wrong. They are based on the values individuals are brought up with and they will influence behaviours and attitudes as well as conscience. Understanding exactly what ethics is can be difficult, as it is based on attitudes, values and beliefs which are hypothetical; that is, based on ideas or thoughts. It is an abstract concept formed in the mind; there is nothing concrete to measure.

Ethics, however, is not always an individual decision. Some groups of people have shared ethics by which they operate. An example of this is the British Psychological Society (BPS) who has a code of ethics and conduct. This code sets out the core values and principles of the society which should guide the professional decisions of its members. It gives clear parameters which help guide members' decision making and the way they deal with ethical issues in the context of research. Further information about this code of ethics can be found at the BPS website (www.bps.org.uk).

Applying ethics when carrying out research

In all types of research, ethics should be applied to the way the research methods are carried out. They will influence what is considered to be good or bad practice in the methodology. Ethics also applies to the way the information that has been gathered is used. This means taking a responsible attitude to the work being carried out and the results obtained.

Deception

Generally, it is good practice to make sure the participant is clear about the aims of the research they are taking part in. However, sometimes it is necessary for some mild temporary deception to avoid participant bias, or avoid influencing a particular type of behaviour in the response. Any deception should be corrected in the debriefing. For example, participants taking part in a trial of new drugs will often be split into two groups, one group having the drug and the other a placebo (a version without the active ingredient), but the participants will not know which group they are in. The results will be monitored and participants told at the end of the trial.

Any deception must not cause danger to the participant – either mentally or physically – for example, it is not ethically correct to tell a participant that someone they know has been fatally injured in order to monitor the response they give.

It is vitally important that throughout the research process the researcher is sensitive to how others may feel. It is also important to remember that some people may feel embarrassment and/or distress at questions that wouldn't embarrass

the researcher personally. Researchers therefore need to be alert to the signals they receive from participants during the research.

Maintaining confidentiality

Often people are giving you personal and sensitive information and therefore they and their information should be treated with respect. Remember that different people have different opinions on what is sensitive information, so the best approach is to treat any information which is given to you in any research as confidential. Do not repeat to anyone any information in a form which can be traced back to the person who gave it.

Confidentiality is an important issue to be aware of. Any information which is collected through different primary research methods should be confidential. Therefore, it is important that specific details of what individuals have said or put in questionnaires are not discussed with family or friends. It can be very easy to do this when chatting casually, but researchers could find themselves in a very difficult situation if they were overheard or if someone repeated their comments. Researchers should be prepared to give an overview or general findings to those interested but not to attribute comments to individuals.

All research should show an awareness of culture, race, family circumstance, gender, disability, age and sexual orientation. Respect for others includes respect for their customs and beliefs. For example, it would be inappropriate to

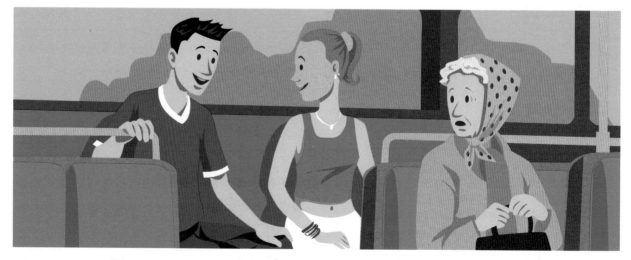

FIGURE 21.8 *Confidentiality is essential*

insist on interviewing a Muslim at a time when they may need to pray. Muslims pray at specific times of the day – a researcher should either avoid these times or be sensitive enough to leave the room so that praying can take place.

In order to maintain confidentiality, it is important that the participants, the people used in the research, remain anonymous. This can be achieved by using first names only. If the first name is unusual, and the person could easily be identified, the name used can be changed or participant one, participant two, participant three and so on can be used.

Seeking informed consent

People involved in research have a right to understand the purpose of the research and how the information which is being collected about them will be used. If participants understand this, they are able to give informed consent to the research. Permission may be needed before some information can be collected, especially if the research involves gaining information from children, or researching in a particular organisation or establishment. It is also worth remembering that participants have the right to withdraw from research at any point if they feel uncomfortable about the process and no longer want to be involved.

Maintaining neutrality

It is important that researchers do not influence the participants with their own views and opinions through the way they ask questions or respond to responses given. It is highly likely that participants will have different views and ideas from those of the researcher. The researcher must appear neutral and non-judgemental if they are to gain open responses from their participants.

Think it over

List the different ways in which a researcher may suggest they do not agree with the responses a participant gives – think about tone of voice, body language and facial expressions.

Debriefing

It is important to 'debrief' the participant as soon as possible after the research has been carried out. This usually happens immediately after the process. The debriefing should tell the participant what the research was about and what will happen with the results. They may also wish to ask questions, which may include questions on how they performed. The researcher should use their own judgement as to whether they should reveal individual 'scores'. It may be appropriate to tell individuals the 'raw results' but not to interpret them or pass judgement as to whether they scored well or badly.

Summary

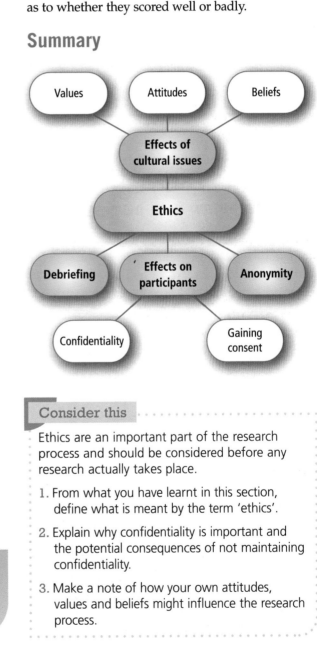

Consider this

Ethics are an important part of the research process and should be considered before any research actually takes place.

1. From what you have learnt in this section, define what is meant by the term 'ethics'.

2. Explain why confidentiality is important and the potential consequences of not maintaining confidentiality.

3. Make a note of how your own attitudes, values and beliefs might influence the research process.

21.4 Data processing and presentation

An important aspect of the research process is the way you choose to present the information or data you have collected. How you choose to present the data can affect the manner in which information is collected, so you should consider your method of presentation before you undertake your research.

What is data?

Research produces a lot of information and this is known as data. This 'raw data' is then interpreted in a manner which best presents the findings. Raw data is not usually presented as part of the finished project, but it is retained for a period of time after the project is finished in case the findings are queried. Quantitative research methods generally produce a large amount of numerical data which is usually best presented using graphs, pie charts or diagrams.

How should raw data be presented?

Presenting research findings in clear and concise formats such as tables or graphs make the information far easier to read and more accessible. There are a number of different ways in which data could be presented:

* sociograms
* Venn diagrams
* tables
* pictograms
* bar charts
* pie charts
* line graphs
* histograms
* scatter grams.

Some data is better presented in certain formats, but generally the choice of presentation is down to the person writing the report and their own preferences. Make sure the method chosen presents the information in the clearest manner. Graphs and charts can easily misrepresent data and therefore it is important to choose the method of presentation carefully.

Tables

Tables are a useful way to present a range of information in a neat, clear format, particularly where comparisons are made. For example, if you wanted to look at information over a number of years and look for changes and trends, you might use a table. The information in Table 21.4 shows the number of parents using different forms of full-time childcare in a particular housing estate over a period of time.

You can draw conclusions from this in relation to which types of care are growing and declining. You could decide to analyse in further depth by exploring if there is any difference in the ages of the children who attend the different types of care. A table can include a lot of information in a small area. It is therefore important that tables are clearly labelled so the reader can see what is being depicted. Units of measurement must also be clearly stated.

Graphs

There are a number of different types of graphs which can be used to present data; the one chosen will depend on the type of data being presented.

TYPE OF CHILDCARE	2000	2001	2002	2003	2004
Childminding	20	22	24	25	25
Private nurseries	18	21	24	26	28
Nanny based in own home	10	10	8	7	7
Family or friends	6	6	6	5	5

TABLE 21.4 *Types of childcare*

There are several points to note whatever type of graph is being used:

* graphs usually have vertical and horizontal axes
* axes should be clearly labelled
* any units of measurement must be very clear
* graphs should have a clear title which clarifies what they depict for the reader
* graphs should be presented on graph paper – not lined or plain
* the source of any data should be given at the bottom of the graph.

Bar charts

Bar charts are easy to draw and understand. Therefore, they are the most common type of graph. They are particularly useful for presenting data with descriptive categories. Bar charts may be presented with the bars close together, or with a space between each one. Bar charts have a number of common features including:

* all bars are the same width
* bars may be horizontal or vertical
* the length of the bar will indicate the frequency
* one axis has the scale and the other the descriptive category
* bar charts are often coloured to improve the presentation
* a code may be used to label the bars as long as a clear key or legend is included on the graph which explains the codes.

Line graphs

Line graphs are often used when changes over time need to be shown, as they can show fluctuations in values clearly. They are good for plotting more than one line to show differences, or how two variables might compare, e.g. changes in heart rate and breathing rate during exercise over a period of time. Generally, you need a lot of data to produce a line graph which is meaningful. Limited data used in line graphs can easily give the wrong impression. Line graphs are produced by plotting points of data on a graph and then joining the points to produce a line. Features of a line graph are:

* the horizontal axis has a continuous variable such as time, temperature or number
* the vertical axis has the scale.

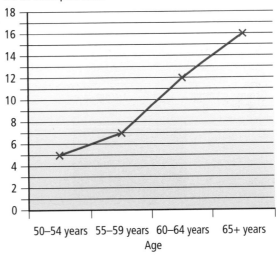

Travel pass users – by age
Sample size = 40

FIGURE 21.10 *A line graph*

Histograms

Histograms look very similar to bar charts but are in fact very different. The main differences are that:

* they are generally used for grouped data, i.e. data that covers a band
* columns are not the same width – they vary according to the proportion of the size or class they represent in relation to the total
* there are no gaps between the columns
* the frequency of the class is indicated by the size of the column
* the horizontal axis has a scale similar to any other graph, in that the interval represents the same number of units.

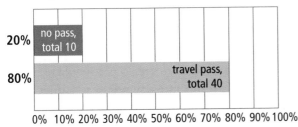

Travel pass usage
Sample size = 50

FIGURE 21.9 *A bar graph*

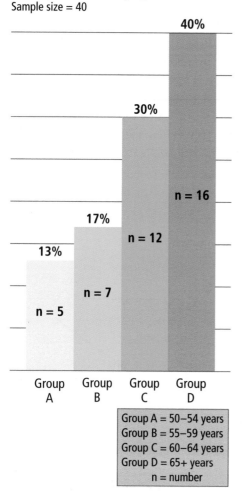

Travel pass users – by age
Sample size = 40

40%

30%

n = 16

17%

13%

n = 12

n = 7

n = 5

Group
A

Group
B

Group
C

Group
D

Group A = 50–54 years
Group B = 55–59 years
Group C = 60–64 years
Group D = 65+ years
n = number

FIGURE 21.11 *A histogram*

Scatter graphs

Scatter graphs are generally used where data showing two corresponding variables needs to be presented in order to see if there is a pattern or correlation, e.g. the relationship between blood pressure and age of a group of people. Scatter graphs will show a positive correlation where if one variable increases, so does the other; a negative correlation where if one variable increases, the other decreases, or no significant correlation. A pattern or correlation does not always mean there is cause and effect but it will indicate that changes in one variable have an effect on the other.

When the data has been plotted on the scatter graph, it is useful to draw a line of best fit which is where the main cluster of the data occurs. This line can then be used as the starting point for devising any formulas or hypotheses to link the two

variables, and to make predictions of one value given the value of the other.

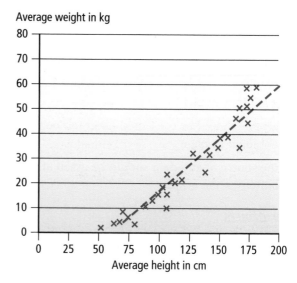

FIGURE 21.12 *A scatter graph*

Pie charts

Pie charts are a way of presenting data that shows each category's share of the total. It involves converting the results into percentages. A simple way of doing this is to divide the component by the total and multiply by 100. Pie charts should be presented on plain paper, not lined or graph.

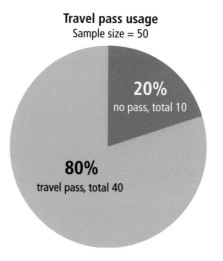

Travel pass usage
Sample size = 50

20%
no pass, total 10

80%
travel pass, total 40

FIGURE 21.13 *A pie chart*

Once you have calculated the percentage, you need to convert this into degrees to construct a pie chart. Imagine you have collected the data shown in Table 21.5 on how students in three classes get to college.

FORM OF TRAVEL	NUMBER OF PEOPLE	%	DEGREE
Bus	10	17	61
Train	4	7	25
Walk	15	25	90
Car	25	43	155
Bike	3	5	18
Moped	2	3	11
	59	100	60

TABLE 21.5 *How students get to college*

To work out the percentage of the different forms of travel, the following calculation is made:

Students that walk $\frac{25}{59} = 0.43 \times 100 = 43\%$

To find the degree for the pie chart, you divide 360 by 100 which equates to degrees per percentage. Then multiply the percentage by this. Therefore:

$$\frac{360}{100} = 3.6 \text{ degrees per percentage}$$

$$43 \times 3.6 = 155 \text{ degrees}$$

Try it out

Using the information in Table 21.5, construct the pie chart.

Carry out a survey of how your own class get to school or college and present it as a pie chart.

When using pie charts, remember to:

* show any calculations
* colour each segment to improve the presentation
* label each section with the percentage it represents
* provide a clear key or legend so the reader knows what each section represents
* give the pie chart a title
* present pie charts on plain paper.

Pictograms

Pictograms can be a very creative way of presenting information in a pictorial format rather than lines or bars. Information is usually presented using lines of pictorial icons. For example, if doing a survey into how people travelled to a health centre for a particular surgery session, you could present the findings by drawing the modes of transport (see Figure 21.14).

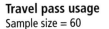

Travel pass usage
Sample size = 60

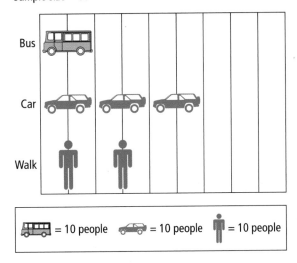

FIGURE 21.14 *The different ways patients travelled to Newtown Surgery on 20 March 2005*

Calculating data – basic statistics

Analysing data using a range of different calculations means you can draw more conclusions. The most common calculations are mean, median and mode. The following data will be used to demonstrate how to calculate each. The ages of the children in an after-school club were recorded as follows:

10, 12, 11, 11, 13, 9, 12, 13, 10, 11, 10, 9, 11, 12, 11, 11, 9.

Mean

The mean is the average of the group of numbers given. To calculate the mean, add all the numbers together, and then divide by the total number in the sample. Therefore, the mean age is represented as:

$$\frac{\text{Sum of all numbers}}{\text{total in sample}} = \text{mean}$$

$$\frac{185}{17} = 10.9$$

The mean age in the after-school club is 10.9.

Mode

The mode is the figure in the data collected that appears the most often. For example:

Age 9	3
Age 10	3
Age 11	6 ◄──── mode value
Age 12	3
Age 13	2

This means that age 11 is the mode value, as it occurs six times. If another figure also scored six, both would be the mode and known as bi-modal. Tri-modal is also possible if there are three numbers which appear the same number of times.

Median

The median is the figure which falls exactly in the middle of a set of numbers. To find the median, set out the fingers in order from lowest to highest.

9
9
9
10
10
10
11
11
11 ◄──── median value
11
11
11
12
12
12
13
13

Age 11 is the one that falls in the middle and is therefore the median value. With an even number of figures, the median will fall between two figures. For example, if there data were as follows:

9
9
10
10
10
11 ◄──── median value
12
12
13
13

The median here falls between two figures, 10 and 11. To find the median, add the two together and divide by 2.

$$10 + 11 = 21$$
$$21 \div 2 = 10.5$$

Therefore the median is 10.5.

Range

The range is the difference between the lowest and highest number in the data set. To find the range, subtract the lowest figure from the highest, in this case $13 - 9 = 4$. The data has a range of 4.

Mean and mode are generally used most as a tool to analyse data as they identify the most common characteristic (mode) and the average (mean). They are useful as they can lead to valid conclusions to be drawn. The median can sometimes be misleading if one or two very high or very low numbers are present in the sample.

Errors when presenting data

Errors can occur when presenting data. They can be made during the calculation process and therefore it is wise to estimate what you think a graph or chart should look like as a way of checking the results. It is also common to find errors in the way statistics are used. It is easy to find correlations but often much more difficult to explain them. When reporting findings, it is important to interpret only what you can see and be sure of. What appears to be a correlation between two factors may be because of another factor unknown to the researcher. Broad and wild predictions are likely to be inaccurate and make the project invalid, so stick to what is clear and obvious. To reduce the chance of error, be as accurate as possible at each stage of the process. Check and recheck each stage from the trial of the different research methods to the calculations from the results. Always be honest about the shortcomings of your work in your evaluation.

Using the computer to calculate and present data

It is common for researchers to use computer programmes such as Microsoft Excel to help them analyse and present data. Computers can calculate the data accurately, provided it has been input correctly. It can also present the data in a number of formats at a touch of a button to allow the researcher to choose the most appropriate. It is extremely quick and the presentation looks very professional. It is worth learning how to use Excel to be able to present your data.

Summary

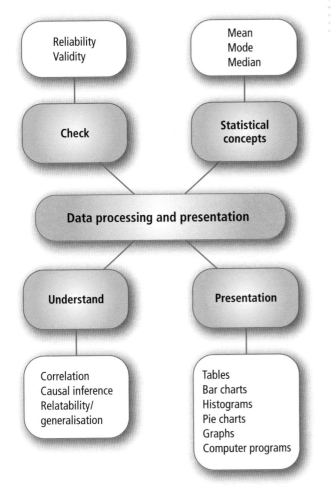

UNIT 21 ASSESSMENT

How you will be assessed

You need to select a topic in health and social care, find out about previously published studies into this area, then design, carry out and report your own empirical study, which should collect numerical data.

You can work in groups of up to three investigating the same topic in order to collect data from a larger sample, but your report must be written and presented on your own. It must be your own work.

Work which does not show independence cannot be awarded high marks.

To gain high marks in this unit you should plan your study carefully, possibly by trying out parts of the procedure beforehand.

You should be familiar with examples of published research, and you should demonstrate a good grasp of scientific method, methodological terminology and the ethics of research.

Your report must be written in the following sections:

Assessment preparation

A Introduction
This should briefly state the aim(s) and the research hypothesis if this is relevant.

B Background
In this section, you need to carry out some secondary research into your chosen topic area. It is likely that you will find that others have carried out research in the area you are going to look at.

It is common for several researchers to have carried out work in the same or similar areas. Repeating research can bring advances in thinking or understanding. It can also highlight new areas which need investigation.

You may be lucky and find a lot of published material on your chosen topic. The key will be to decide what is relevant and of value to your work. It will also be necessary to assess the quality of the information you have found. Just because it is printed does not mean it is accurate or correct. Look at how the information was collected and decide if you feel the material is good.

This section should outline the topic area, relevant theory and previous studies, making clear how it is related to health and well-being, explain the rationale for the study and its relationship (if any) with previous studies (for example, whether it is a modified replication, a study with similar aims but using a different method, etc.).

Referencing
Good referencing will be important in this section. Referencing is useful as it allows the reader to check the source if they wish.

If you are writing other authors' ideas in your own words, you must acknowledge this by giving their name and the date of the publication in which you have read their ideas.

There are a number of different ways to reference; however, the Harvard system is most commonly used (see page 306).

C Method

This section should include the following subsections:

Design
This should state and justify the method of study chosen, state clearly what is to be measured and how.

Materials
This should list any apparatus and measuring instruments used.

Participants
This should briefly describe the sample (indicating size, age range, location and other factors relevant to the study) and should state and justify the sampling method used.

Ethical issues
This should draw the reader's attention to the specific ethical issues raised by the study, for example temporary mild deception or the risk of a participant's embarrassment on performing poorly in some measure of skill.

Procedure
This should be a description of the procedure experienced by the participant in the order in which it happened (not the process by which you planned or designed the study). It should include reference to the initial request, a detailed description of what was done to obtain the data and reference to debriefing.

D Results

This should include a graphical summary of results (such as a table of means, or percentages), and/or appropriate chart(s) properly labelled, and an analysis of the implications of the findings in relation to the aim or hypothesis.

E Discussion

This should include an evaluation of your study from a methodological viewpoint, commenting on the advantages and disadvantages of the method chosen, strengths or weaknesses of the design, sample and measures used, any risks of bias and unforeseen flaws.

Evaluation
Evaluation of the study will form part of the discussion. To evaluate the work, you need to show you appreciate the factors that have affected the effectiveness of the project. As you evaluate, think about each section of the work and comment on any issues which could have affected the validity and reliability of the findings.

Asking yourself questions may help you evaluate effectively. For example:

Planning
Did you plan the project well?
Did you keep to the plan?
How did this affect your work?

Secondary research
Did you use an effective range of research methods?
Were the sources up to date?
Were the sources valid and reliable?
Did you carry out enough secondary research before you designed the primary research?
How did the results for the secondary research help you with the primary research?

Primary research methods

You need to evaluate each primary research method you used. The following questions can be applied to most research methods as a way of starting the evaluative process.

Was this an effective choice of research method for the chosen topic?

Did you plan the method well?

Was the sample used appropriate?

Did the method gain the information you hoped for – if not, why not?

Were the result presented appropriately?

F Appendices

This should include examples of materials used, raw data together with calculations and a reference section, using the conventional form and giving references for all studies and authorities cited in the report.

It is not useful to put in reams and reams of notes, but do include a bibliography of the text books and other sources you have used. You should use the Harvard method of referencing.

The appendices should be set out in an organised manner giving details of the work carried out. Each section of the appendix should be labeled with a letter or number. In general, each section will represent a method of research. Each appendix allows you to show off the full extent of the work you have done in each research method you have used, as you may not draw on all of it for the report.

Referencing and writing the bibliography

There are conventions for writing a bibliography, which should be followed. The Harvard method for writing a bibliography is commonly used. It has the following headings:

Author (surname, initial)

Date

Title

Publisher

Place where published

Generally, the title of the book is written in *italics* or **bold** or <u>underlined</u> to make it stand out.

The date is the published date of the edition you have used and this should be in (brackets).

When using a number of books, they are recorded in the bibliography in alphabetical order according to the author.

Author	Date	Title	Publisher	Place
Apple, J.	(1998)	*Sociology*	Lonlish	London
Davies, A.	(1999)	*Women's roles*	Penguin	New York
Summers, G.	(1997)	*Social Lives*	Lonlish	London

Tassoni, P. and Hucker, K. (1999) *Planning Play and the Early Years* Heinemann Oxford

When you refer to these books in the text of your report, you should simply write 'Apple (1998)' or 'Davies (1999)'. If two authors have written a book, then the referencing is slightly different: 'Tassoni and Hucker (1999)'.

If a text has been written by more than two authors, then the bibliography should list all the names of the authors, but if making reference to it in the text, you only need to use the full list of authors the first time you refer to the text. After that, you can just write the name of the first author followed by *et al* and the date (in brackets). *Et al* means 'and the others' and this form of shorthand saves you time in writing all the names out. Also, long lists of authors names will affect the flow of the text and make it more difficult for the reader.

Davies, L., March, P. and James, T. (1987) *People Talking*   Penguin, London

The first reference in to this work in the text would read Davies, March and James (1987). Subsequent references would read Davies *et al* (1987).

Magazine articles and journals are referenced in a particular way as well. This is not as straightforward as text books, as they are not all the same. Also, a magazine article is likely to be only part of the magazine and therefore, the exact pages must be indicated. For example:

'Bottled water on test' *Good Food* August 2005 page 117

References and further reading

Bell, J. (1999) *Planning your research project,* Open University Press, Buckingham

Green, S. (2000) *Research Methods,* Stanley Thorne, Cheltenham

Hucker, K. (2001) *Research Methods in Health, Care and Early Years* Heinemann, Oxford

Useful websites

www.statistics.gov.uk

www.stats.gla.ac.uk

www.ons.gov.uk
    Office for National Statistics

www.updates.co.uk
    Sociology Update (good source of statistics for social issues)

Answers to Assessment Questions

UNIT 12

1. Shevita's musical skills might be influenced by:

   * genetic inheritance

   * socio-economic factors including a good education in music, sufficient income to pay for private tuition, parental interest

   * the development of a sense of self as a person who plays music.

2. An individual's phenotype is the outcome of the interaction of the person's genotype with the environment that they experience.

3. A low income housing estate might be associated with a risk of increased crime; risk of increased litter, vandalism and graffiti; risk of increased congestion and difficulty with travel; overcrowding.

4. Piaget's demonstration of conservation of volume is being tested.

5. Children using pre-operational logic will say that the amount of water (volume) has changed. Children who have developed concrete logical thinking will understand that the amount of water stays the same – they can 'conserve volume'.

6. Object permanence is the ability to understand that objects exist independently (they are permanent) of the infant's ability to sense – e.g. see, hear or touch – them. Within Piaget's theory children in the sensorimotor period were believed to be unable to conserve objects. Object permanence began in the pre-operational period of development.

7. Decentring is the ability to imagine the thoughts and feelings of other people when they are experiencing different feelings or perceptions. Being able to decentre is the opposite of egocentricity. Within Piaget's theory children in the pre-operational stage of intellectual development were believed to be unable to decentre their assumptions about other people's perceptions.

8. Some limitations of Piaget's developmental theory are that:

   * there is evidence that infants may conserve objects long before the age of one and a half years

   * children may be able to demonstrate conservation of number, mass and volume well before six years of age if problems are put to them in an informal and playful manner

   * there is evidence that very young children can decentre and imagine the perceptions and emotions of other people long before six years of age

   * many adolescents and adults fail to use formal operational thinking in real life. The development and use of formal operational thinking may be strongly influenced by education rather than an outcome of general maturation.

9. Ross is receiving a better outcome (reinforcement) for getting out of his seat than he would if he concentrated on his work. A classroom assistant might try to provide attention and other forms of social reinforcement when Ross has been concentrating on his work. The classroom assistant would try to ensure that 'concentrating' behaviours achieved more reinforcement than disruptive behaviours.

10. Bandura's research suggests that children can learn just by watching events. People can therefore learn from other people's experiences. Bandura's research suggests that people are more likely to imitate behaviour if they pay attention to the behaviour; remember what they have witnessed; if they have the ability to imitate the behaviour and the motivation to imitate the behaviour. Mark may have copied the behaviour because he was motivated to pay attention, remember and act the behaviour out. Mark may have perceived the characters as relevant to his own life. Sarah may not have copied the behaviour because of gender differences. Sarah may have paid less attention, remembered less and not have been motivated to copy the behaviour.

11. In Freudian theory, the Id is unconscious and represents animal instincts. The ego is the decision-making 'self' that enables a person to cope with external reality. The ego has both conscious and unconscious aspects. The superego represents the internalised value system of one's opposite sex parent.

12. Tom is addressing his need for self-actualisation. His interest in making wooden furniture may suggest that he has engaged the aesthetic and cognitive aspects of self actualisation. The four deficit needs of physical, safety, belonging and self-esteem all have to be successfully met in a person's development before becoming needs associated with self-actualisation can be addressed. Maslow's later work suggested that cognitive and aesthetic needs were potential steps in the process of self-actualisation.

13. Short-term effects of separation may include protests and anger, depression and sadness, and detachment from the mother. Longer term effects may involve separation anxiety resulting in a personality that is vulnerable to loss. Separation in infancy might result in people who are possessive towards their partner in later life, or people who cannot commit themselves to an intimate relationship because of the fear of separation.

14. Monotropic attachment is the theory that an infant will seek to make only one main attachment to his or her principal carer. Usually this principal carer will be the child's mother. Michael Rutter quotes research that many children make multiple attachments and one study where one third of children made their principal attachment to the father rather than to the mother.

UNIT 13

1. Wellness can be viewed as our approach to personal health that emphasises individual responsibility for well-being through the practice of health-promoting lifestyle behaviours. These include regular physical activity, a healthy diet, and the maintenance of good emotional and spiritual health. There are strong interactions between the different components of wellness; none of these work in isolation. Total wellness is achieved by balancing physical, social, emotional and spiritual health.

2. Any benefits identified under the following headings providing some explanation of each benefit identified.

   * physical

   * social

   * psychological

   * economic

   * environmental.

3. It is essential that health and lifestyle screening takes place prior to fitness testing and prior to exercise prescription, preferably by a medical or fitness practitioner. with all who are contemplating starting an exercise programme. Health and lifestyle screening is usually carried out in the form of an interview or questionnaire. Comprehensive lifestyle and pre-exercise screening will help to identify medical conditions that may prevent the participant from exercising safely. It will also highlight the participant's objectives and ensure that the exercise prescription fulfils their needs.

4. One mark for each of the following and one mark for providing some explanation of relative merits of each for application to the sedentary population.

   * skinfold thickness

   * underwater or hydrostatic weighing

   * body impedance analysis

   * near infrared interactence

   * body plethysmography.

5. VO_2 max is a measure of the endurance capacity of the cardiorespiratory system and exercising skeletal muscles.

6. Rockport walk test; Cooper's 1.5 mile run; three minute step test.

7.

   * warm-up and warm-down

   * clothing and footwear should be appropriate for the specific activity or exercise to be undertaken. This will minimise the risk of injury or illness, help the participant perform better and facilitate the enjoyment of the activity or exercise.

   * adequate hydration should be maintained by drinking plenty of fluids before, during and after the activity or exercise. Exact amounts will depend on factors such as the length of the activity or exercise, temperature and humidity.

   * interactions between medication and exercise should be monitored carefully, such as medications to control diabetes.

   * if the exercise requires the use of equipment this should be only used in the appropriate manner for which it was designed and be well maintained.

8. Enjoyment and smart goal setting

Specific	–	to wants or needs
Measurable	–	fitness test
Agreed	–	and recorded
Realistic	–	achievable
Time framed	–	to keep you on track

9. Frequency of exercise refers to the number of times, usually expressed in times per week, that the exercise is to be undertaken.

   Intensity of exercise refers to how hard, or the amount of stress or overload that is to be applied.

   Time (duration) of exercise refers to how long the activity is to be carried out.

   Type of exercise refers to the mode of exercise performed.

   Adherence to the programme should produce the desired adaptations in response to the prescribed training programme.

10. To achieve a higher level of fitness it is necessary to stress the body systems and place them in a state of ***overload*** a point that reaches above and beyond that which is usually achieved. If this greater level is not achieved adaptation will not occur.

11. Three of:

    * long, slow distance training

    * interval training

* varied pace or fartlek training

* circuit training

* cross training.

12. Three of:

* improved shape and tone

* improved posture

* improved co-ordination

* increased metabolic rate.

13. Any risk factor identified under the following headings providing some explanation of how a programme of regular physical activity and exercise can benefit each risk factor identified:

* raised blood cholesterol

* raised blood pressure

* cigarette smoking

* inactivity

* obesity

* diabetes.

14. Stress can be considered a physiological and mental response to things in our environment that make us feel uncomfortable. Chronic stress is thought to lower our resistance to disease and increase our risk of emotional disorders. Although high-intensity, prolonged exercise can be seen to impose physical and mental stress on the body, there is evidence to suggest that low-to moderate-intensity physical activity and exercise can reduce some types of stress. Those activities proposed to have a beneficial effect include aerobic activities such as walking, swimming and cycling, but other activities focused on relaxation such as tai-chi, pilates and yoga are also beneficial.

15. To gain health benefits the Department of Health recommends us to do at least 30 minutes of moderate exercise on five, if not all days of the week. This 30 minute a day recommendation should probably be viewed as the minimum required to gain health benefits, but the good news is it does not have to be achieved in a single bout. Several short bursts of activity can count towards the total. This approach may make it easier for some individuals to meet their daily physical activity target. Greater benefits will be gained from increasing the amount to 40–60 minutes each day, especially for those that are at risk of weight gain. The same recommendations apply to older people dependent on ability, but children are encouraged to achieve at least one hour every day of moderate-intensity activity. By moderate this means that you must get a little warmer and slightly out of breath. The more vigorous the activity the greater the gains in terms of cardiovascular health. In terms of type, it can be anything that raises your energy expenditure above resting level, enough to expend about 200 calories, and bring about the symptoms already described, for example brisk walking, swimming, cycling, jogging, dancing, or heavy housework or gardening.

16. Reasons include:

* increased fitness and stamina

* increased muscle tone, strength and shape

* decreased body fat

* protection from osteoporosis

* decreased cardiovascular risk

* improved immune system

* increased psychological well-being

* increased social interaction.

17. Any five barriers identified under the following headings providing some explanation of each barrier identified:

* money and finances

* time

* location and environment

* transport

* responsibilities including family and work commitments

* attitude and motivation

* religious beliefs and practices

* peer pressure

* illness, disease or disability

* education

* current skill and fitness level.

18. Monitoring progress in attaining and maintaining physical fitness is a vital factor in providing motivation to stick to an exercise regime. Progress can be monitored by keeping training logs or diaries which record the distance walked or run, or the amount of weight lifted for example. Another means of monitoring fitness progress is by fitness testing. Fitness testing can provide very strong positive feedback when fitness levels are improving, but may be demotivating when they are not.

19. The warm-up should be included at the beginning of **all** exercise programmes to achieve the following objectives:

* prepare the body for exercise

* maximise performance

* prevent injury.

The warm-down should be included at the end of **all** exercise programmes to achieve the following objectives:

* return the body to the pre-exercise state

* relax the body and reduce tension

* realign muscle fibres and prevent muscle soreness and injury

* promote circulation and motor fitness.

20. Since the early 1990s many areas in the UK have operated 'exercise on prescription', also known as GP referral schemes. This is where a medical practitioner may refer an individual for exercise programming as a way to speed rehabilitation after illness and hopefully encourage the exercise habit. GP referral schemes work as partnerships between medical practitioners, including GP's practice nurses and other health care professionals, with local authority or private sector fitness facilities. The types of patient that might be referred for exercise on prescription include those with high blood pressure, obesity,

depression and low back pain. Within such a scheme the patient would undergo a thorough health, fitness and lifestyle screening. If they were deemed to be low risk their physical activity and exercise programme would reflect this in terms of minimal supervision. Those deemed to be high risk would require greater supervision while carrying out their physical activity and exercise programme.

UNIT 15

1a. Alzheimer's (accept dementia)

b. Any of the following are acceptable:

* GP
* community nurse
* health visitor
* social worker
* day unit manager.

c. The 1995 Carers (Recognition and Services) Act entitles Selina to an assessment of her own needs.

Organisations such as Carers UK provide advice, help and support to carers. Help is also available from dedicated organisations such as the Alzheimer's Society.

d. People with Alzheimer's have a great need for physical and emotional comfort. They need to experience attachment in the form of meaningful relationships. They also need to feel included by the people they relate to. Reinforcement of a sense of personal identity is also important.

2a. Angela's employer might make 'reasonable adjustments' with respect to access to the building and the office. These might include ramps, lifts, electronically-activated doors. An ergonomically designed workstation would allow Angela to operate IT and telephone equipment in comfort. Voice-activated software would allow her to continue to use the computer when her hands and arms became tired. Provision for flexible working hours would allow Angela to work during the hours that she is most productive.

b. Angela may encounter attitudes ranging from indifference to over-protectiveness. Her line manager has a key role to play, and the attitude of her colleagues is also critical. If her line manager is unsympathetic, Angela may be faced with unrealistic demands or time-schedules; conversely, if the manager is over-protective, she may be given very boring, routine tasks that do not use her skills to the full.

Colleagues can also help or hinder Angela's enjoyment of her working life, either by failing to respond to her needs, or by trying to protect her from 'difficult' situations or problems. She may also be excluded from team decision-making.

Angela may also experience some unhelpful attitudes from the council's service users that she works with. This problem may not be so evident during telephone calls, when Angela's disability is not evident; however, service users who meet with her face-to-face may be shocked or uncomfortable to find that they are being advised by a person with a disability. They may be unused to the idea that disabled people can make excellent employees, with skills, knowledge and experience to match those of non-disabled workers. Non-disabled people tend to stereotype disabled people as being helpless and dependent, and these stereotypes are often a very real barrier to the inclusion of disabled people into society.

3a. People with Down's syndrome have an extra copy of chromosome 21. There are three variants. The extra chromosome may come from either the father or the mother.

b. Any of the following are acceptable: distinctive physical characteristics such as reduced muscle tone, flat facial profile, distinctive eyes, small mouth and protruding tongue, 'sandal gap' between toes, short fingers, broad palms, single palm crease, below average birth weight and length; associated developmental problems, e.g. learning difficulties, reaching key 'milestones' later than other people.

c. Screening for Down's syndrome can be done prenatally. Tests include blood test, ultrasound, chorionic villus sampling and amniocentesis. After birth, testing is by blood test, to produce a karyotype analysis of chromosomes.

Parents whose unborn baby is suspected to have Down's syndrome may be given counselling to help them decide whether or not to proceed with the pregnancy. However, this raises some ethical questions about the right to life of the foetus, and whether or not abortion is in reality a form of killing and therefore unethical. There is also the risk that the parents may experience emotional harm, whichever decision they make. People with Down's syndrome may feel that this approach devalues them as human beings, and that aborting a foetus because it has Down's syndrome is an extreme form of discrimination against people with disability conditions.

d. About 30 years ago, the medical model of disability was dominant. This model sees disability as a 'problem'; people with physical and cognitive impairments cannot function in society like everyone else because they are not 'normal'.

In contrast, the social model of disability says that it is society's attitude that truly disables a person. The inevitable consequence of this model is that society should make every effort to regard disabled people as equal to everyone else; this should be reflected in law, and in practical day-to-day life.

Developments such as the DDA 1995 and DDA 2005, the Valuing People initiative, and the move to empower all disabled people to speak for themselves and to take part in decisions that affect them, are a consequence of this change in attitude.

However, there is still a long way to go before all barriers to inclusion are removed for disabled people.

4a. Any two of the following are acceptable:

Consultant: will assess Lilian's state of health and medical condition.

Physiotherapist: will assess Lilian's ability to move around, both indoors and out, and suggest aids to mobility that she might need. Ability to perform personal care tasks may also be assessed.

Occupational therapist: will assess Lilian's ability to perform tasks such as cooking, washing, dressing.

Social worker: will assess Lilian's needs at home, and should take an all-round view of her physical, intellectual, emotional and social needs. The social worker may be from a specialist Older Person's Team.

b. Any of the following are acceptable:

Provision of daily hot meal (from a private supplier or council facility); daily domiciliary help to assist with dressing, personal tasks, cleaning etc.; regular visits from Health Visitor or Community Nurse; support to Lilian's daughters to see if they need any assistance in caring for their mother.

c. If Lilian remains in her own home, she retains her independence and can continue to run her life as she wishes, without the constraints that come with living in residential care. She can see friends and family when she wishes, and can retain aspects of her existing social life. Many of the necessary psychological lifefactors such as choice, autonomy, dignity and privacy are assured.

d. If Lilian goes into residential care, many of her physical needs will be met. There will be regular and well-balanced meals, physical comfort and safety, assistance with personal tasks such as bathing and dressing. There should also be provision for exercise, and regular intellectual stimulation. If she requires regular medication, qualified staff will be on hand to administer this.

Glossary

A

accommodation a process which happens when existing knowledge is changed to fit with new learning. Alternatively, something that happens when a child takes in new information which causes a change to an existing schema.

acetylcholine (ACN) a common neurotransmitter.

adaptation a term normally reserved for the process of making significant structural alterations to buildings, or mechanical alterations to cars, normally to make them more user-friendly to people with disabilities.

adrenaline a hormone with similar effects to the sympathetic nervous systems that boosts these effects.

advocate a person who speaks on the behalf of someone else who is unable to voice their views because of learning difficulties, mental health problems or other reasons. The advocate can be a professional, a volunteer or a relative.

aerobic energy processes that take place in the presence of oxygen.

aid any device used to assist a disabled person with daily life, work, personal tasks, etc.

amoeba a microscopic single-celled organism capable of changing shape.

anaerobic energy processes that take place in the absence of oxygen.

angina pain in the chest resulting from inadequate blood supply to the heart.

antibodies a blood protein induced in response to an antigen (a foreign substance).

antigens a foreign substance that causes an immune response in the body.

aortic body clusters of chemoreceptors located on the arch of the aorta.

arteriosclerosis hardening of the arterial walls associated with ageing.

assessment a formal method of identifying the health and social care needs of a person in order to set up a care plan.

assimilation changing our understanding of an issue in the light of new knowledge; taking in and understanding new information.

assistive technology expertise which makes possible the provision of practical support to disabled people using a wide range of technologies, including electronic and computerised equipment.

associative play interacting and cooperating with others.

asthma difficulty in breathing resulting from respiratory disease.

atherosclerosis the formation of plaque on the artery wall restricting blood flow.

attachment the emotional process that results in a loving relationship between people. John Bowlby emphasised the importance of attachment during the early years of a child's development.

attitude a mental pattern or posture which can influence thinking, emotions or behaviour.

autonomic nervous system a system of nerves associated with automatic control of internal organs.

axilla technical term for the armpit.

B

bioelectrical impedance analysis a method of body composition assessment using electrical resistance.

body composition the ratio of lean body mass to fat mass in an individual.

body image the image or impression an individual has of their own body.

body mass index an index of body fatness used as a measure of obesity.

body plethysmography a method of body composition assessment using air displacement.

bonding the emotional tie between an infant and his or her mother.

bronchitis inflammation of the bronchial tubes of the lungs.

C

calibration the determining, adjustment or marking of scale graduations.

care plan a formal document that sets out everything that needs to be done to meet someone's needs. This will include the objectives or goals of the plan, together with the services that will be provided to meet these objectives.

care provider any organisation that delivers a service e.g. a home meals delivery company, an NHS Trust, a voluntary organisation.

care purchaser the organisation that controls the funding to buy care – usually the local authority or the PCT.

carer anyone who looks after someone who is ill, disabled, or otherwise unable to look after him or herself. The term usually refers to someone who provides informal (unpaid) care, rather than to a paid worker.

carotid body clusters of chemoreceptors located on the fork of the carotid bodies.

central nervous system (CNS) the brain and the spinal cord.

charities non-profit making organisations set up to support different groups, and they may also lobby on behalf of certain groups.

chemoreceptor a sensory part that responds to a chemical, molecule etc.

cholesterol a fat-like substance implicated in the development of heart disease.

chronic a term used to describe a condition that persists over a long period of time.

Clinical Governance action taken by NHS trusts to ensure that clinical standards are maintained in hospitals and in the community.

code of conduct professional code of behaviour and practice drawn up by a professional body in order to set standards, e.g. General Medical Council, the Nursing and Midwifery Council.

cognition a term which covers the mental processes involved in understanding and knowing.

cognitive development the development of understanding and concepts.

Commission for Social Care Inspection (CSCI) a statutory body set up in 2004 to register and inspect all social care organisations.

concrete operations the third stage of intellectual development In Piaget's theory. At this stage, individuals can solve logical problems, provided they can see or sense the objects with which they are working. At this stage, children cannot cope with abstract problems.

conservation no matter what shape something is made into, unless it is added to or something is taken away, the amount remains the same. The ability to understand the logical principles involved in the way number, volume, mass and objects work.

co-operative play playing with others.

coronary heart disease a degenerative disorder of the heart primarily caused by atherosclerosis.

critical period/sensitive period John Bowlby believed there was a sensitive period between six months of age and three years of age when infant humans needed to form an attachment. This 'sensitive period' might be similar to the 'critical period' identified in animal studies.

D

decentring involves the ability to imagine the thoughts and feelings of other people, when they are different from the thoughts and feelings that you are currently experiencing.

defence mechanisms in Freudian theory ego defence mechanisms are ways in which people distort their understanding and memory in order to protect their ego.

deficit needs the physiological needs, safety needs, belonging needs and self-esteem needs that represent the four deficit needs described in Maslow's hierarchy of need.

diabetes a disorder of carbohydrate metabolism as a result of a lack of or insufficient production of insulin resulting in high blood glucose levels.

diastole, diastolic state of relaxation of cardiac muscle.

diet a term to describe the usual eating habits and food consumption of an individual.

diffusion passage of molecules (of gases or liquids) from a high concentration to a low concentration.

diplegia paralysis in both legs.

district nurse a qualified nurse who works closely with the GP and is employed by the PCT.

dysfunction impairment of function.

E

Early Learning Goals outcomes required in the foundation stage by the age of five.

ego a term used in psychodynamic theory to describe the decision-making component of the mind. Ego has some similarity with the notion of 'self' used in other perspectives.

elaborate code the language code of wider society.

eligibility criteria the rules that explain a person's entitlement to receive services. The greater a person's needs and risks to their independence, the greater is that person's entitlement to receive services.

emotional development the development of emotions and how to control these.

empathy an attitude of mind that involves recognising someone's needs, whilst at the same time respecting the ways in which a person may wish to have those needs met. This attitude is empowering rather than disempowering.

emphysema lung disease that causes breathlessness.

empowerment giving power to others.

enactive thinking involves being able to remember and perform physical actions.

endocrine describing a gland that secretes hormones into the blood.

equilibration something that occurs when all pieces of information fit into the schemata a child has developed.

ethics study of the moral value of human conduct.

evaluation to evaluate something is to assess it, in particular its worth, value or importance.

Excellence Clusters provide additional support for children in deprived areas and help them overcome these associated barriers to learning and opportunities.

experiential learning learning by doing.

F

facilitating helping and encouraging children.

fastlek a method of training in athletics that mixes fast and slow work.

fatigue a generalised or specific feeling of tiredness.

fine motor skills smaller, precise skills such as drawing, cutting, painting or colouring.

fixation in Freudian theory fixation is when life energy (called libido) remains attached to an early stage of development. Life energy can also become fixated on objects and people in a person's life.

formal operations the fourth stage in Piaget's theory of intellectual development. People with formal logical operations have the ability to solve abstract problems.

Foundation Stage Profile the statutory assessment for children in the final year of the foundation stage.

Foundation stage the section for the national curriculum covering ages 3–5.

G
genes units which contain the information and instructions that control the development of living organisms.

genetic code a set to of instructions passed on from one generation to another for building a living organism.

genotype the type of genetic pattern that an individual inherits. Your genotype will influence issues such as your height hair and eye colour and so on.

governance the way organisations in health and care ensure the quality and safety of the services they provide.

gross motor skills larger muscle movements and control such as running, throwing, hopping and skipping.

H
health care assistant a health worker who is not a registered nurse but is working towards, or has achieved, either a Level 2 or Level 3 NVQ award. HCAs work in a variety of settings in hospital and in the community.

Healthcare Commission an organisation set up in 2004 to encourage and monitor improvement in public health and health care in England and Wales.

health visitor a registered nurse with additional training who works in the community with children under eight years of age.

healthy eating a term used to describe the pursuit of a balanced diet to support health and reduce the risks of chronic disease.

hemiplegia paralysis of one side of the body.

high density lipoprotein a protein-lipid complex found in the blood that transports fats.

homeostasis process of maintaining the constancy of the internal environment around cells despite external changes.

hydrocephalus an accumulation of cerebrospinal fluid around the brain.

hypertension high blood pressure.

hypotension low blood pressure.

hypertrophy enlargement of an organ through an increase in the size of its cells.

I
iconic means picture, remembering events in pictures.

id a term used in psychodynamic theory to describe the 'powerhouse' of drive energy that motivates the behaviour. Instinctive drives develop from the Id.

identity the understanding of self which an individual needs to develop in order to cope with life in modern society.

imitation learning learning to imitate or copy the behaviour of others.

immunisation stimulation of the body to create antibodies to a disease, by introducing a weak or inactivated version of the disease organism.

income money that an individual or household gets from work, investments or other sources

Independent Complaints Advocacy Service (ICAS) a statutory service offering free, impartial and independent support to people who wish to complain about their hospital care or treatment. They are situated in all areas of the UK.

independent sector agencies that provide health and social care independently from statutory providers. They could be private or voluntary agencies.

in-group a social group which an individual identifies with. A group that individual is 'in with'.

insulin the hormone produced by the pancreas important in the control of carbohydrate metabolism.

internal working model in Bowlby's theory, an internalised set of assumptions about the way in which we relate to other people. This internal working model develops from our attachments to other people from early years onwards.

intussusception telescoping of the bowel.

K
key worker/lead professional a named person who ensures that the care plan is followed and care is given to the user. In health care this would be a named nurse.

kilogram a unit of mass from the metric system equivalent to 2.2 pounds.

L
labelling classifying someone in a fixed way that refers only to one aspect of that person, e.g. physical appearance, ethnicity, disability, etc.

LAD language acquisition device something humans are born with to enable them to learn language.

language development the development of the way we communicate.

lean body mass body weight minus body fat primarily composed of muscle, bone and other non-fat tissues.

low density lipoprotein a protein-lipid complex found in the blood that transports fats.

M
maturation the process of physical growth.

means testing assessing the income of a person and deciding how much they will pay for a service provided by social services.

medical model of disability a scientific view of health and body functioning; this view sees disability as a 'problem' because a disabled person is prevented from doing everything a non-disabled person can do. Disabled people are thus not 'normal'.

mixed economy of care the notion that care can be provided by a range of different service providers, e.g. statutory agencies, private and voluntary organisations, informal carers.

modelling imitation of behaviour. People often imitate or copy others without direct reinforcement taking place.

monitoring to monitor something is to make regular checks on progress.

monoplegia paralysis of one leg.

monotropic attachment John Bowlby believed that every infant needed to attach to, or bond with just one principle caregiver. Usually this would be the child's mother.

MRSA a kind of antibiotic–resistant bacteria.

multi-disciplinary teams teams of professionals who are qualified in different disciplines who work together in the community or in hospital.

multi-disciplinary working the practice whereby professionals from different disciplines work together to provide care to individuals and/or groups.

N
National Curriculum the curriculum set out by the government which all state schools must follow.

National Patients' Survey annual surveys that take place every year to monitor patient's satisfaction with the services they receive.

National Service Frameworks (NSFs) national standards in certain conditions, or focussing on particular age groups that have been set by government in order to improve standards.

nature influences on development that are biological.

near infrared interactance a method of body composition assessment using infrared technology.

negative energy balance a situation where energy output exceeds energy input and weight is lost.

neonatal relating to newly born infants.

neurological pertaining to the body's nervous system.

neurotransmitter chemical substance that pours into a synapse to enable nerve impulses to progress onwards.

NHS national staff survey an annual survey of staff working in the NHS.

NHS trusts NHS hospitals and Primary Care Trusts (PCTs) which are independent bodies and employ staff to deliver health care.

noradrenaline hormone that acts as a neurotransmitter at the postganglionic synapse of the sympathetic nervous system and helps to maintain blood pressure.

norms patterns of behaviour that are expected to be followed by the members of a particular society or group.

nurture influences on development that are socially learned or as effect of the environment.

O

object permanence the understanding that objects exist whether they can be seen or not.

observational learning learning by watching.

occupational therapist a therapist working in health or social care who assists people to be more independent through the use of aids and appliance.

OFSTED (the Office for Standards in Education) a statutory body set up in 1993 to monitor all educational provision. It also monitors child minding and out of school provision for children up to the age of eight.

operant conditioning conditioning caused by reinforcing outcomes which cause a behaviour to become strengthened.

out-group a social group which is the opposite of an 'in-group'. A group an individual is not a member of; which the individual may feel hostile towards.

overload a state in which the body is pushed to achieve a high level of fitness.

P

palpitations quick, irregular heartbeats.

parallel play playing alongside another child.

parasympathetic nervous system a branch of the autonomic nervous system associated with peace and contentment.

Patient Advice and Liaison Service (PALS) departments within every NHS trust that advise patients on the services and they may deal with queries and complaints.

peak flow maximum speed of a forced expiration.

Person Centred Care care that places the person at the centre of decision-making activities, thereby valuing the individual 'personhood' of service users.

phenotype an individual's phenotype is the outcome of the interaction of the person's genotype with the environment that they experience.

physical development the development of fine and gross motor skills.

play a child's 'work'.

positive energy balance a situation where energy input exceeds energy output and weight is gained.

PPI forums Patient and public involvement forums which replaced CHCs (Community Health Councils) in 2004. They are patients and members of the public who have a special interest in the NHS. They are attached to PCTs and hospital trusts and they monitor services and represent the public.

pre-operational the second stage of Piaget's theory of intellectual development, a pre-logical period when children cannot reason logically.

Primary Care Trusts (PCTs) bodies set up after 1999 to commission services from hospitals and other agencies to deliver care.

primary care health care that takes place in the community.

primary health care team members of the health care team that are usually based at a health centre or surgery, including practice nurses, health visitors and GPs.

primary research where you collect your own original data using one of the primary research techniques.

psychodynamic a psychological perspective which interprets human behaviour in terms of a theory of the dynamics of the mind.

Q
quadriplegia (see also tetraplegia) paralysis of all four limbs.

R
reflection accommodating ideas and concepts by thinking about them; the act of thinking about something objectively.

registration the process through which the CSCI, OFSTED, and other bodies assesses whether institutions offering services are suitable to do so.

regression in Freudian theory regression is when a person's behaviour can be explained in terms

of a return to behaviours associated with the first three psychosexual stages.

reinforcement learning through their actions being reinforced either positively or negatively.

reinforcer anything that causes behaviour to be repeated.

restricted code a limited vocabulary which means general communication is difficult.

risk assessment procedure that assesses the risks in the environment to the service user (unsafe homes). It can also be applied to people with mental health problems when a doctor will decide whether they are a risk to themselves or to others.

S
S–A node *see* sino-atrial node.

schema an organised pattern of thought.

schemata patterns of behaviour or actions.

school nurse registered nurses who visit schools and advise on health issues. They may also be attached to family planning clinic for young people.

scoliosis curvature of the spine.

secondary research matured that has already been written on the topic you are researching.

self-actualisation an important need identified by Maslow which explains that individuals need to fulfil their potential. Most people spend their life focused on deficit needs and do not achieve self actualisation.

self-advocacy the service user is encouraged to speak on their own behalf about the services they need.

sensorimotor the first stage in Piaget's theory of intellectual development. Infants learn to co-ordinate their muscle or motor movements in this stage.

sino–atrial node the pacemaker of the heart, sets the heart rate by sending periodic waves of excitation over the heart.

skinfold thickness a method of body composition assessment using skinfolds.

social class the status given to different types of occupation or work.

social development learning the norms and values of society.

social exclusion being excluded from opportunity – people with fewer life chances to become economically prosperous than the majority of people.

social impact theory we respond to the 'social impact' of the people that surround us. Our behaviour is strongly influenced by our perception of others. We go with the crowd and seek to fit in with the social norms of others.

social learning theory learning by observing and imitating the behaviour of others.

social model of disability this view stresses that it is the attitude of society that disables people, preventing or limiting disabled people from doing what they want to.

social role a set of expectations which guide an individual's behaviour in specific circumstances.

socialisation the process by which we learn the norms, values and behaviour that makes us a member of a particular group.

solitary play playing alone.

somatic nervous system nervous control of the body (wall) but not including the internal organs.

spectator play watching others play.

speech and language therapist a professional who helps adults and children with communication problems and also with swallowing difficulties.

sphygmomanometer device for measuring blood pressure.

spirometer (spirometry) an instrument for measuring lung volumes.

statemented child a child who has had a statement of special educational needs made about him or her.

statementing the process of making an assessment of special educational needs for a child, under the provisions of legislation.

statutory sector services provided by the state either directly or indirectly. The statutory sector includes services provided by the NHS and by the local council.

stereotyping a fixed way of thinking that involves generalisations about an issue or a group of people (e.g. all older people like to sit around all day, etc.).

structured tasks very directed activities.

Sure Start Centres a programme set up by national government to improve life chances for children and families in deprived areas.

Sure Start a government programme which aims to achieve better outcomes for parents, children and communities.

symbolic thinking involves the use of language and other symbolic systems.

sympathetic nervous system a branch of the autonomic system associated with fear, stress and muscular activity.

synapse a minute gap between the end of one neurone and the next or muscle/gland.

systole, systolic associated with the contraction phase of cardiac muscle.

T

tetraplegia (*see also* quadriplegia) paralysis of all four limbs.

thalidomide a drug which causes malformation of a foetus if taken by a pregnant woman.

tidal volume the volume of breath entering and leaving the lungs in one respiration.

topical treatment a treatment that is applied to the body as the site of the problem, e.g. as a cream or gel.

U

unconscious mind within psychodynamic theory the unconscious mind contains drives and memories that influence our behaviour. An individual is not conscious of these influences on his or her behaviour.

underwater weighing also referred to as hydrostatic weighing a method of body composition assessment using water displacement.

V

vaccination the procedure by which a dead or weakened version of a disease organism is injected into a person, to challenge the immune system to produce antibodies to fight that particular disease.

verbal instruction learning from being told.

vital capacity the maximum volume of air that can be expelled after a maximum inspiration.

VO_2 max the maximum amount of oxygen used in one minute per kilogram of bodyweight.

voluntary sector organisations that provide services to bridge gaps in statutory provision. These organisations sometimes provide services without charge. They are non-profit-making organisations.

voluntary services services that are independent of the statutory sector and provide a range of services commissioned by local councils, PCTs and Health Trusts. They also represent the interests of certain sections of the community and lobby government on their behalf (e.g. Age Concern, Mencap, National Children's Home).

W

waist circumference a measure of obesity using the circumference of the waist at its most narrow point.

Index

Note: Page numbers in *italics* refer to figures and tables. Page numbers in **bold** are key concepts.

1RM (1 repetition maximum) **129**
3-minute step test 96

A

A-V (atrio-ventricular) node 264
abstract thinking **64**
access
  for disabled people 175–7
  to early years education 195–6
active transport **103**
adaptations, for disabled people **180–2**
adrenaline 249, 250
advocacy **26**
aerobic, definition of **100**
aerobic fitness 94–7
  training techniques for 127–8
aerobic system responses 99
Age Concern 10–11
Agenda for Change (NHS, 2004) 15
aids, for disabled people **180–2**
Ainsworth, Mary, attachment theory 82–3
Allied Health Professionals **4**
Alzheimer's disease (AD) 145–7
anaerobic **100**
anti-discrimination policies 182–5, 201–2
anti-social behaviour 71–2
antibodies 262
arteries 258, 260–1
arteriosclerosis 233
arthritis 158–60
assessment
  care management process 170–2
  disability needs 169–70
  early years education 218–22
  of needs 23–9
  SEN children 170
assistive technology **180–2**
associative learning 206
attachment theories 81–4
attitudes **295**
autonomic nervous system 249,
    263–4, 265
axilla (armpit), body temperature 236

B

backward chaining 69
Bandura, Albert, social learning theory 71–5, 208
becoming needs **85**
behaviour, learning by imitation 72–5, 200, 207–8
beliefs **295**
Berko, Jean, language theorist 215
Best Treatments (website) 144, 159
BIA *see* body impedance analysis
blood cells, type and function 261–2
blood pressure measurements 238–40
blood vessels 260–1
BMI *see* body mass index
body composition 97–8
  assessing 107–10
body impedance analysis (BIA) 109
body mass index (BMI) 107
body plethysmography 109
body temperature
  maintenance of 245–8
  measurement of 235–8
body weight, measuring 106–7
bonding, theories of 81, 83–4
Bowlby, John, attachment theory 81–2
brain functioning 141–3, 250–1, 266–7
breathing *see* respiration
Brown, Roger, language development 214
Bruner, Jerome, cognitive development 212–13

C

CAMs *see* complementary therapies
cancer, exercise reducing risk of 123
carbon dioxide levels 250–2
cardiac cycle 262–4
cardiac output **115**, 263
cardiovascular system
  arteries and veins 260–1
  blood cells 261–2
  cardiac cycle 262–4
  function of 262–3
  heart 258–60
  see also heart rate
care management 170–2

care planning 23–5, 169–74
  care plans **169**
  health care 27–8
  social services 25–7
care providers & purchasers **183**
carers **164–5,** 167
Carers (Recognition & Services) Act (1995) 183
central nervous system (CNS) 141–3, **156,** 264–7
cerebral palsy (CP) 147–9
chaining, teaching complex behaviours 68
chemoreceptors 251–2
children
  assessment of needs 28–9
  attachment types 83
  development 193–7
  effect of poverty on 53
  encouraging play 202–4
  interaction with others 58
  language acquisition 69–70
  maturation of 193–4
  Piaget's stages of development 60–4, 209–11
  quality in early years' services 35–6
  with special educational needs (SEN) 170
  testing, pressures of 223–4
  ways of learning *200*
  see also early years education
Children Act (1989) 201
Children Act (2004) 31
Chomsky, Noam, language theorist 214–15
circuit training 128
closed questions 38–9, 287
cognitive development
  Bandura's theory 72–5
  Bruner's theories 212
  Piaget's theories 59–66, **208–11**
  through play 199
  Skinner's theories 66–70
  social learning theories 70–2
  Vygotsky's theories 211–12
Commission for Social Care Inspection
  (CSCI) 35
commissioners of services **12**
Common Assessment Process (CAP)
  for children 28–9
community care/services *166–7,* 183
complaints, NHS patients 34
complementary therapies (CAMs) **146,** 156, 157–8
concrete operational stage, child
  development 63–4, 211
conditions of employment 17–18
confidentiality
  interviews 42
  observations 283
  in research 296–7

conservation, of number/volume/weight 62, 63,
  65, **210**
control mechanisms 245–53
Cooper's 1.5-mile run test 95–6
coronary heart disease (CHD) 121–2
crime, link to poverty 53, 55
critical period, attachment theory **81**
cross training 128
cultural issues
  access to health services 56–7
  recruitment of overseas staff 6
cystic fibrosis (CF) 149–51

D

data collection surveys 289–91
data presentation 298–303
day care provision 35–6
decentring **62–3,** 65
deception 296
defence mechanisms 79–80
deficit needs **84–5**
demand characteristics **277**
demographics and job availability 15
Desirable Learning Outcomes 218
diabetes, link to obesity 122–3
diastolic blood pressure 238
diffusion **256**
diplegia **149**
disability
  access issues 175–7
  assessment of needs 169–70
  assistive technology **180–2**
  barriers 174–9
  care management 170–2
  care provision *168*
  causes of 141–3
  children with SEN 170
  conditions 144–61
  definitions of 139
  detection/prevention 162–3
  discrimination 177–9
  employment issues 175
  financial provision *167*
  legislation 140, 182–6
  models of 139–40
  support services 164, *165*
  treatment decisions 144–5
Disability Discrimination Act (1995 & 2005) 140,
  176, 183–4
Disabled Persons Act (1986) 169, 183
discrimination 177–9, 201–2
double-blind techniques, experiments 277
Down's syndrome (DS) 151–4
Duchenne muscular dystrophy (DMD) 154–6
dynamic strength **97**

E

Early Learning Goals 219–20
  assessment of learning 221
  planning 220–1
early years education
  assessment 218–22
  developmental stages 201
  factors affecting 192–7
  influential theorists 215–17
  issues of contention 223–5
  jobs in 10
  play experiences **197–8**
  role of adults in 198–9, 202–4, 211–12
  see also education
economic factors
  effect on early education 196–7
  effect on job availability 15
education
  barriers to 174–5
  by ability group 223
  family influences 195
  impact of poverty 55–6
  importance of play 198
  planning the curriculum 220–1
  SEN children 170
  Sure Start 8–9
  see also early years education
Education Act (1996) 170
Education Act (2002) 219
egg-screening 162, 163
ego defence mechanisms **79–80**
egocentricity **62–3**
eligibility criteria 25, **169,** 170
emotional development, importance of play 201
emotional relationships, attachment
    theories 82–3
empathy **178–9**
employment
  barriers to 175
  conditions 17–18
  private sector 9–10
  qualifications 18–20
  skills needed 3–4
  statutory sector 4–9
  voluntary sector 10–11
  see also jobs
empowerment **179**
'enactive thinking' 212
endurance training 127–8
environmental factors, early education 195–7
equal opportunities 184, 185, 201–2
ethical issues 295
  confidentiality 283, 296–7
  debriefing 297

deception 296
  disability prevention 162–3
  interviews 42–3
  observations 282–3
evaluation, care plans **171–2**
exercise 99, **101**
  aerobic system responses 99
  body responses to 98–9
  and disease prevention 121–4
  government guidelines 131–2
  government promotion of 119–20
  health benefits of 101–2, 103–4
  health screening 113–14
  intensity, measures of 111–12
  muscular system responses 99–100
  for osteoarthritis sufferers 160
  programme structure 114
  reasons for avoiding 118–19
  for rehabilitation 132
  risks involved in **113**
  safety issues 117
  societal benefits 102–3
  warm-down 116
  warm-up 115–16
  and weight control 104–5, 132
exercise-related fitness 93–4
  aerobic fitness 94–7
  body composition 97–8
  flexibility 97
  motor fitness 97
  muscular fitness 97
exercise programmes
  aerobic fitness 127–8
  constructing 125–6
  FITTA principles 126–7
  for flexibility 131
  muscle fitness 128–30
  for older adults 130–1
  for stress management 131
existentialism 84–7
expenditure, local authority 9
experiments
  quasi- 279
  scientific 277
  social 278
  stages of 277–8

F

FACS *see* Fair Access to Care Services
Fair Access to Care Services (FACS) 23, 25,
    169, 170, 183
family influences on early education 194–5
fartlek training 127–8
fine motor ability **159,** 201

fitness
  components of 94–7
  guidelines 131–2
  monitoring 106–12
  monitoring progress 116
  testing 114
FITTA principles, exercise
    programming 126–7
fixation **78**
flexibility 97, 130
flight/fright/fight response 250
formal operational stage, child
    development 64, 65–6, 211
forums, patient 33–4
Foundation Stage, early years
    education 219, 222
Foundation Stage Profile 221–2
Freud, Sigmund 76–81
Froebel, Friedrich 216
funding
  local authority *9*
  private sector 14
  statutory sector 11–13
  voluntary sector 13–14

G

gender roles 72
genes/genotype **51**
genetic counselling 162, 163
genetic factors in development 51, 193
governance **32**
graphs 298–300
gross motor ability **159,** 201
groups, identifying with 71–2

H

health, definition of **93**
health and lifestyle screening **113–14**
health and safety
  blood pressure (BP) 239
  body temperatures 237–8
  during exercise 116–17
  electrical equipment 234
  lung function tests 243
Health and Social Care
    Act (2001) 34, 35
health care assistants (HCAs) 6–7
Health Care Commission 33
Health Status Questionnaire 135
heart rate **115,** 263
  homeostatic regulation of 248–50
  monitors 112
  see also cardiovascular system
height and weight charts 106–7

hemiplegia **149**
homeostasis **245,** 257
  body temperature 245–8
  heart rate 248–50
  respiratory rate 250–2
hospitals
  discharge scheme 11, 12
  in-patient survey 34–5
  recruitment issues 5–6
housing
  effects on health 53–5
  rising costs of 15
human development
  genetic factors 51, 193
  learning theories 59–75
  personality theories 76–87
  sense of self 57–8
  socio-economic factors 52–7
humanistic theories of
    personality 84–7
hydrocephalus **161**
hydrostatic weighing 108
hypertension 122
hypertrophy 100
hypotheses 278

I

ICES (Integrated Community
    Equipment Services) 37
'iconic thinking' 212
identity, development of 70–1
imagination 57
immunisation **153**
'Improving Working Lives' (IWL),
    NHS Plan 5
income 52–3
  and early education 196–7
  impact of low 53–8
Independent Complaints Advocacy
    Service (ICAS) 34
independent sector *see* private sector;
    voluntary sector
informed consent 43, 297
intellectual development
    see cognitive development
interaction with others 58
interval training 127
interviews 283–4
  conducting structured 38–41
  ethical issues 42–3
  interview schedules **38,** 41
  types of 284–5
'inverse prevention law' 56–7
Isaacs, Susan 217

J

job satisfaction 21–2
  measuring 38–40
jobs
  in early years education 8–9
  factors affecting availability of 14–16
  job descriptions 18
  job status 22
  in the NHS 6–7
  qualifications required 19–20
  roles and responsibilities **17,** 19–20, 166–7
  skills needed for 3–4
  in social care 7–8
  see also employment
'joined-up' services 163

L

labelling **178**
language acquisition device (LAD) 215
language development 69–70, 194,
    199–201, 212
  stages of 213–14
  theories of 214–15
'Law of Effect' 206–7
learning, early years 199–205
  assessment of 218–22
learning disabilities **139**
learning theories 65, 205–208
  cognitive development 59–66, 208–9
  operant conditioning 66–70, 206–7
  social learning 70–5, 207–8
legislation 26, 30–2, 169, 170, 182–6
'libido' 76, 78
life expectancy, link to poverty 53
life quality factors 25, 172–3
lifestyle screening 113–14
local authorities
  employment 7–9
  funding 12–13
  income/outgoings 9
long, slow distance training 127
lung function, measuring 110–11, 240–4

M

Maslow, Abraham, hierarchy of needs 84–7
maternal deprivation theory 81
maturation **193–4**
maximum strength **97**
medical model of disability 139
mental health, improved by exercise 124
mental mechanisms, Freudian 77–8
metabolism 253
midwifery 6
minute volume **110**

mixed ability groupings, education 223
mixed economy of care 12, **163–4,** 182–3
Modernising Social Services
    (white paper, 1998) 31
monitoring of services 33, **171–2**
monoplegia **149**
monotropic attachment **81**
Montessori, Maria 216
motivation, Maslow's theory of
    needs 84–7
motor fitness 97
movement, control of 266–7
multi-disciplinary teams 9, **31**
multi-disciplinary working
  children 28
  disability **163–4**
  Sure Start 8–9, 31
multiple sclerosis (MS) 156–8
muscle endurance **99,** 128–9
muscle fitness 97
  training techniques for 128–30
muscle strength **99,** 128–9
muscular dystrophy (MD) 154–6
muscular system responses 99–100

N

National Assistance Act (1948) 169, 183
National Curriculum 218–19, 224–5
National Health Service (NHS)
  access to services 36–7, 56–7
  employment 4–7
  funding 11
  key professionals *166–7*
  monitoring of 34–5
  quality of services 33–4
National Institute for Health and Clinical
    Excellence (NICE) 157
National Patients' Surveys 35
National Service Frameworks (NSFs) 16, 31,
    153, 161, 170, 183
National Strategy for Carers (DoH) 165
nature versus nurture debate 193
near infrared, body fat measure 108
needs assessment 23–9, 169–72
neighbourhoods, effects of living in
    deprived 53–8
neonatal **149**
nervous system 264–6
  central nervous system (CNS) 141–3, **156**
  voluntary movement 266–7
neurotransmitters 249, 266
NHS and Community Care Act (1990) 10, 12,
    23, 30, 169, 183
NHS Plan (2000) 4, 5, 16, 57

non-participant observation **280–1**
noradrenaline 249, 250
'normality' 180–1
not-for-profit service providers 10
nursing, recruitment issues 5–6
nutrition, impact of low income 55

O

obesity
  link to poverty 55
  and physical inactivity 121
object permanence **61–2**
observations
  ethical issues 282–3
  limitations 282
  methods 281–2
  types 280–1
Office for Standards in Education
    (OFSTED) 35–6, 218
older people
  benefits of exercise 130–1
  voluntary services 10–11
onion theory 70–1
open questions 38–9, 287
operant conditioning **66**, 206–7
osteoarthritis 158–60
osteoporosis, benefits of exercise 123–4
overload **100**, 126

P

P-I-E-S, categories of needs 172
PALS (Patient Advice and Liaison Services) 34
parasympathetic nervous system 249–50,
    263–4, 265–6
participant observation **280–1**
Patient and Public Involvement Forums
    (PPIFs) 33–4
PCTs *see* Primary Care Trusts
peak expiratory flow (PEF) 242–3
peak flow measurements 110–11, 242–3
person-centred care 25, 172–3
Person Centred Planning (PCP) 173
personal qualities, for working in health/social
    care 3–4
personality, theories of 76–87
phenotype **51**
physical access issues, disabled people 175–7
physical activity *see* exercise
physical development 201
physical disabilities **139**
physical life quality factors 23, 172–3
Piaget, Jean, learning theory 59–66, 208–11
pictograms 301
pie charts 300–1

play in childhood 58, **197–8**
  enabling learning 199–205
  theorists 215–17
political factors, effect on job availability 16
positive feedback, helping children
    learn 204
poverty 53–6
Practical Guide for Disabled People and
    Carers (DoH) 170
pre-operational stage, cognitive
    development 62–3, 65, 210
prenatal screening 151, 154, 162
Primary Care Trusts (PCTs)
  patient prospectuses 35
  working conditions 5
primary reinforcers 207
primary research **275**
private sector
  employment 9–10
  funding 14
pro-social behaviour 71–2
providers of services **12**
psychodynamic theories 76–81
psychological life quality factors 25, 172–3
psychosexual stages of development 76–7, 78
public sector *see* statutory sector
pulse rate measurements 111–12, 233–5
punishment **67–8**, 207

Q

quadriplegia **149**
qualifications 18–20
qualitative research 276
quality assurance 32–7
quality control **33**
quality of early relationships 83–4
quality of life factors 23, 25, 172–3
quantitative research 276
quasi-experiments 279
questionnaires 38–41, 285–6
  designing 286–9
  health/lifestyle screening 113–14

R

rate of perceived exertion (RPE) 111
rating scales 39–40
recruitment issues
  overseas staff 6, 16
  rising housing costs 15
  shortage of nurses 5–6
referrals, needs assessment *24*, 25
reflection **172**, 200
regression **78–9**
rehabilitation, exercise aiding 132

reinforcement **66–9,** 200, 207
reliability **275**
research methods
  correlation 279–80
  experiments 277–9
  interviews 283–5
  observations 280–3
  primary 275
  qualitative 276
  quantitative 276
  questionnaires 285–9
  secondary 275
  surveys 289–91
respiration
  blood exchange 257
  breathing 253–6
  factors affecting 257
  functions of 257–8
  gaseous exchange 256–7
  homeostatic control 250–2
  internal **257**
  rate, measurement of 240
responsibilities, duties of job roles **17,** 18
Rockport 1-mile walk test 95
roles
  gender 72
  job **17,** 19–20, 166–7

S

S-A (sino-atrial) node 248–50, 264
sampling 292–4
SATS (standard assessment tests) 218, 224
schemata 59–60, **208,** 209
scoliosis **155**
secondary care *see* hospitals
secondary reinforcers 207
secondary research **275**
self, developing sense of 57–8
self-actualisation **85–6**
SEN *see* special educational needs
sensitive period, attachment theory **81**
sensorimotor stage, cognitive
    development 60–2, 64–5, 210
sensory disabilities **139**
separation, effects of mother-infant 81–2
services
  for disabled people 164, *165*
  factors affecting access to 36–7, 56–7
  monitoring delivery of 33
skills
  effect on job availability 15
  for jobs in health/social care 3–4
  needed by care workers 27

skinfold thickness 108
Skinner, B.F., operant conditioning 66–70, 207
'smart houses' 180
social care workers 8, 18
social development 201
social expectations, conforming to 71
social factors in early development 194–5
social identity 70–1
social impact theory 71–2
social learning theory 70–1, 207–8
social model of disability 139–40
social services
  children and families department 7
  community access to 37
  funding 12–13
  jobs in 7–8
  key professionals *166–7*
  quality assurance 35–6
social workers 7–8
socio-economic factors
  early years education 196–7
  housing 53–5
  income 52–3
somatic nervous system 264, 265
Special Educational Needs and Disability Act
    (SENDA) 170, 184
special educational needs (SEN) 10, 170
sphygmomanometers 238–9
spina bifida (SB) 161–2
spirometry 110, 240–2
staff
  factors affecting job availability 14–16
  at GP surgery 5
  shortage of midwives and nurses 5–6
Standard Spending Assessment (SSA) 12
standards **32–3**
statementing/statemented
    child **170**
statistics 301–2
statutory sector
  employment 4–9
  funding 11–13
Steiner, Rudolph 217
stereotyping **178**
stress
  and high-density housing 54
  reduced by exercise 124, 130
stroke 122, 143, 144
stroke volume 115, 263
structured interviews 38–41, 284
structured tasks, early years
    learning 204
Sure Start Centres 8–9

surveys
  data collection 289–91
  hospital 34–5
'symbolic thinking' 212
sympathetic nervous system 249–50,
    263–4, 265–6
synapses 249
systematic observation 280–3
systolic blood pressure 238

T

technological advances, effect on job availability 15
'telecare' 180
temperature 235–8, 245–8
tetraplegia **149**
thermometers 235–7
Thorndike, E.L. 'Law of Effect' 206–7
tidal volume 240, 241, 242
topical treatments **160**
training 8, 18
triangulation **276**

U

'UK In-patient Survey' 34–5
unconscious mind 77–8
underwater weighing 108
unemployment 55
urban environment 196
user involvement, NHS services 33–4, 34–5

V

vaccination **154**
validity **275**
values **295**
Valuing People 153, 170, 173
variables **277**
veins 260–1
vital capacity (VC) 240–2
VO_2 max **95**
voluntary movement 266–7
voluntary sector
  employment 10–11, 12, *13*
  funding 13–14
Vygotsky, Lev, cognitive
    development 211–12

W

waist circumference 107
warming down, following exercise 116
warming up, prior to exercise 115–16
weight control, role of exercise
    in 104–5, 132
weight height charts 106–7
wellness **93**

Z

zone of proximal development 211

Your Notes

Your Notes

Your Notes

Your Notes

Your Notes

Your Notes

Your Notes

Your Notes